Colorectal Cancer: Diagnosis and Clinical Management

Colorectal Cancer: Diagnosis and Clinical Management

Edited by Horton Murphy

STATES
ACADEMIC PRESS
www.statesacademicpress.com

States Academic Press,
109 South 5th Street,
Brooklyn, NY 11249, USA

Visit us on the World Wide Web at:
www.statesacademicpress.com

ISBN: 978-1-63989-117-7

Cataloging-in-Publication Data

Colorectal cancer : diagnosis and clinical management / edited by Horton Murphy.
p. cm.
Includes bibliographical references and index.
ISBN 978-1-63989-117-7
1. Colon (Anatomy)--Cancer. 2. Colon (Anatomy)--Cancer--Diagnosis.
3. Colon (Anatomy)--Cancer--Treatment. I. Murphy, Horton.

RC280.C6 C65 2022
616.994 347--dc23

Table of Contents

Preface

This book aims to highlight the current researches and provides a platform to further the scope of innovations in this area. This book is a product of the combined efforts of many researchers and scientists, after going through thorough studies and analysis from different parts of the world. The objective of this book is to provide the readers with the latest information of the field.

The development of cancer in the rectum or the colon is termed as colorectal cancer. It originates in the epithelial cells. It generally occurs due to factors related to lifestyle or old age. Its major symptoms are blood in the stool, fatigue, weight loss and a change in bowel movements. It might begin as a benign tumor, and could become cancerous as time passes. It can be diagnosed through a colonoscopy or a sigmoidoscopy. The treatment of colorectal cancer is done through various methods such as radiation therapy, chemotherapy, surgery, targeted therapy, etc. There are various methods of reducing the risk of colorectal cancer such as through exercise, quitting smoking and reducing alcohol intake. The objective of this book is to give a general view of the diagnosis and management of colorectal cancer. It brings forth some of the most innovative concepts and elucidates the unexplored aspects of research on this disease. The book is appropriate for students seeking detailed information in this area as well as for experts.

I would like to express my sincere thanks to the authors for their dedicated efforts in the completion of this book. I acknowledge the efforts of the publisher for providing constant support. Lastly, I would like to thank my family for their support in all academic endeavors.

Editor

1

Diagnostic Modalities in Colorectal Cancer – Endoscopy, CT and PET Scanning, Magnetic Resonance Imaging (MRI), Endoluminal Ultrasound and Intraoperative Ultrasound

Valentin Ignatov, Nikola Kolev, Anton Tonev, Shteryu Shterev, Elitsa Encheva, Tanya Kirilova, Tsvetelina Teneva and Krassimir Ivanov

1. Introduction

Colorectal cancer (CRC) is the third most diagnosed cancer in men, next to prostate and lung cancer. In women it is the second most diagnosed cancer, next to breast cancer. In a time of limited resources in health care, there has been considerable debate which imaging modality offers the best non-invasive examination of colorectal cancer, offering both detection and characterization. The use of multiple diagnostic modalities is both costly and time-consuming. Clinical evidence amassed over the last several decades indicates that routine colorectal cancer (CRC) screening, compared to no screening, detects CRC at an earlier stage, reduces the incidence of CRC or the progression early CRC through polypectomy, and reduces CRC mortality.

2. Endoscopy

The first complete examination of the colon using a flexible fiber optic endoscope is reported by Wolff and Shinya in 1971 [42]. Nowadays colonoscopy is the gold standard for evaluation of the entire colonic mucosa with therapeutic capability of resecting detected malignancies.

In the last years the colonoscopy is the modality of choice to detect and correct the adenomatous polyps and colorectal cancer. The diagnosis CRC can be confirmed after biopsy in a known malignant pathology and by obtaining more tissue sampling and/or a second opinion from a consulting pathologist in none diagnostic, highly suspected colon lesion. Besides the role as a diagnostic tool in CRC, colonoscopy identifies subsequent lesions at the time of surgery, which is called preoperative endoscopic marking. It is performed through metallic clip placement and endoscopic tattooing.

The colonoscopic equipment consists of camera and four-way tip controls [43]. The camera can produce images of high-definition quality. The four way tip controls include (1) examination of a found patch to confirm an abnormal growth; (2) insufflating air to dilate the lumen for mucosal inspection and relieving air after examination, (3) irrigating a suspected region; (4) suctioning to avoid missing lesions under fluid, and (5) inserting biopsy devices.

The patient must undergo bowel preparation - taking clear liquid diet and ingesting laxative solutions for colon cleansing the day before examination. Sedation is needed to relieve the discomfort during the procedure, but it increases the costs. The complication of sedation are different cardiac disturbances such as hypotension, arrhythmias,oxygen desaturation, and others. The preparation with purgatives may cause abdominal discomfort, nausea, and other symptoms. The colonoscopy continues from 30 minutes to an hour. The risk during colonoscopy consists in colonic perforation in 0,1 % of cases. Colonoscopy fails to visualize the entire colon in 10–15% and it may miss up to 10–20% of polyps fewer than 10 mm.

Colonoscopy is golden standard for diagnosing of CRC but there are more symptoms which could be evaluated and appreciated by endoscopic examination, for example- abdominal pain, unexplained gastrointestinal bleeding, diarrhea of unexplained origin, chronic inflammatory bowel disease, etc. It is also the most common interventional modality for polypectomy, hemostasis, balloon dilation, foreign body removal, palliative treatment of neoplasms, etc. Colonoscopy could be the best screening option for all none specific underdiagnosed gastrointestinal symptoms.

Colonoscopy removes all detected polyps, regardless of histology type- adenomatous or hyperplastic. Not all of them must undergo resection. The polyps vary in size and polyps under 5 mm are not detected endoscopic. For detection of polyps smaller than 5 mm the virtual colonospcopy is the alternative to the conventional colonoscopy.

3. Virtual colonoscopy

Virtual Colonoscopy uses computed tomography (CT) imaging virtual- reality technology for the purpose of screening the entire colon which is reconstructed from abdominal CT images.

The technique starts after cleansing of the colon with oral laxatives with inflation of air or CO2 introduced through rectal tube [71]. Then abdominal CT images are taken during a single breath holding with sub mm resolution in axial and transverse directions. The volume model of the colon is constructed from the spiral CT images. Image segmentation is necessary for the reconstruction of an accurate colon model [72]. Computer graphics navigate inside the 3D colon model, the navigation is called fly through model. For validating the detection in the 3D colon model, interpretation of the 2D image slices at transverse, sagital and coronal directions is often included in the procedure.

The virtual colonoscopy achieves higher sensitivity and specificity rates compared to conventional colonoscopy for detecting polyps, which are 8 mm and larger by the same bowel preparation, and for polyps larger than 10 mm they have a comparable performance. CTC can be a potential screening tool to supplement OC for colorectal cancer. CTC is refused to be included in Medicare coverage because of its radiation risk- in about 50 mAs or 2 rads. Reducing the radiation could be achieved by decreasing of the mAs level optimization of kVp value, X-ray flux beam collimation, filtering, etc. The low-mAs strategy will lead to higher noise in the acquired data which results in steak artifacts. The significant amount of X-ray radiation exposure and the data noise cannot be disregarded and allowed to the CTC to be a preferred screening modality.

An alternative method to minimize the radiation is to use magnetic resonance imaging (MRI), i.e., MR colonography (MRC). However, this MRC has several limitation compared to CTC- high costs, sensitiveness to motion and other artifacts, and has lower spatial resolution. Modern CT can reach sub-millimeter spatial resolution and acquire a volumetric image of the abdomen, detecting polyps which are smaller than 5mm.

There are other reasons responsibe for missing small polyps.

The main reason is due to the partial colon cleansing and air/CO2 inflation and this will not generate a good interface between the colon wall and the lumen. Others include loss of image information in post-imaging processing, different anatomical characteristics in the bowel mucosa, residual fluid or stool covering the polyps. The solution could be virtual or electronic colon cleansing (ECC) - special type of software programming for virtually cleansing of the colon. It consists of three main components - (1) fecal tagging, (2) image segmentation for classifying the tagged image voxels, and (3) post-segmentation operation for cleansing the colon. ECC works virtually on the residual faecal materials with or without adequate bowel preparation with purgatives (the so called cathartic-free CTC). The ECC must handle with the partial volume (PV) effect and with the non-uniformly altered image intensity distribution. Partial volume (PV) effect is the interface between the colon wall and the fecal materials with heterogeneously enhanced image intensities. The PV effect blurs the interface over several image voxels, causing the loss of details about the interface what results in the misdetection of small polyps. A dual energy scans of a modern CT device or a dual X-ray source scanner is a new challenging imagining modality. Two volumetric images can be acquired simultaneously at two energy levels. It is expected that the polyps would have different image contrasts in the two scans and if the contrasts are insufficient for segmenting the image voxels, oral contrast media may be utilized to increase the density of the polyps. The ECC role in this dual energy strategy is to segment the colonic materials from multi-spectral CT images. After ECC-cleansing the colon lumen could be easily inspected for abnormalities and polyps along the long colon during the fly-through navigation.

Variation among readers with different experience has been noticed. Computer-aided detection (CAD) can minimize the variation among readers' assessments. CAD system's disadvantages are many false positives (FPs), such as partial bowel cleansing, image noise, motion artifacts, colon fold structures, etc. High sensitivity CAD with minimal number of FPs and development of various texture features and virtual biopsy features remains an innovative research goal.

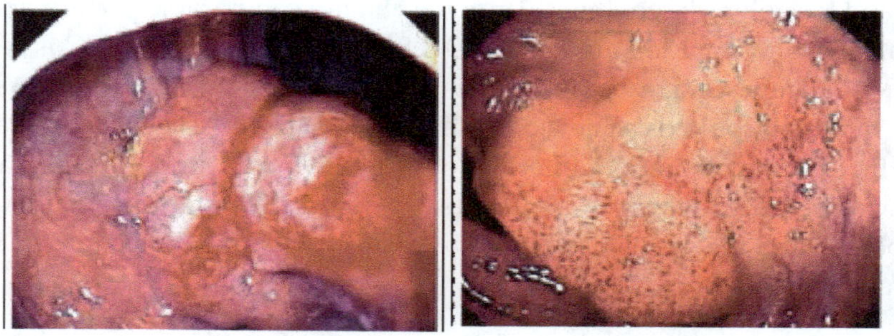

Figure 1. Endoscopic view of corectal tumor – conventional endoscopy

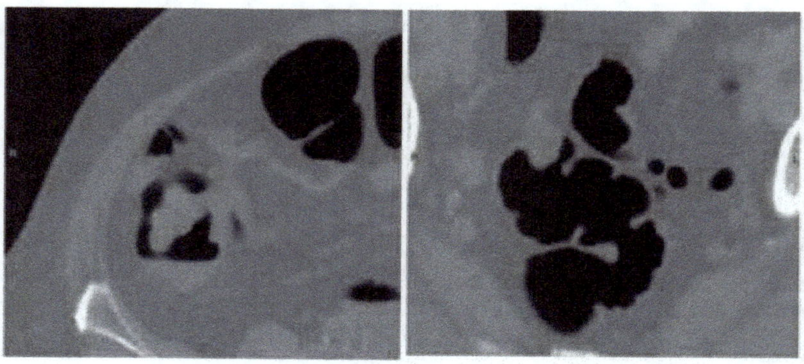

Figure 2. Virtual colonoscopy – a view of pediculaneted polypus and a small carcinoma - CT images.

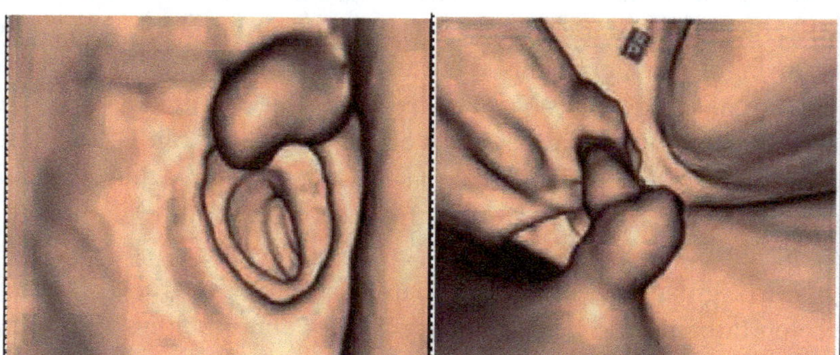

Figure 3. Virtual colonoscopy – a view of pediculaneted polypus and a small carcinoma - a 3-D reconstruction after software rendering.

4. Imaging diagnostics in rectal cancer

Staging of rectal cancer is of great importance before the surgical treatment, because staging predicts the management, prognosis, recurrence and/or metastatic disease risk (13). Staging is divided into local and distant staging. Local staging points at wall invasion, resection margin involvement and the nodal status for metastasis and distant staging refers to presence or absence of metastatic disease. Rectal examination using proctoscopy may be considered as an important tool for newly diagnosed rectal cancers. Proctoscopy may determine better visualization, localization and fixity of the tumor, including taking biopsy, which may affects positively the staging of the rectal cancer.

Nowadays several imaging modalities or combination of these are available for evaluating preoperative staging of colorectal cancer- computed tomography (CT), magnetic resonance imaging (MRI), and/or endorectal ultrasonography (EUS). EUS and MRI of the pelvis are used to appreciate the local dissemination while CT defines systemic dissemination. PET is indicated when there is clinical, biochemical or radiological suspicion of local recurrence or systemic disease. Functional imaging such as diffusion weighted MRI imaging (DWI) and CT/PET are used to distinguish fibrosis from tumor [33].

The T staging accuracy in more advanced cancer is achieved by using MR imaging modality because MRI can distinguish between mesorectum and mesorectal fascia. The N staging accuracy is also provided by MRI particularly using superparamagnetic iron oxide particles.

4.1. Endorectal ultrasound

The advancing of imaging technologies has made endoscopic ultrasound a modality of choice in gastrointestinal diseases, regarding diagnosis, staging and prognosis stratification. These novel techniques assign excellent to rectal tumors.

Endorectal ultrasound (EUS) is useful in evaluating early rectal cancers (T1 and T2 lesions) and post transanal surgery. EUS can visualize the rectal wall without distinguishing of mesorectal fascia, peritumor inflammation, or faeces collections. The accuracy of the T stage evaluation varies from 60%-90% [45].

In comparison to MRI EUS was found to be highly accurate in early lesions (for T1 and T2 the accuracy can reach to 100%), as well as for nodal metastases. For evaluation of metastatic disease neither MRI nor EUS enable reliable diagnosis.

Besides the misleading lymph node assessment, EUS has its disadvantages in detecting T3 lesions (advanced, stenotic, bulky lesions) or tumors after neoadjuvant therapy, and the technique is operator dependent.

Hypoechoic appearance, size > 5 mm, round shape, peritumoral location are characteristics suggestive of malignant involvement of lymph nodes [45,46,51-53]. EUS-guided fine-needle aspiration can be carried out from the lesion or suspiciously looking lymph nodes.

An newer technique is the three-dimensional ERUS (3D-ERUS). It consists of transverse, coronal and sagittal scan and has been found to be more reliable in staging colon cancer to two-dimensional EUS and CT. The accuracy of 3D-ERUS for assessing the depth of cancer infiltration and for nodal involvement is with 10% more than the other imaging modalities. 3D images have proved a better visualization of the mesorectal margins. With 3D-ERUS the surgeon can perform endoscopic mucosal resections of early tumors. A reliable predictor for response after chemoradiation therapy are the accurate volumetric measurements achieved by 3D-ERUS. Using Doppler signal enhancers tumor perfusion can be determine, coming to better results in neoadjuvant therapy and antiangiogenesis treatment.

3D-ERUS, elastography, and contrast enhancement might bring additional information, increasing diagnostic accuracy of ERUS and amplifying its roles in the complex management in rectal cancer.

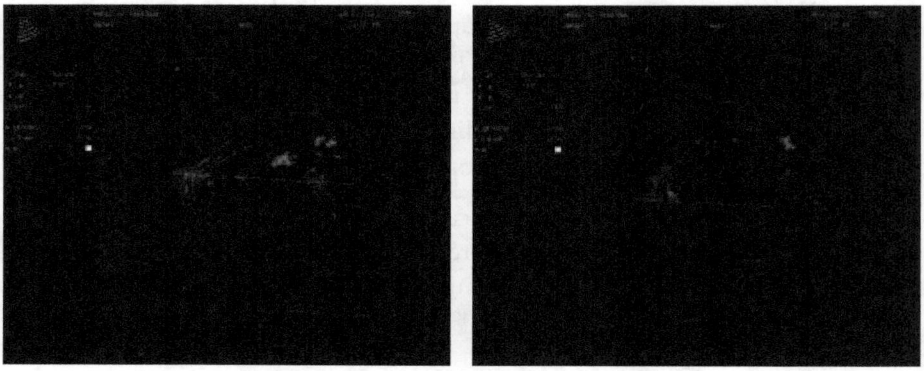

Figure 4. Endorectal ultrasonography – a view of T-3 carcinoma - 3-D reconstruction after real-time software rendering.

T and LN staging

In colon cancer patients it is essential to correctly determine the TNM stage. The modalities of choice are CT, MRI and, as mentioned above, the novel technique ERUS.

ERUS shows high sensitivity and specificity in T-staging and is prior to CT and MRI for staging superficial rectal tumors, with accuracy in evaluating rectal wall invasion to 97% [23,24]. For T1, T2, T3 and T4 staging accuracy of ERUS is more than 80%. One common finding is a lower accuracy for T2 tumors, because the impossibility in distinguishing those tumors that have deep invasion into the muscularis propria from those with microscopic invasion into the perirectal fat.

Transanal endoscopic microsurgery (TEM) and endoscopic submucosal dissections are novel important strategies which directs the mode of surgery because of the ability to visualize the submucosa. This can lead to down- or upstaging of the detected rectal cancer. Besides ERUS can detect recurrence at the anastomosis site and to differentiate between postoperative scars and local recurrences. Unfortunately assessment for nodal metastases is less accurate than that for tumor depth and reaches 75%. For rectal cancer in particular, over half of the metastatic nodes are less than 5 mm and are located within 3 cm of the primary tumor [31]. Metastatic disease was shown to predict local recurrence.

The sensitivity of ERUS in detecting LN metastasis ranges from 50% to 83%, because small lymph node (less than 5mm) is not observed with ERUS and it has limited field of view. Factors for malignancy in lymph node besides node size, echogenicity, shape, border, include: hypoechogenicity, short axis ≥ 5 mm, long axis length greater than 9 mm.

Detecting of iliac adenopathy is crucial because it goes after total mesorectal excision. This is possible through flexible not rigid probes. In general, ERUS is better at detecting lymph nodes in the distal and middle thirds of the rectum [21,33]. The reactive swollen lymph nodes, small blood vessels, urethra, and seminal vesicle often are mistaken for malignant lymph nodes and these results in over staging of the disease. On the other hand, the major reason for nodal status under staging is misdetecting of very small involved nodes (less than 2 mm) and nodes outside the perirectal tissue [21,33].

Preoperative chemoradiation is a limiting factor affecting accurate staging of rectal cancer. There are associated reactive and inflammatory changes in the rectum wall after radiotherapy. However, radiotherapy affects the wall thickness but does not change the five-layered image.

The 3D reconstruction allows improved T and N staging through direct visualization of subtle protrusions of tumors infiltrating into adjacent tissues and organs.

Limitations of ERUS are several. Firstly it is operator's experience dependent; it varies after partial excision or neoadjuvant chemoradiation. It has poor patient acceptability and it has limited depth of penetration; Another disadvantages are those that it cannot be performed in obstructive tumors [16,21]; it is unable to visualize tumors located higher with a rigid probe. It is insufficient in detecting lymph nodes outside the range of the transducer, or visualize mesorectal fascia because of its limited field of view. In addition, accuracy is affected by villous or pedunculated tumors, inflammation, hemorrhage [22,31].

MRI

MRI obtain image identification of the distance of the CRM to the tumor, the relation to pelvic floor and anal sphincter complex, differentiation between mucinous and none mucinous neoplasia. T staging accuracy of MRI is 52% when compared to histology, because of the interface between muscularis propria, perirectal fat and mesorectal fascia. MRI cannot distinguish between T1 and T2 lesions, as well as between T2 and T3 cancer.

T staging

The depth of invasion through the muscle wall is one important element seen on MRI that can help guide clinical decision making for patients with rectal cancer. Not only does the incidence of nodal involvement increase with increasing tumor penetration [19,20], but clinical studies have shown that patients with stage ◎ (T1-2 N0) rectal cancer do not benefit from neoadjuvant radiotherapy [21] and may be amenable to a less than radical surgical treatment [22]. Patients with clinically staged T3-4 tumors typically require preoperative CRT since it reduces the rates of local recurrence more effectively than either postoperative CRT or preopera-

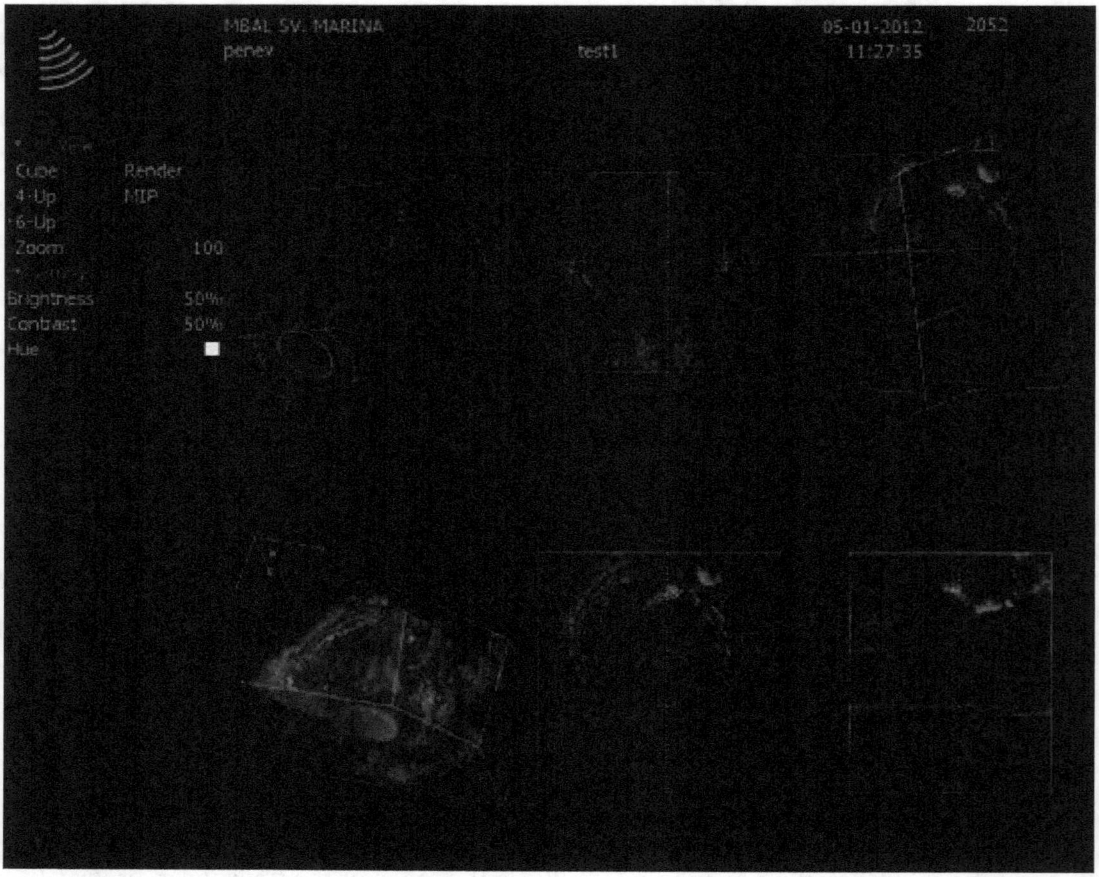

Figure 5. Endorectal ultrasonography – a real time 3-D reconstruction with different options for endorectal evaluation of the tumor process.

tive radiotherapy alone [23-25]. However, some problems remain with T stage determination on MR imaging. Overall, the agreement between MRI and histology for T staging has ranged from 66%-94% [18,26-28]. One of the main problems of T staging on MRI is the distinction between T2 and T3 tumors. In fact, investigators have shown that the negative predictive value for invasion beyond the muscularis propria varied from 93% (expert reading) to 76% (general radiologist reading) [26]. This difficulty is attributed to the presence of desmoplastic reactions around the tumor. This reaction makes it difficult to distinguish between spiculation in the perirectal fat caused by fibrosis alone from that caused by fibrous tissue that contains tumor cells [26]. In contrast, MRI has been shown to be more accurate in imaging the more advanced tumors (T4) [27,29]. According to a metaanalysis, MRI for T4 lesions has a specificity of 96% [30].

CRM

The CRM (lateral, radial) is defined as the surgical cut surface of the connective tissues (i.e. lymphovascular, fatty and neural tissue) that circumferentially encase the rectum. It equates to the mesorectal fascia that forms the plane of dissection in rectal cancer surgery. It is assessed by marking the outer surface (i.e. the CRM) with ink, taking serial cuts through the specimen and examining the macroscopic and microscopic relations between the tumor and the inked margin. The CRM gives significant information not only about the quality of the performed operation but also prognosis of the disease. Indeed, in a recent study based on the data from a randomized clinical trial, Nagtegaal *et al* [31] demonstrated in a multivariate model that the CRM is more important than the T stage for the prognosis of rectal cancer. The definition of a positive CRM remains a matter of debate. A review of the literature in 2006 showed that the majority of studies that dealt with CRM status used the ≤ 1 mm definition for positive CRM (91.1%; 7373 of 8094 patients) [32].

Six distinct types of CRM involvement have been described; direct tumor spread which occurs in 18% to 29% of cases; discontinuous tumor spread in 14% to 67% of cases; lymph node metastases in 12% to 14% of cases; venous invasion in 14% to 57% of cases; lymphatic invasion in 9% of cases; and perineural tumor spread in 7% to 14% of cases [32]. In approximately 30% of patients, there is more than one type of margin involvement. In contrast to direct tumor spread, the involvement of the CRM by lymph node metastases is not associated with local recurrence [32]. MRI is highly accurate and reliable for prediction of the CRM [33,34]. In their most recent study of 98 rectal cancer patients, Brown *et al* [27] reported a 92% agreement between MRI images and histologic findings for prediction of CRM involvement. In another study assessing the tumor relationship to the mesorectal fascia, two observers independently scored the tumor stage and the distance to the mesorectal fascia on MRI and compared these observations with the final histological findings [26]. For twelve tumors with involved mesorectal fascia, and thus, a CRM of 0 mm, the accuracy in predicting the CRM was 100% for both readers. In 29 patients with a wide CRM (10 mm), the accuracy for predicting the negative margin was 97% (27 of 28) for one reader and 93% (26 of 28) for the other [26]. It is relevant to point out that 5 mm of mesorectal tissue surrounding the lateral tumor edge on MRI was shown to equal a CRM of 2 mm in the surgical specimen [26]. In the report by Nagtegaal *et al* [35], a linear regression curve showed that the crucial distance of at least 2 mm could be predicted with 97% confidence when the distance on MRI is at least 6 mm. Therefore, the safe rule to predict CRM involvement on MRI is considered to be an MRI measurement minus 4 mm due to shrinkage of the specimen with fixation [6]. Of note, the CRM becomes more difficult to identify in low, anterior tumors and in patients with a limited amount of perirectal fat [36]. In a recent study by Frasson *et al* [37], the 5-year local recurrence rates for patients with a preoperative CRM of < 2 mm on MRI or EUS who did not receive preoperative chemoradiation was 19.4% compared to 5.4% for patients with a non-threatened margin. It is important to realize that a short course of preoperative radiotherapy has limited ability to control positive CRM. An analysis of more than 17 500 pathologic specimens by Nagtegaal *et al* [32] revealed that the chance of local recurrence was higher for patients with a positive CRM after neoadjuvant treatment (both radiotherapy and radiochemotherapy) than those with a positive CRM following immediate surgery (Hazard ratio 6.3 *vs* 2.0, respectively). Similar results have been reported following postoperative treatment [38]. In the MRC CR-07 trial, patients with positive radial margins who were selected to receive postoperative chemoradiation had a 21% local recurrence rate [39]. Thus, in cases where the tumors are close (< 2 mm) or through the mesorectal margin on preoperative MRI, a more aggressive treatment regimen is required with neoadjuvant CRT or an upfront regimen of chemotherapy before chemoradiation prior to operation. In contrast, patients with a free margin > 2 mm from mesorectal fascia may undergo surgery [total mesorectal excision (TME)] alone, avoiding preoperative chemoradiation. Interestingly, MRI-based therapy for CRM positive tumors was able to reduce the frequency of neoadjuvant therapy for rectal carcinoma by 35% without the risk of worsening the oncological results [40]. However, omitting preoperative chemoradiation for all CRM-negative tumors on MRI needs to be further investigated in prospective clinical trials before it is adopted as standard therapy.

N staging

The presence of involved lymph nodes is an indicator for the likelihood of systemic disease and local recurrence [41]. Therefore node-positive disease is generally an indication for preoperative chemoradiation. However, radiological evaluation of lymph node metastatic involvement remains a challenge. Results of anatomic studies show that over half of the metastatic nodes from rectal cancer are within 3 cm of the primary tumor and are smaller than 5 mm in size [42]. With a standard TME, the perirectal nodes are removed with the primary tumor, but the internal iliac and obturator nodes are left in place. Moriya *et al* [43] reported that as many as 28% of lymph node-positive distal rectal cancers have involvement of lateral nodes and in 6% of cases, these were the only nodes involved. This means that in 6% of patients, the disease was incorrectly staged postoperatively as node-negative at TME. For pre-operative lymph node imaging, MRI at present is only moderately accurate, although this could change with advances in new MR techniques. Currently, the reported accuracy rate of MRI for nodal staging ranges from 71% to 91% [42]. On MRI, lymph nodes typically have lower signal intensity than the perirectal fat but higher signal intensity than arteries and veins. In patients with mucinous carcinoma, metastatic lymph nodes are visualized as hyperintense nodules alone or as hyperintense areas within hypointense nodules. A node is considered enlarged if the major axis length is more than 5 mm (mesorectal), 7 mm (internal iliac), 10 mm (external iliac), or 9 mm (common iliac) [44]. However, the morphological features or signal intensity of the nodes on MRI may more accurately determine metastatic involvement rather than measurement of size. Brown *et al* [45] demonstrated that an irregular border or mixed signal intensity of lymph nodes on MRI improved the specificity of predicting nodal status from 68% (based on size alone) to 97%. One of the more promising advances of MRI may be the use of new lymphographic agents that help assess tumor spread to lymph nodes. In a recent study, gadofosveset-enhanced MRI improved the specificity of nodal staging from 82% achieved with standard MRI to 97% [46]. Fusion of diffusion-weighted MR with T2-weighted images improves identification of pelvic lymph nodes compared with T2-weighted images alone. Using fusion images, 29% additional nodes were detected compared with T2-weighted images alone [47]. The improved nodal identification may aid in treatment planning.

For the vast majority of rectal carcinomas, MRI is currently the most accurate modality on which to base treatment decisions for patients with rectal cancer. Traditionally, the decision to apply preoperative treatment for rectal cancer patients has been based on the T- and N-stage. Lately, other MRI findings such as the radial distance of the tumor to the CRM and extramural vascular invasion score have been identified as important risk factors for local failure and survival. Every center that treats patients with rectal cancer should develop a multidisciplinary team featuring a description of the MRI findings and their implementation in the treatment strategy with the aim of increasing resectability, reducing the local recurrence and treatment morbidity, and improving the quality of life.

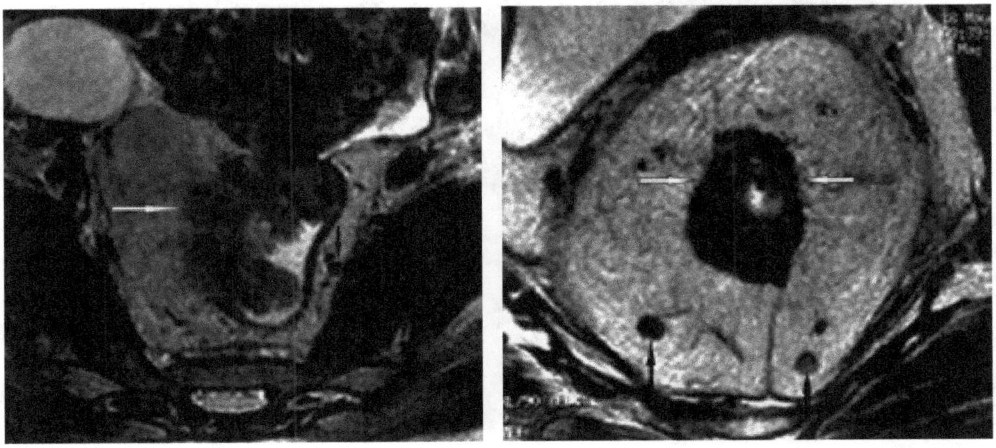

Figure 6. MRI – a view of T-3 carcinoma - 3-D reconstruction after real-time software rendering.

CT, MRI and intraoperative ultrasound for evaluation of the systematic progression in colorectal cancer

The morbidity rate for patients with cancer depends on the early detection of liver metastases. The presence of liver metastases makes of the primary tumour non-resectable for oncologic reasons, except for tumour palliative treatment (for example resection for obstruction of the gastrointestinal tract). For a few malignancies, as in colorectal carcinoma, resection of liver metastases has been shown to improve the survival of the patients. The hepatic metastases are divided into synchronous (i.e. occurring at the time of diagnosis of the primary tumour) and metachronous (occurring after diagnosis of the primary tumour). The surgical resection of the metastases depends on the division, number, size, regional distribution and all clinical parameters of the patient, which makes resectable only 30% of all colorectal patients with metastases. The 5-year survival rate of these patients is more than 30% in comparison to a survival of less than 5% of patients with liver metastases not amenable to liver surgery [1–4].

The goal of imaging modalities is to assess the presence or absence of liver metastases in surgical candidates. Different studies indicate ferumoxide-enhanced magnetic resonance (MR) imaging as more sensitive and specific than contrast-enhanced computed tomography (CT) in detection of hepatic metastases. The different MR pulse sequences and MR contrast media agents makes MRI the modality of choice for non-invasive lesion characterization.

Preoperative assessment of surgical candidates

Preoperative assessment of metastatic liver involvement should be performed for all surgery candidates. This preoperative staging is conceivable by contrast-enhanced CT and/or MRI in

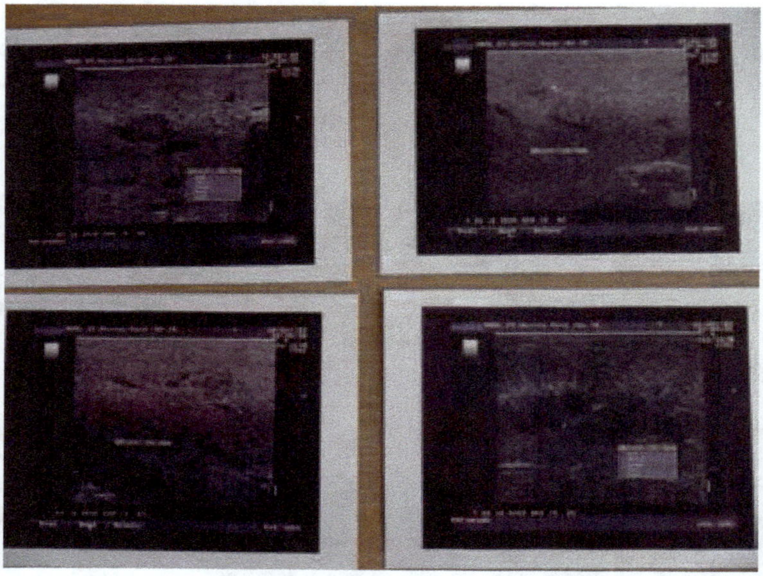

Figure 7. Intraoperative ultrasound of the liver

most oncologic centers. All imaging modalities present different false-positive or false-negative diagnoses- for helical CT- in 42%, intraoperative US- in 22.8%, mangafodipir-enhanced MRI- in 10%, ferumoxide-enhanced MRI technique is accurate as CT during arterioportography (CTAP)- in 19%. Another study found that FDG-PET CT is the most sensitive method for detection of metastases. There is no firm statement which is the best imaging modality, further more the choice depends on local equipment, availability, and operator expertise. MDCT is preferred as a screening method for hepatic lesions because of its ability to reduce respiration-related artifacts, to shorten scan time, to perform multiphase scanning. The disadvantage is the high radiation exposure.

Clinical Role of Intraoperative US

Intraoperative US provide more diagnostic and staging information to the surgeon during hepatic resection. Intraoperative US supplies 35% more information about the lesion type, localization and expansion to adjacent tissues, relation to vascular structures, providing more specificity in the evaluation of liver lesions. In addition intraoperative US represent 25% more lesions than did preoperative US, CT, or angiography. This results in correction in disease staging, which affects the surgical management and postoperative treatment. The intraoperative US has a positive effect on patient care, surgical planning, and clinical outcome.

Magnetic resonance imaging

The standard phased array MRI produces good quality images with good contrast resolution and a relatively large field of view, so it is the modality of choice for preoperative staging of rectal primary tumor. MRI is reliable for assessment of the tumor and its locoregional extension, for identifying recurrence and for planning radiation therapy. The disadvantage of MRI is impossibility in evaluation nodal metastases.

Deciding in management of rectal cancer is the differentiation of the mesorectal fascia-circumstance, which is possible using phased-array coils (confirmed from the multicentre European MERCURY study)(21,23).

MRI may not be the examination of choice for every patient. Patients with contraindications to MRI (e.g. implantable pacemakers), or unable to tolerate MRI (e.g. due to claustrophobia) would preferably undergo preoperative imaging with CT. Motion related imaging artifacts that can severely dampen the diagnostic quality of MRI will occur in patients who are unable to breath hold for longer than 20 seconds.

FDG PET in the Initial Staging of CRC

FDG PET is not a routine investigation for primary cancer due to its limited spatial resolution. PET cannot define the T-category of the primary tumor, but PET is superior to other imaging modalities in detecting of lymph node and distant metastases- an important prognostic factor. After PET-CT investigation the patient could be upstaged in 17% because of identifying unsuspected systemic and lymph node metastases. But the specificity of PET in nodal staging does not be higher than multi-detector CT scan (MDCT).

The principle of positron emission tomography (PET) (and Fluoro-deoxy-glucose (FDG) used as tracer or enhancer) is based on the differential metabolic profile of tumors - higher metabolic activity, change in the tumor biology. FDG/PET is mainly useful in the assessment of local recurrence and metastases. Besides in neoplastic cells FDG accumulates in areas of inflammation, infection, in organs of increased metabolic activity such as brain, myocardium, liver or kidneys leading to false positive results. Interpretation of PET without anatomic correlation is difficult which results in necessity of fusing PET with CT images-PET-CT fusion scans are invented. This offers a detailed anatomical and functional imaging. The combination provides additional value to localize the hot spots. The false positive rates are due to other diseases and physiological processes. PET scans improve the management plan for rectal cancer. The addition of FDG-PET changes patient management in up to 30% of patients with potentially resectable liver metastases, mainly by detecting previously unknown extrahepatic disease. Furthermore, FDG-PET is useful in the follow-up of patients who underwent surgical procedures of the liver, since it is sensitive in detecting residual or relapse malignancy in scarred liver tissue following both resection and local ablative techniques. For follow-up during systemic therapy, early FDG-PET appears predictive for response to therapy. FDG-PET, computerized tomography and magnetic resonance imaging are complementary techniques in staging and restaging patients with advanced colorectal cancer. A combination of FDG-PET and CT scanning characteristics seems promising, and integrated PET/ CT is becoming more widely available, although the exact clinical value and efficacy is not yet fully established. In addition, assessment of these modalities in joint reading sessions with radiologist, nuclear medicine physician, medical and surgical oncologists significantly impacts upon patient management. This review evaluates the potential of FDG-PET and combined PET/CT in patients with colorectal liver metastases and discusses potential future possibilities.

Suggested investigations for tumor staging of rectal cancer

CT scanning is still the current standard for distant staging, but not to stage the local neoplasm. The combination of CT and PET offers both anatomical and functional imaging, so it is sufficient for recurrent rectal cancers. MRI and EUS should be considered as the initial modalities to stage the local tumor. For T1-T2 lesions EUS is more appropriate, whereas MRI is used in advanced rectal cancer. MRI has been shown to be highly accurate in predicting a clear circumferential resection margin in patients undergoing TME.

Suggested investigation for nodal staging of rectal cancer

Significant malignant lymph nodes (more than 1cm in diameter), in conjunction with size, shape and morphology, are identified through MRI, CT and EUS studies. The enlarged lymph node can be as a result of the inflammatory process but normal size nodes can have micrometastases. Moreover the halves of nodes less than 5 mm are proved to be malignant. One novel technique involves use of a contrast media containing superparamagnetic iron oxide particles SPIO which accumulates in normal lymph nodes, but not in malignant nodes due to poor uptake. Then, using T2 weighted imaging, these nodes can be identified. Initial studies are promising but further research is needed [35].

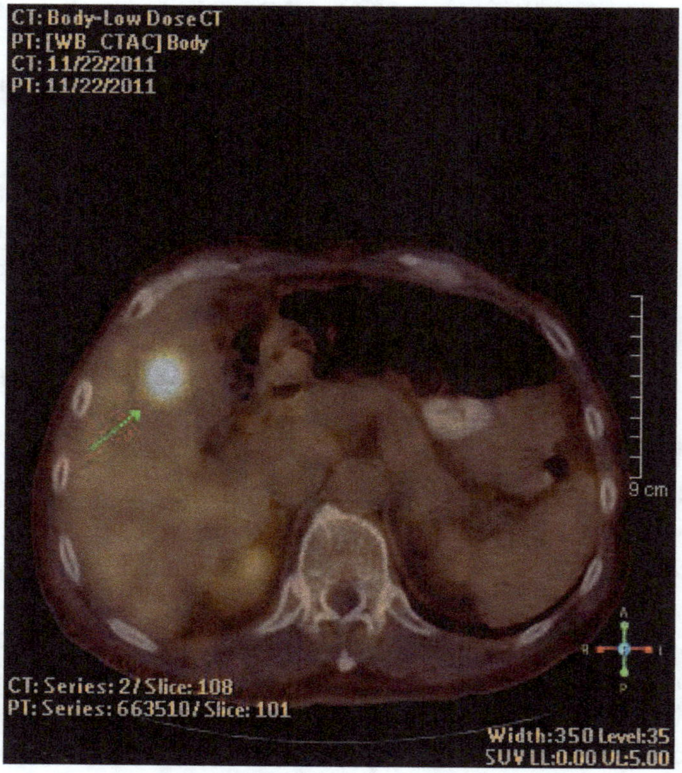

Figure 8. Positron emission tomography of the liver – an observation of metastasis from colorectal origin

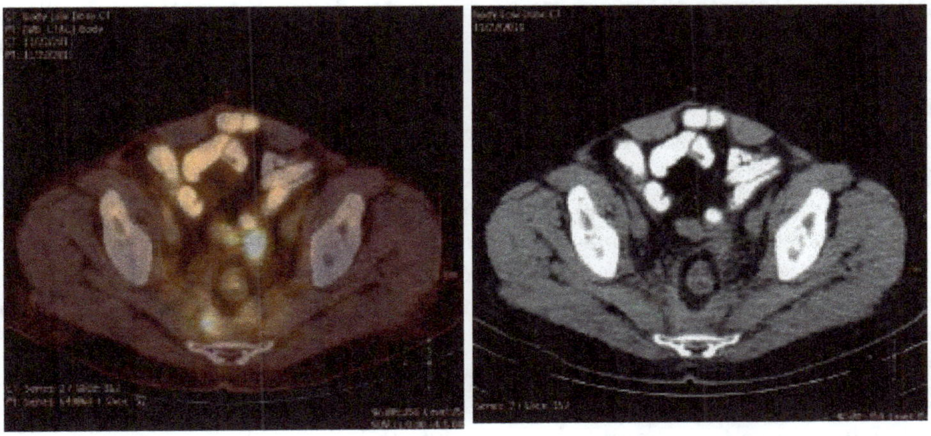

Figure 9. Positron emission tomography of the body – an observation of perirectal lymphadenopathy

5. Conclusion

Optical colonoscopy (OC) and virtual colonoscopy (VC) (i.e. CT colonoscopy and MR colonoscopy) are constantly developing and adapting to the new clinical needs. The optical colonoscopy has the advantage of being both diagnostic and therapeutic procedure for patients with positive findings on screening tests. The virtual colonoscopy is much less invasive method and can be used for mass screening because of the high prevalence of the colorectal cancer. As a screening test the VC has advantages over OC and other options such as FOBT, FIT, stool DNA testing, and DCBE. These methods can make a good combination of VC screening with OC follow-up on the positive findings. The current imaging modalities for VC are CT and MRI and in the future other modalities might be available.

The imaging standard for accurate diagnostics for colorectal cancer includes ultrasound (US), CT and MRI. The nuclear medicine has its role in finding extra-regional localization of the main disease by FDG-PET and FDG-PET/CT. The protocol for liver metastases includes CT as a first choice, which is followed by US. Lung-metastases are evaluated by X-ray or chest CT. The extrahepatic metastases are assessed by CT. The present guidelines could be adjusted by conducting comparative studies on different strategies for colon and rectal cancer, such as CT liver/abdomen vs. MRI liver/abdomen for liver and extrahepatic metastases, X-ray chest and CT chest for lung metastases.

The screening of asymptomatic patients is justified due to the high prevalence of colon carcinoma and the mortality can be effectively reduced by removing adenomatous polyps. Although effective, this method consumes large resources if applied to the whole target population. The currently available screening options have limitations. The VC has the option to identify patients with adenomatous polyps. The combination of VC screening and OC follow-up might prove as a cost-effective measure against colorectal cancer.

The challenges of VC are the associated radiation and the differentiation of the colonic materials from the colon wall. The MRI-based VC has no radiation and has better potential in differentiation of colonic materials from the colonic wall, but it has lower spatial resolution and is prone to motion artifacts. CT and MRI VC require sophisticated software processing to construct the colon model and real-time fly-through inside the lumen. More sophisticated image processing is important for the differentiation of adenomatous from hyperplastic ones. The extraction of the colon wall can be performed by the new method of electronic colon cleansing and analysis of texture features from image intensity of the wall. These processing methods are step toward computer-aided detection and diagnosis. Despite recent advances in chemotherapeutic agents, the prognosis for metastatic colon cancer remains poor. Over the past two decades, hepatic metastasectomy has emerged as a promising technique for improving survival in patients with metastatic colon cancer and in some cases providing long-term cure. To maximize safety and efficacy of metastasectomy, appropriate pre-operative imaging is needed. Advancements in computed tomography (CT), magnetic resonance imaging (MRI) and positron emission tomography (PET) have led to improved detection of occult lesions and better definition of surgical anatomy. While CT, PET and MRI have a comparable sensitivity for detection of large liver metastases, MRI excels at detection of subcentimeter liver metastases compared to CT and FDG-PET, especially with the combination of diffusion weighted imaging (DWI) and hepatocyte-specific contrast agents. CT may be useful as a screening modality or in preoperative planning such as volumetric estimation of the remnant liver size or in defining preoperative arterial anatomy for hepatic artery infusion pump placement. While technologic advancements have led to unprecedented image quality and clarity, this does not replace the need for a dedicated, competent radiologist with experience in hepatic imaging.

Author details

Valentin Ignatov[1], Nikola Kolev[1], Anton Tonev[1], Shteryu Shterev[1], Elitsa Encheva[4], Tanya Kirilova[2], Tsvetelina Teneva[3] and Krassimir Ivanov[1]

1 Department of General and Operative Surgery, University Hospital "St. Marina" – Varna, Bulgaria

2 Department of Gastroenterology, University Hospital "St. Marina"- Varna, Bulgaria

3 Department of Image diagnostics, University Hospital "St. Marina"- Varna, Bulgaria

4 Department of Radiology, University Hospital "St. Marina" – Varna, Bulgaria

References

[1] American Cancer Society. Cancer Facts & Figures 2008. Atlanta: American Cancer Society; 2008.

[2] Jemal A, Siegel R, Ward E, et al. Cancer Statistics – 2008. A Cancer Journal for Clinicians 2008;58 (1):71–96.

[3] Hill M, Morrison B, Bussey H. Etiology of Adenoma Carcinoma Sequence in the Large Bowel. Lancet 1978;1(2):245–247. [PubMed: 74668]

[4] Rickert R, Auerbach O, Garfinkel L, et al. Adenomatous Lesions of the Large Bowel – An autopsy survey. Cancer 1979;43(11):1847–1857. [PubMed: 445371]

[5] Grandqvist S. Distribution of Polyps of the Large Bowel in Relation to Age: A colonoscopic study. Scandinavian Journal of Gastroenterology (SJG) 1981;16(11):1025–1031.

[6] Stryker S, Wolff B, Culp C, et al. Natural History of Untreated Colonic Polyps. Gastroenterology 1987;93(5):1009–1013. [PubMed: 3653628]

[7] Winawer S, Zauber A, Diaz B. The National Polyp Study – Temporal sequence of evolving colorectal cancer from normal colon. Gastrointestinal Endoscopy 1987;33(2): 167.

[8] Fearon E, Vogelstein B. A Genetic Model for Colorectal Tumorigensis. Cell 1990;61(5):759–767. [PubMed: 2188735]

[9] Johnson D, Gurney M, Volpe R, et al. A Prospective Study of the Prevalence of Colonic Neoplasms in Asymptomatic Patients with an Age-Related Risk. American Journal of Gastroenterology (AJG) 1990;85(6):969–974.

[10] Simons B, Morrison A, Lev R, Verhoek-Oftendahl W. Relationship of Polyps to Cancer of the Large Intestine. Journal of the National Cancer Institute (JNCI) 1992;84(5): 962–966.

[11] Potter J, Slattery M. Colon Cancer: A review of the epidemiology. Epidemiologic Reviews 1993;15 (3):499–545. [PubMed: 8174669]

[12] Byers T, Levin B, Rotherberger D, et al. ACS Guidelines for Screening and Surveillance for Early Detection of Colorectal Polyps and Cancer: Update 1997, CA. A Cancer Journal for Clinicians 1997;47(1):154–160.

[13] Winawer S, Fletcher R, Mayer R. Colorectal Cancer Screening: Clinical guidelines and rational. Gastroenterology 1997;112(3):594–642. [PubMed: 9024315]

[14] Robbins D, Itzowitz S. The Molecular and Genetic Basis of Colon Cancer. Medical Clinics of North America (MCNA) 2002;86(6):1467–1495.

[15] Church J. Clinical Significance of Small Colorectal Polyps. Diseases of the Colon and Rectum 2004;47(4):481–485. [PubMed: 14994108]

[16] Lieberman D, Holub J, Eisen G, et al. Prevalence of Polyps Greater Than 9 mm in a Consortium of Diverse Clinical Practice Settings in the United States. Clinical Gastroenterology and Hepatology 2005;3(8):798–805. [PubMed: 16234009]

[17] Odom S, Duffy S, Barone J, et al. The Rate of Adenocarcinoma in Endoscopically Removed Colorectal Polyps. The American Surgeon 2005;71(12):1024–1026. [PubMed: 16447472]

[18] Jass J. Classification of Colorectal Cancer based on Correlation of Clinical, Morphological and Molecular Features. Histopathology 2007;50(1):113–130. [PubMed: 17204026]

[19] Yoo T, Park D, Kim Y, et al. Clinical Significance of Small Colorectal Adenoma Less Than 10 mm: The KASID study. Hepatogastroenterology 2007;54(74):418–21. [PubMed: 17523287]

[20] Smith L. Fibreoptic Colonoscopy: Complications of colonoscopy and polypectomy. Diseases of the Colon and Rectum 1976;11(1):146–150.

[21] Kronberg O, Fenger C, Olsen J, et al. Randomized Study of Screening for Colorectal Cancer with Fecal-Occult-Blood Test. Lancet 1996;348(12):1467–1471. [PubMed: 8942774]

[22] Mandel J, Church T, Bond J, et al. The Effect of Fecal Occult Blood Screening on the Incidence of Colorectal Cancer. The New England Journal of Medicine 2000;343(22): 1603–1607. [PubMed: 11096167]

[23] Allison J, Sskoda I, Ransom L, et al. Screening for Colorectal Neoplasms with New Fecal Occult Blood Tests: Update on performance characteristics. Journal of the National Cancer Institute 2007;99 (11):1462–1470. [PubMed: 17895475]

[24] Imperiale T, Ransohoff D, Itzkowitz S, et al. Fecal DNA verse Fecal Occult Blood for Colorectal Cancer Screening in an Average-Risk Population. The New England Journal of Medicine 2004;351 (26):2704–2714. [PubMed: 15616205]

[25] Ahlquist D, Sargent D, Loprinzi C, et al. Stool DNA and Occult Blood Testing for Screen Detection of Colorectal Neoplasia. Annals of Internal Medicine 2008;149(7): 441–450. [PubMed: 18838724]

[26] Fork F. Double Contrast Enema and Colonoscopy in Polyp Detection. Gut 1981;22:971–977. [PubMed: 7308852]

[27] Morosi C, Ballardini G, Pisani P. Diagnostic Accuracy of the Double-Contrast Enema for Colonic Polyps in Patients with or without Diverticular Disease. Gastrointestinal Radiology 1991;16(2):345–347. [PubMed: 1936780]

[28] Brady A, Stevenson G, Stevenson I. Colorectal Cancer Overlooked at Barium Enema Examination and Colonoscopy: A continuing perceptual problem. Radiology 1994;192(2):373–378. [PubMed: 8029400]

[29] Selby J, Friedman G, Quesenberry C, Weiss N. A Case Control Study of Screening Sigmoidoscopy and Mortality from Colorectal Cancer. The New England Journal of Medicine 1992;326(10):653–657. [PubMed: 1736103]

[30] Elwood J, Sli G, Schlup M, et al. Flexible Sigmoidoscopy or Colonoscopy for Colorectal Screening: A randomized trial of performance and acceptability. Cancer Detection and Prevention 1995;19(4): 337–347. [PubMed: 7553676]

[31] Kewenter J, Breringe H, Engaras B, Haglind E. The Value of Flexible Sigmoidoscopy and Double Contrast Barium Enema in the Diagnosis of Neoplasms in the Rectum and Colon in Subjects with Positive Hemoccult: Results of 1,831 rectosigmoidoscopies and double contrast barium enemas. Endoscopy 1995;27(1):159–163. [PubMed: 7601048]

[32] Newcomb P, Storer B, Morimoto L, et al. Long-Term Efficacy of Sigmoidoscopy in the Reduction of Colorectal Cancer Incidence. Journal of the National Cancer Institute 2003;95(8):622–625. [PubMed: 12697855]

[33] Levin T, Farraye F, Schoen R, et al. Quality in the Technical Performance of Screening Flexible Sigmoidoscopy: Recommendations of an international multi-society task group. Gut 2005;54(6): 807–813. [PubMed: 15888789]

[34] Wolff W, Shinya H. Colonofiberoscopy. Journal of the American Medical Association (JAMA) 1971;217(11):1509–1512.

[35] Hafner M. Conventional Colonoscopy: Technique, indications, limites. European Journal of Radiology (EJR) 2007;61(2):409–414.

[36] Winawer S, Zauber A, Ho M, et al. Prevention of Colorectal Cancer by Colonoscopic Polypectomy. The New England Journal of Medicine 1993;329(27):1977–1981. [PubMed: 8247072]

[37] American Society for Gastrointestional Endoscopy. Appropriate Use of Gastrointestional Endpscopy. Gastrointestinal Endoscopy 2000;52(5):831–837.

[38] Seeff L, Richards T, Shapiro J, et al. How Many Endoscopies are Performed for Colorectal Cancer Screening? Results from CDC's survey of endoscopic capability. Gastroenterology 2004;127(6): 1670–1677. [PubMed: 15578503]

[39] Bartram C. Bowel Preparation – Principles and practice. Clinical Radiology 1994;49(2):365–367. [PubMed: 8045057]

[40] Ristvedt S, McFarland E, Weinstock L, Thyssen E. Patient Preferences for CTC, Conventional Colonoscopy, and Bowel Preparation. American Journal of Gastroenterology 2003;98(4):578–585. [PubMed: 12650790]

[41] "A Consensus Document on Bowel Preparation Prior to Colonoscopy," prepared by a Task Force from American Society of Colon and Rectal Surgeons (ASCRS), the American Society of Gastrointestinal Endoscopy (ASGE), and the Society of American Gastrointestinal and Endoscopic Surgeons (SAGES) on April of 2006.

[42] Cai S, Zhang S, Zhu H, Zheng S. Barriers to Colorectal Cancer Screening: A case-control study. World Journal of Gastroenterology 2009;15(12):2531–2536. [PubMed: 19469005]

[43] Stevenson G, Wilson J, Wilkinson J, et al. Pain Following Colonoscopy: Elimination with carbon dioxide. Gastrointestinal Endoscopy 1992;38(3):564–567. [PubMed: 1397911]

[44] Steine S. Which Hurts the Most? A comparison of pain rating during double-contrast barium enema examinations and colonoscopy. Radiology 1994;191(1):99–101. [PubMed: 8134605]

[45] Orsoni P, Berdah S, Verrier C, et al. Colonic Perforation due to Colonoscopy: A retrospective study of 48 cases. Endoscopy 1997;29(1):160–164. [PubMed: 9201463]

[46] Weitzman E, Zapka J, Estabrook B, Goins K. Risk and Reluctance: Understanding impediments to colorectal cancer screening. Preventive Medicine 2001;32(6):502–513. [PubMed: 11394954]

[47] Rex D, Rahmani E, Haseman J, et al. Relative Sensitivity of Colonoscopy and Barium Enema for Detection of Colorectal Cancer in Clinical Practice. Gastroenterology 1997;112(1):17–23. [PubMed: 8978337]

[48] Bressler B, Paszat L, Vinden C, et al. Colonoscopic Miss Rates for Right-Sided Colon Cancer: A population-based analysis. Gastroenterology 2004;127(2):452–456. [PubMed: 15300577]

[49] Pickhardt P, Nugent P, Mysliwiec P, et al. Location of Adenomas Missed by OC. Archives of Internal Medicine 2004;141(2):352–359.

[50] Heresbach D, Barrioz T, Lapalus M, et al. Miss Rate for Colorectal Neoplastic Polyps: A prospective multi-center study of back-to-back video colonoscopies. Endoscopy 2008;40(4):282–290.

[51] Lieberman D, Moravec M, Holub J, et al. Polyp Size and Advanced Histology in Patients Undergoing Colonoscopy Screening: Implications for CTC. Gastroenterology 2008;135(4):1100–1105. [PubMed: 18691580]

[52] Kim D, Pickhardt P, Taylor A. Characteristics of Advanced Adenomas Detected at CTC Screening: Implications for appropriate polyp size thresholds for polypectomy versus surveillance. American Journal of Roentgenology 2007;188(6):940–944. [PubMed: 17377027]

[53] Lieberman D, de Garmo P, Fleischer D, et al. Colonic Neoplasia in Patients with Non-Specific GI Symptoms. Gastrointestinal Endoscopy 2000;51(6):647–651. [PubMed: 10840294]

[54] Gelfand D. Gastrointestinal Radiology: A short history and predictions for future. American Journal of Roentgenology 1988;150(4):727–730.

[55] Vining, D.; Gelfand, D.; Bechtold, R., et al. Technical Feasibility of Colon Imaging with Helical CT and Virtual Reality. Annual Meeting of American Roentgen Ray Society; New Orleans. 1994. p. 104

[56] Hong, L.; Kaufman, A.; Wei, Y.; Viswambharan, A.; Wax, M.; Liang, Z. IEEE Biomedical Visualization Symposium. IEEE CS Press; CA: 1995. 3D Virtual Colonoscopy; p. 26-32.

[57] Hara A, Johnson C, Reed J, et al. Detection of Colorectal Polyps by CTC: Feasibility of a novel technique. Gastroenterology 1996;110(2):284–290. [PubMed: 8536869]

[58] Hong L, Liang Z, Viswambharan A, et al. Reconstruction and Visualization of 3D Models of Colonic Surface. IEEE Transactions on Nuclear Science (TNS) 1997;44(11): 1297–1302.

[59] Reed J, Johnson C. Automatic Segmentation, Tissue Characterization, and Rapid Diagnosis Enhancements to the CTC Analysis Workstation. Journal of Digital Imaging 1997;10(1):70–73. [PubMed: 9268843]

[60] Wan, M.; Tang, Q.; Kaufman, A.; Liang, Z. Proc IEEE Computer Graphics and Applications. 1999. Volume Rendering Based Interactive Navigation within the Human Colon; p. 397-400.

[61] Coin C, Wollett F, Coin J, et al. Computerized Radiology of the Colon: A potential screening technique. Computed Radiology 1983;7(2):215–221.

[62] Shinners T, Pickhardt P, Taylor A, et al. Patient-Controlled Room Air Insufflation versus Automated Carbon Dioxide Delivery for CTC. American Journal of Roentgenology 2006;186(10):1491–1496. [PubMed: 16714635]

[63] Liang Z, Chen D, Li B, et al. On Segmentation of Colon Lumen for VC. Proc SPIE Medical Imaging 1999;3660:270–278.

[64] Fenlon H, Nunes D, Schroy P, et al. A Comparison of Virtual and Conventional Colonoscopy for the Detection of Colorectal Polyps. The New England Journal of Medicine 1999;341(11):1496–1503. [PubMed: 10559450]

[65] Fletcher J, Johnson C, Welch T, et al. Optimization of CTC Technique: Prospective trial in 180 patients. Radiology 2000;216(4):704–711. [PubMed: 10966698]

[66] Yee J, Akerkar G, Hung R, et al. Colorectal Neoplasia: Performance characteristics of CTC for detection in 300 patients. Radiology 2001;219(4):685–692. [PubMed: 11376255]

[67] Johnson D, Harmsen W, Wilson L, et al. Prospective Blinded Evaluation of CTC for Screen Detection of Colorectal Polyps. Gastroenterology 2003;125(2):311–319. [PubMed: 12891530]

[68] Pickhardt P, Choi R, Hwang I, et al. Computed Tomographic VC to Screen for Colorectal Neoplasia in Asymptomatic Adults. The New England Journal of Medicine 2003;349(12):2191–2200. [PubMed: 14657426]

[69] Johnson C, Chen MH, Toledano A, et al. Accuracy of CTC for Detection of Large Adenomas and Cancers. The New England Journal of Medicine 2008;359(12):1207–1217. [PubMed: 18799557]

[70] Regge D, Laudi C, Galatola G, et al. Diagnostic Accuracy of Computed Tomographic Colonography for the Detection of Advanced Neoplasia in Individuals at Increased Risk of Colorectal Cancer. The Journal of the American Medical Association 2009;301(23):2453–2461.

[71] Brenner D, Georgsson M. Mass Screening with CTC: Should the radiation exposure be of concern? Gastroenterology 2005;129(2):328–337. [PubMed: 16012958]

[72] Neri, E.; Faggioni, L.; Cerri, F., et al. CTC versus Double-Contrast Barium Enema for Screening of Colorectal Cancer: Comparison of radiation burden. 2009. Published online by September 24:

[73] Brenner DJ, Hall EJ. Computed Tomography – An increasing source of radiation exposure. The New England Journal of Medicine 2007;357(11):2277–2284. [PubMed: 18046031]

[74] Lu H, Li X, Li L, Chen D, Xing Y, Wax M, Hsieh J, Liang Z. Adaptive Noise Reduction toward Low-Dose CT. Proc SPIE Medical Imaging 2003;5030:759–766.

[75] Wang J, Li T, Lu H, Liang Z. Penalized Weighted Least-Squares Approach to Sinogram Noise Reduction and Image Reconstruction for Low-Dose X-ray CT. IEEE Transactions on Medical Imaging (TMI) 2006;25:1272–1283.

[76] Wang J, Wang S, Li L, Lu H, Liang Z. VC Screening with Ultra Low-Dose CT & Less-Stressful Bowel Preparation: A computer simulation study. IEEE Transactions on Nuclear Science 2008;55 (5):2566–2575. [PubMed: 19169383]

[77] Rust G, Aurich V, Reiser M. Noise/Dose Reduction and Image Improvements in Screening VC with Tube Currents of 20 mAs with Nonlinear Gaussian Filter Chains. Proc SPIE Medical Imaging 2002;4683:186–197.

[78] Purkayastha S, Tekkis P, Athanasiou T, et al. Magnetic Resonance Colonography versus Colonoscopy as a Diagnostic Investigation for Colorectal Cancer: A meta-analysis. Clinical Radiology 2005;60 (6):980–989. [PubMed: 16124980]

[79] Laks S, Macari M, Bini E. Positional Change in Colon Polyps at CTC. Radiology 2004;231(4):761–766. [PubMed: 15163817]

[80] Liang, Z.; Yang, F.; Wax, M., et al. Inclusion of A Priori Information in Segmentation of Colon Lumen for 3D VC. Conf Record IEEE NSS-MIC, in CD-ROM; 1997.

[81] Liang, Z. Electronic Colon Cleansing Techniques: Past, present, and future. The 11th International Conference on Medical Image Computing and Computer Assisted In-

tervention (MICCAI) Workshop – "New Era of Virtual Colonoscopy"; New York City, NY. September 6; 2008. p. 26-32.

[82] Liang Z, MacFall J, Harrington D. Parameter Estimation and Tissue Segmentation from Multispectral MR Images. IEEE Transactions on Medical Imaging 1994;13(3): 441–449. [PubMed: 18218519]

[83] Summers R, Johnson C, Pusanik L, et al. Automated Polyp Detection at CTC: Feasibility assessment in a human population. Radiology 2001;219(1):51–59. [PubMed: 11274534]

[84] Yoshida H, Nappi J. Three-Dimensional Computer-Aided Diagnosis Scheme for Detection of Colonic Polyps. IEEE Transactions on Medical Imaging 2001;20(8):1261–1274. [PubMed: 11811826]

[85] Wang Z, Liang Z, Li L, et al. Reduction of False Positives by Internal Features for Polyp Detection in CT-Based VC. Medical Physics 2005;32(12):3602–3616. [PubMed: 16475759]

[86] Zhu H, Liang Z, Barish M, Pickhardt P, et al. Increasing Computer-aided Detection Specificity by Projection Features for CTC. Medical Physics, to appear. 2010

[87] Liang Z, Lakare S, Wax M, et al. A Pilot Study on Less-Stressful Bowel Preparation for VC Screening with Follow-up Biopsy by OC. Proc SPIE Medical Imaging 2005;5746:810–816.

[88] Pickhardt, P.; Kim, D. CTC: Principles and practice of virtual colonoscopy. Saunders, Elsevier; Philadelphia, PA, USA: 2009.

[89] Park S, Lee S, Choi E, et al. Flat Colorectal Neoplasma Definition, Importance, and Visualization on CTC. American Journal of Roentgenology 2007;188(5):953–959. [PubMed: 17377029]

[90] Liang Z, Wang S. An EM Approach to MAP Solution of Segmenting Tissue Mixtures: A numerical analysis. IEEE Transactions on Medical Imaging 2009;28(2):297–310. [PubMed: 19188116]

[91] Wang S, Li L, Cohen H, Mankes S, Chen J, Liang Z. An EM Approach to MAP Solution of Segmenting Tissue Mixture Percentages with Application to CT-based VC. Medical Physics 2008;35(12):5787–5798. [PubMed: 19175136]

2

Management of Non-Hepatic Metastatic Disease in Colorectal Cancer

C. Alberto Blanco, R. Sánchez, F. Piniella,
D. Pescador, G. Borobio, A. García and C. Cano

1. Introduction

Colorectal cancer is one of the most frequent malignant tumors and a leading cause of cancer-related death. One third of the patients develop a metastasis during the course of the disease. Because of that, it is very important to know about the evolution of the illness, how to make a quick diagnosis and how to provide an appropriate treatment depending on the tumor and the location of the metastases.

Management of patients with colorectal metastases without the intervention of a multidisciplinary team specialized in the liver can lead to patients being denied potentially curative treatments.

1.1. Metastatic disease

It´s necessary to have a protocol before the treatment of metastatic disease:

- Physical examination
- Laboratory test: The serum carcinoembryonic antigen (CEA) level is a valuable marker in patients with recurrent colorectal cancer. It must be remembered that about 25% of tumors do not secrete CEA.
- Imaging: Radiologic imaging is a critical component of the preoperative research on a patient with colorectal liver metastasis. In fact, it is often used to determine whether the patient should be further considered for resection.
- Surgical indications: the patient must be in acceptable health to tolerate the physiologic consequences of the surgery. Next, the primary colorectal cancer must be resected and the

presence of other extrahepatic disease must be ruled out. Preoperative workup should include a recent colonoscopy, chest X-ray and chest CT.

- Complications: Successful outcome in hepatic surgery depends largely upon minimizing intraoperative blood loss. Excessive blood loss is not only associated with increased perioperative morbidity but also with a shorter time to recurrence and decreased survival rates after resection of colorectal liver metastases.
- Survival

2. Non hepatic disease in colorectal cancer

2.1. Lung metastases

2.1.1. Lung metastases in CRC

Colon cancer is a systemic disease in 19% of the patients, and the liver and lungs are the most common locations for a metastasis. Colorectal adenocarcinoma is the most common cancer leading to pulmonary metastasectomy

2.1.1.1. Symptoms

Most pulmonary metastases are asymptomatic and they are detected incidentally during the initial diagnostic staging study for a primary tumor or in the monitoring imaging studies afterwards, generally during a thoracic CT scan. Symptoms such as coughing, pain or hemoptysis mainly appear in patients with hilar involvement.

2.1.1.2. Preoperative evaluation

A solitary pulmonary nodule in a patient with a previous cancer can be bening or malignant (primary or secondary); although in most cases will be malignant (Mery et al. 2004). When there are multiple nodules, the probability of metastatic disease increases significantly.

There are no pathognomonic radiological features that distinguish the metastasis of primary tumors, even though metastasis is generally well circumscribed, spherical with smooth margins and are mainly subpleurales or periferics. However, primary lung cancers are single lesions, with irregular edges, asociated linear densities and are often more central.

Although the background and radiographic features of a lesion can provide clues as to whether an individual lesion is bening or malignant, it is not posible to distinguish reliably a metastasis from a primary lung cancer. The resection of the nodule is the most reliable method to establish the diagnosis.

The presence of pulmonary metastasis makes it necessary to carry out a complete staging. The extent of the required pulmonary resection will guide the preoperative evaluation of the patients: patients who require a pneumonectomy will need a higher level of cardiopulmonary reserve compared with patients who only require wedge resections (Villeneuve and Sundaresan 2009). The key for a successful surgical resection of pulmonary metastases is an adequate selection of the patient through a preoperative evaluation and a precise surgical planning. To do so, we can use the following diagnostic tests:

High-resolution helical CAT scan is a basic tool which detects approximately 20-25% more nodes that standard CT, and the detection is reliable in nodes of 2-3 mm (Remy-Jardin et al. 1993; Collie et al. 1994).

PET – An examination with Positron Emission Tomography (PET-FDG) is recommended to optimize the selection of patients who are candidates for pulmonary metastasectomy. However, we have to take into account the fact that PET has a limited sensitivity for lesions <1 cm in size (Reinhardt et al. 2006). It is very useful to assess the intra-thoracic node involvement (hilar or mediastinal), local hidden recurrence of the primary tumor or in other locations such as the abdomen or the pelvis (Villeneuve and Sundaresan 2009).

The main value of PET is its high sensitivity to detect an extra-thoracic disease. In general terms, metastasectomy must not be performed unless all the deposits or foci of the disease are treatable (except when the patient is included in a specific protocol such as a clinical trial for a vaccine or symptomatic lesions that cannot be treated otherwise). In any case, a positive extra-thoracic result in a PET examination is not enough evidence to rule a patient out from surgery for pulmonary metastases. All suspicious extra-thoracic FDG-highlighted areas must be biopsied before surgery.

Preoperative biopsy – In patients with highly suspicious lesions in imaging tests, the final diagnosis is often achieved after the surgical removal of the metastases. However, in many cases, a preoperative biopsy with CT-guided fine needle aspiration is a useful and less invasive method to obtain a pathological diagnosis, particularly if the diagnosis of the metastatic disease is not clear, if the patient is not a good candidate for surgery or if the patient has a primary tumor (such as testicular germ-cell cancer or lymphoma) for which surgery may not be required.

Bronchoscopy (with or without endobronchial ultrasound) is indicated as part of the evaluation in cases of lesions that are centrally located in the CT scan, patients with symptoms of involvement of the respiratory tract and some types of tumors prone to endobronchial involvement, such as breast cancer, colon cancer and renal cell carcinoma [36]. Bronchoscopy is performed before surgery, when a positive result may contraindicate an operation.

The presence of pathological mediastinal adenopathies requires a **biopsy** with a mediastinoscopy or ultrasound-guided endobronchial needle **aspiration cytology**. Most authors consider mediastinal node involvement (N2) as a contraindication for resection.

2.1.1.3.Treatment

Management of patients with pulmonary metastases, according to the guidelines of the National Comprehensive Cancer Network (NCCN) will depend on the form of presentation along time and on whether the metastases can be resected or not. Synchronous resectable metastases are treated with chemotherapy with or without later resection; and if they cannot be resected, then chemotherapy is indicated. Metachronous resectable metastases can be resected with or without neoadjuvant chemotherapy, and chemotherapy is indicated when they cannot be resected. The evaluation of patients in treatment with chemotherapy that can be transferred to surgery is carried out every 2 months in the selected cases (2013).

Although the quality of the currently available evidence on pulmonary **metastasectomy** in cases of colorectal cancer is not enough to draw conclusions on the effectiveness of this kind of surgery (Pfannschmidt et al. 2007; Fiorentino et al. 2010; Pfannschmidt et al. 2010; Salah et al. 2012; Gonzalez et al. 2013), pulmonary metastasectomy in cases of selected patients with metastatic colorectal cancer is a general practice and it is included in the clinical guidelines (Poston et al. 2011). The objective is to limit surgery only for patients who have the highest chances to benefit from it, either with longer survival rates or symptom relief, and to optimize the time of the operation.

The **resectability criteria** admitted by the main groups are the following (Ehrenhaft et al. 1958; Martini and McCormack 1998; Greelish and Friedberg 2000; Jaklitsch et al. 2001; Pfannschmidt et al. 2003; Kondo et al. 2005):

- Complete anatomical resection maintaining an adequate pulmonary function (McAfee et al. 1992; Regnard et al. 1998; Inoue et al. 2000; Sakamoto et al. 2001)
- Removal of the primary tumor without persistence of residual disease (R0)
- The existence of resectable extra-pulmonary metastases does not contraindicate pulmonary resection (Yano et al. 1993; Ambiru et al. 1998; Irshad et al. 2001; Rena et al. 2002); in this case, the metastases must be treatable with surgery or other therapeutic approach.
- Resectable metastases can be treated with a synchronous resection or a sequential approach.

The resection of one or more pulmonary lesions may also be indicated in a patient with a known malignant tumor when:

- A new primary lung cancer cannot be ruled out
- There are symptomatic metastases (such as bronchial obstruction with distal suppuration) that cannot be treated in any other way
- Tissue is required for a new therapeutic strategy (such as an autologous vaccine), preferably in the framework of a clinical trial.

The approach depends on the number, size, location and estability during the time in TC. In general, Video-assisted thoracoscopic surgery (VATS) is ideal for peripheral metastases single or few, stable and smaller than 3 cm. The central lesions are likely to require a segmentectomy or lobectomy and is best addressed by open thoracotomy.

Video-assisted thoracoscopic surgery has the advantage that it is less painful, postoperative recovery is faster, hospitalization is shorter and lower long-term morbidity, especially intrathoracic recurrences (Saisho et al. 2009). Recurrence rates appear to be similar to the approach using thoracotomy (Saisho et al. 2009). There are no randomised trials comparing results between open resections and thoracoscopic surgery, although retrospectively patients treated by VATS have similar results to patients treated by conventional open thoracotomy (Carballo et al. 2009)

Concerning the number of metastasis, it is clear that technically the fewer there is, the better. Although there is no general consensus, ideally from technical and oncologic point of view, it would be less than five (Hellman and Weichselbaum 1995; Weichselbaum and Hellman 2011) however it is true that in the majority of cases, unique pulmonary metastasectomies are conducted and in these patients there is a greater survival advantage (Fiorentino et al. 2010). Metastases in both lungs are not a contraindication for surgery.

For some patients with metastatic CRC, repeated pulmonary metastasectomy offers an excellent opportunity for long-term survival, and it is associated with a low operative mortality rate. Patients with more than 2 metastatic nodes and a maximum diameter of the metastatic pulmonary node of more than 3 cm present a significantly lower survival rate (Hendriks et al. 2001; Salah et al. 2013).

In the case of patients who do not meet the criteria for a metastasectomy, there are alternative ablative techniques to locally control the lesion, such as **stereotactic radiotherapy** and **radiofrequency ablation** or **cryoablation**. The experience with these ablation techniques is limited, but the initial results look promising (Pennathur, Abbas et al. 2009). The role of **chemotherapy** is not yet defined for pulmonary metastases with a colorectal origin, because traditionally, these lesions do not show a good response to adjuvant treatments. Currently, chemotherapy has shown very good responses in primary CRC with regimens such as FOLFOX (fluorouracil, leucovorin and oxaliplatin) and FOLFIRI (fluorouracil, leucovorin and irinotecan), with or without the addition of biological agents such as bevacizumab (anti-vascular endothelial growth factor, VEGF), cetuximab and panitumumab (anti-epidermal growth factor, EGFR). These therapies have not yet been systematically studied, and they may become the most effective treatment for pulmonary metastases. As a last resort, patients whose functional state is poor are candidates for palliative treatment only (Villeneuve & Sundaresan 2009).

External radiotherapy can be an option in very specific cases or in clinical trials, provided that the tumors are not potentially resectable.

2.1.2. Prognostic factors

There are many factors that have an influence on survival after a metastasectomy. The presence of one or more factors for poor prognosis does not represent an absolute contraindication for a metastasectomy (Quiros and Scott 2008). Unfavourable prognostic factors include number and size of the metastasis, inability to completely resect the entire metastatic disease, a short disease-free interval after treatment for the primary tumor and thoracic node involvement. For its part, the histology of the tumor also influences the results.

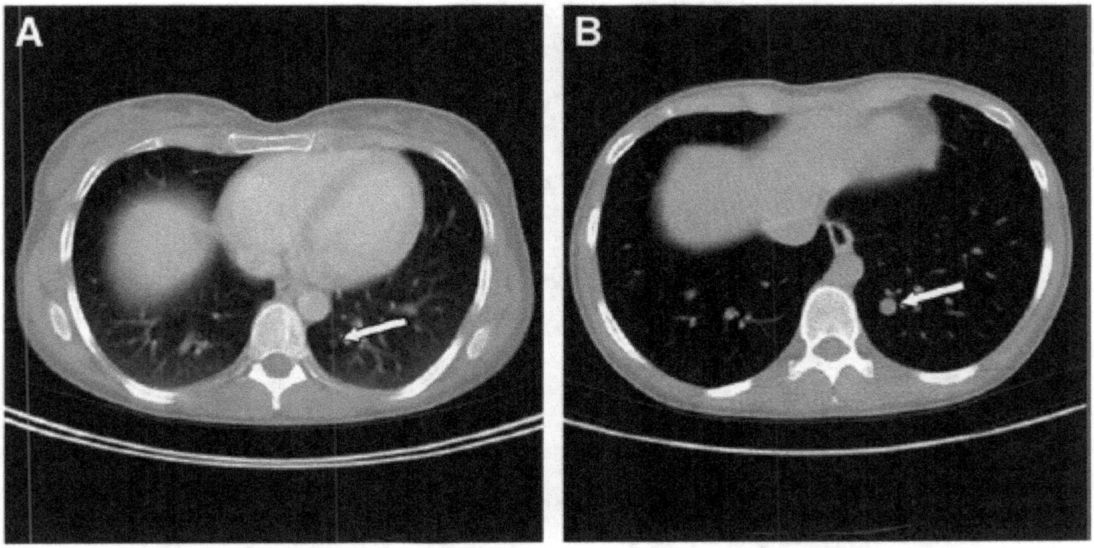

Figure 1. Comparison of chest scanning during shallow breathing (A) and chest scanning with additional low-dose CT during maximal inspiration (B). (A) Lung metastasis from colorectal cancer is only barely visible during shallow breathing (arrow). Also note blurred lung vessels and congested lung parenchyma in this image. (B) Metastasis can be clearly detected by low-dose CT during maximal inspiration (arrow). Additionally, lung parenchyma is well inflated, and lung vessels are displayed sharply. http://jnm.snmjournals.org/content/48/1_suppl/45S/F2.expansion.html

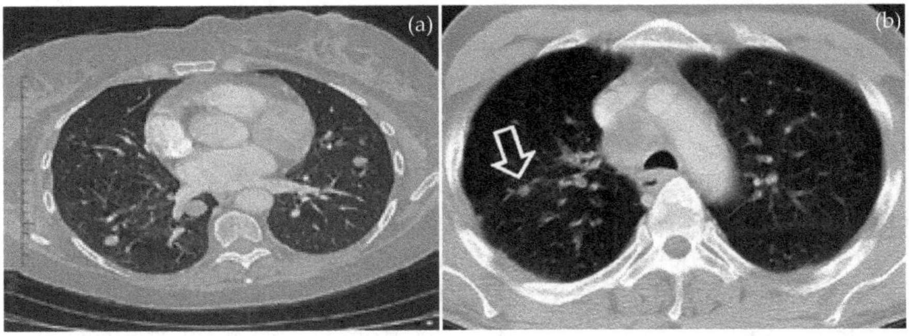

Figure 2. Multiple metastases Multiple pulmonary metastases from colorectal carcinoma. http://radiopaedia.org/articles/pulmonary-metastases, TC/PET metastases from colorectal cancer

3. Node metastases

3.1. Definition and physiopathology

Node metastases are, like with other cancers, the most important dissemination route for colorectal cancers. This makes lymph node involvement the most important factor in the prognosis and therapeutic approach for colorectal cancer.

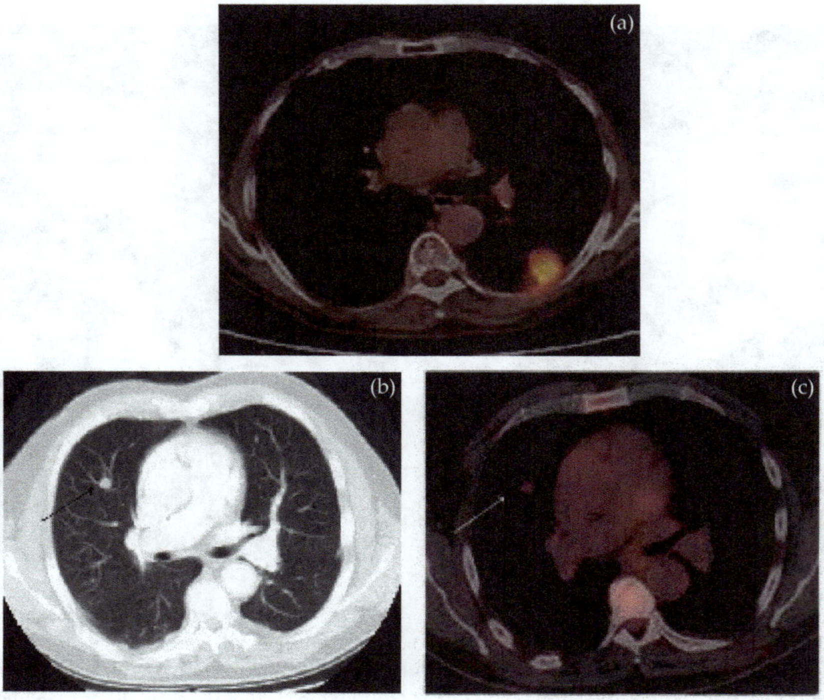

Figure 3. Patient with rectal carcinoma and mildly FDG avid metastases to lung. (a) There is a suspicious right upper lobe lung nodule (arrow) on CT in a patient with prior history of rectal carcinoma. (b) The lesion is only mildly FDG avid (arrow) on fused PET-CT. Based on these images the lesion is not definitively malignant. This may be due to the limited resolution of PET and the small lesion size or reduced cellularity. (c) Lung biopsy was subsequently performed confirming that the lesion (arrow) represented a metastatic deposit from rectal carcinoma. http://www.hindawi.com/journals/ijso/2011/846512/fig7/

The first metastases usually appear in the paracolic nodes closest to the primary tumor they are draining, and frequently only one or two nodes close to the tumor are involved. However, as the disease evolves, node propagation is larger and affects a variable amount of nodes located further away, on the arteriovenous system that depends on the intestinal segment involved. As the neoplasm moves forward, nodes from the main colic vessels that drain the intestinal neoplastic area are invaded, and the process gradually spreads upwards through the node chain that accompanies the vessels until it finally reaches the nodes that depend on the large mesenteric vessels (and, in the case of the rectum, the nodes that depend on the iliac vessels through the hemorrhoidal venous system). In short, it is known that here is a correlation between each segment of the colon and its venous and lymphatic drainage which, although there may be individual alterations, essentially depends on the superior mesenteric venous system up to the splenic flexure of the colon and, from there, up to the superior rectal vein which depends on the inferior mesenteric vein. Both are affluent to the portal vein and the structure of the lymph drainage system is essentially the same. In the area of the rectum, it has been traditionally accepted that the superior rectal venous system depends on the inferior mesenteric system, that the middle rectal system depends on the inferior mesenteric system and the internal iliac system, and that the inferior rectal system depends on the internal and external iliac system.

On the other hand, there are evidences that show that there are factors of the tumor cells which increase angiogenesis and lymphomagenesis, and which lead to an increased rate of node metastasis and a worse prognosis. Specifically, vascular endothelial growth factor C (VEGF-C) and cyclooxygenase-2 (COX-2) (Coexpression of VEGF-C and Cox-2 in Human Colorectal Cancer and its Association With Lymph Node Metastasis Soumaoro et al. Dis Colon Rectum, March 2006 392-398).

Node involvement plays a fundamental role in the correct definition of the extent of tumor spread, together with the depth of the involvement through the wall of the colon or the rectum, the size of the tumor or the presence of metastases. The number of involved nodes and their distance to the tumor is the basis of some classic classifications, such as Dukes, Astler and Coller and the more modern TNM, whose description is already analyzed elsewhere. All decisions on the treatment must be adopted with reference to the TNM classification, instead of the old Dukes system or the modified Astler-Coller staging system (Colon and rectum. In: Edge SB, Byrd DR, Compton CC, et al., eds.: AJCC Cancer Staging Manual. 7th ed. New York, NY: Springer, 2010, pp 143-64).

Given the importance of the whole number of involved nodes in a proper staging and in order to obtain a reliable and comparable prognosis, it is necessary to establish a set of minimum quality criteria for lymphadenectomy. Otherwise, the scenario might be undervalued. Patients in stage I or II (that is, without node involvement) show five-year survival rates of 75%; in contrast to survival rates with N1, which are only 45-60%. Also, the higher the number of nodes studied by the pathologist (and indirectly, resected by the surgeon), the higher the staging accuracy; if that number is low, there is an undervaluing of the tumor dissemination state. (Staging accuracy in colorectal carcinoma. Wong et al. Journal of Clinical Oncology. Vol 17. nº 9 1999pp2896-2900).

A panel sponsored by the American Joint Committee on Cancer (AJCC) and the National Cancer Institute of the USA and presented at the World Conference on Gastroenterology of Sydney in 1990 (J. Gastroenterol Heptol 6:325-244. 1991) has recommended that at least 12 lymph nodes be examined in patients with colon and rectal cancer in order to confirm the lack of node involvement due to the tumor. Wong et al. recommend at least the analysis of 14 nodes in pT2 and pT3 tumors.

There is a special situation with staging patients with rectal cancer and neoadjuvant chemotherapy with ypT0-2. In these cases, staging based on the surgical specimen usually shows a decrease in size and in the involvement of the wall of the intestine of the tumor, but if this is taken into account together with the reduction in the number of existing nodes in the specimen removed from the rectum, it could lead to an undervaluing with negative consequences for the patient's survival (Comparative Analisis of Limph Node Metastasis in Patients UIT ypT0-2 Rectal Cancers. Park et al. Disease of the Colon and Rectum. Volume 56: 2 (2013). Here, it is necessary to insist on the fact that, just as the primary treatment of node metastases in CRC must spread as much as possible (total mesorectal excision, or TME); in the case of patients who have undergone neoadjuvant treatment with chemotherapy it is also essential to perform a TME.

The studies that want to ensure the diagnosis of node involvement have researched the presence of micrometastases or metastases that have been diagnosed with immunohistochemical techniques in patients in stages I and II (that is, without node involvement in microscopical terms), and they have found that the presence of micrometastases in these patients does not affect the prognosis and must not be taken into account when treating CRC (Are Lymph Node Micrometastases of any Clinical Significance in Dukes Stages A and B Colorectal Cancer? Oberg et al. Dis Colon Rectum, October 1998 ol. 41, No. 10 1244-1249).

3.2. Sentinel lymph node

In tumors with a metastasis that takes place through the lymphatic system (breast cancer and melanoma, mainly), there has been a great success in mapping the dissemination of the primary tumor with the so called sentinel lymph node biopsy technique. In view of this situation, several studies have started to analyze it, because lymphadenectomy is an important part in the primary treatment of CRC, both from the staging point of view and in order to prevent recurrence of the tumor if there are infiltrated lymph nodes left. Having a map of lymph dissemination similar to the one obtained with breast cancer would mean knowing the minimum required level of lymphadenectomy, or even of visceral resection. This would allow the medical team to apply an adequate surgical treatment from an oncological perspective but with the minimum morbidity and mortality. Unfortunately, it does not seem that this technique shows reliable results with colorectal cancer ("Técnica del ganglio centinela…". Sardon Ramos et al. CIR ESP. 2013 91(6) 366-371.1).

The identification of the sentinel lymph node shows a low sensitivity in the detection of metastasis and micrometastasis. Approximately one half of the adenopathies are lost if a lymphadenectomy is performed based on the results of the sentinel lymph node study. Faerden et al: sentinel node mapping in colonic cancer Disease of the colon & rectum. Volume 51: 891–896 (2008).

3.3. Treatment of lymphatic metastasis

Treatment of lymphatic metastasis, given its close relation with the growth of the primary tumor, is the same as for the original lesion: primary resection with exeresis of the nodes of the lymphatic area that drain the tumor. If there is a tumor recurrence in the nodes, the patient is classified as stage IV, which means that there will be the corresponding treatment: chemotherapy and surgery and radiotherapy, which will be provisionally palliative.

4. Bone metastases

4.1. Introduction

Bone metastases from colorectal cancer are uncommon (10-23% in autopsy cases). They usually appear late in the natural history of metastatic disease and are associated with liver or lung metastasis. Acrometastasis is reported to be 0.3-3% of all bone metastases. Cancers of the rectum and cecum are accompanied by bone metastasis more frequently than cancers of other portions of the colon. Signet ring cell carcinoma shows a high incidence of bone metastasis.

Pain is the most common symptom of bone metastasis. As a result of the loss of bone density affected bones become prone to fracture and injury.

Testing for bone metastasis includes X-ray and bone scanning. Open biopsy is necessary to establish the diagnosis, exclude osteomyelitis and allow treatment. Early diagnosis is important for improving quality of life in these patients.

Therapeutic management of this condition includes chemotherapy, radiotherapy and surgery, but because survival after onset of bone metastasis is very poor, palliative treatment is the main objective.

4.2. Physiopathology

Bone destruction secondary to metastasis is not caused by the tumor cells, but by the activation of the osteoclasts. The tumor cells secrete an osteoclast activating factor, and the osteoclasts induce the loss of cortical bone and trabecular bone. This process is divided in four stages (Mundy & Yoneda, 1995):

1. The tumor cells adhere to the basement membrane (laminin, E-cadherin, integrins).
2. The tumor cells produce proteolytic enzymes that damage the basement membrane.
3. The tumor cells migrate via the basement membrane under the specific control of chemotactic factors.
4. The tumor cells can stimulate the activity of the osteoclasts.

Clohisy et al. have described four mechanisms that stimulate osteoclast-mediated bone destruction (Clohisy et al., 2000):

a. Stimulation of the union between the osteoclasts and the bone.

b. Stimulation of the osteoclast-mediated bone resorption.

c. Extension of the survival time of osteoclasts.

d. Acceleration of the production of osteoclasts by precursor cells.

4.3. Clinical presentation

a. *Constitutional symptoms*: Some patients report anorexia, nausea, vomiting, asthenia, malaise, and weight loss.

b. *Symptoms derived from the primary location*: Colorectal carcinoma usually presents itself accompanied by an alteration of the intestinal rhythm and by the expulsion of blood originated in the rectum. In advanced stages of the disease, the patient presents constipation, and a transabdominal mass can be perceived on palpation. A rectal examination needs to be performed, because tumors of the lower part of the rectum can be easily found.

c. *Symptoms derived from the metastatic disease*: Regardless of the symptoms that metastases may produce on other regions, bone metastases can lead to:

a. PAIN in the affected area, or referred pain, which may be of insidious, and either progressive or sudden onset, and it may be slight and intermittent or continuous and activity-related. Night pain is a typical symptom, and it does not always disappear with oral analgesics, unlike the pain that derives from degenerative processes, such as osteoarthritis, which increases with loads and articular mobility. When pain affects a long bone, it is easily located by the patient, but when it affects the pelvis or the spinal column, the pain makes it difficult to properly locate the lesion. When it affects the femur or the tibia (load-bearing bones), patients report pain when walking, although the pain usually appears when the bone destruction levels are over 50% and they indicate an imminent fracture.

b. SWELLING: It may be a sign of lesion aggressiveness when the tumor invades the cortical bone and affects soft tissue. This presentation is characteristic from colorectal carcinoma, renal carcinoma and melanoma.

c. FUNCTIONAL DEFICIT: it appears as a consequence of pain. It may be a result of a medullary or radicular involvement in the case of spinal metastases.

d. IMMINENT FRACTURE: It is a fracture that can appear as a result of a physiological load. Anamnesis and plain X-ray are necessary for the diagnosis, and the cortical involvement, the location and characteristics of the lesion (lytic, sclerotic or mixed) and the existence of fracture lines must be assessed. Permeating and lytic lesions of the proximal third of the femur are prone to fractures. Pain after radiation is also a sign of an imminent fracture. In cases in which an imminent fracture is expected on an active patient, a prophylactic fixation is recommended, especially in load-bearing bones.

4.4. Diagnostic assessment

In the context of colorectal carcinoma, bone metastases normally appear when the disease is already in an advanced stage (with metastases on other areas), and when the diagnosis has already been established. For this reason, a histological diagnosis is not usually necessary, and a treatment can be planned in advance. However, we must also take into account the fact that in 1-2% of the cases, the osteolytic lesion is unrelated to the primary tumor, which means that a biopsy is advisable.

4.4.1. Complete physical examination

Including the thyroid gland, breasts, lungs and digestive system.

4.4.2. Laboratory analyses

1. COMPLETE BLOOD COUNT: Anemia, leukopenia or thrombocytopenia may be a sign of medullary involvement.

2. ESR: High levels may indicate a myeloma or an active process.

3. ELECTROPHORESIS OF SERUM PROTEINS: They can show a monoclonal gammopathy and they can confirm a possible myeloma diagnosis.
4. BIOCHEMICAL ANALYSIS: It can rule out hyperparathyroidism.
5. ALKALINE PHOSPHATASE: It shows high levels in cases of advanced metastatic disease. Very high levels show an unfavourable prognostic factor.
6. CARCINOEMBRYONIC ANTIGEN: Its levels are high in digestive or hepatocellular carcinomas.
7. PROSTATE-SPECIFIC ANTIGEN: It can detect a prostate carcinoma.
8. HEPATIC ENZYMES AND SERUM ELECTROLYTES: They can show bone and liver involvement.

4.4.3. Imaging tests

1. ANTEROPOSTERIOR AND LATERAL X-RAYS OF THE LESION: In order to assess an imminent fracture and to analyse the information they provide.
2. THORACIC X-RAY: In order to see the existence of carcinoma or lung metastases.
3. THORACIC AND ABDOMINAL CT SCAN: In order to assess the existence of possible visceral metastases.
4. Tc99m BONE SCINTIGRAPHY: In order to assess bone lesions.

Data from the clinical record, an exhaustive physical examination, blood tests and imaging tests identify more than 85% of all the primary tumors that appear as a bone metastasis. The following tests could also be performed, albeit only when required:

- NMR: It is seldom recommended in cases of isolated bone lesions (fig. 1), but it may be useful in cases of a single metastasis in which a resection can be performed, in order to rule out *skip metastases* or metastases inside the bone and on the vertebrae, due to its excellent properties for the exploration of the bone marrow.
- POSITRON EMISSION TOMOGRAPHY (PET): This imaging technique is becoming more and more important in the field of orthopaedic oncology. It uses [18F]2-fluoro-2-deoxy-Dglucose (FDG) as a tracer. This is a glucose analog which is taken to the cells by a group of proteins. This marker is absorbed by malignant tissue with an increased metabolic activity. PET scans have a very high sensitivity, and it is an important technique for the identification of primary lesions and other metastases. It can establish the difference between a local recurrence and a scar, and it is also useful in the assessment of response to treatment.

4.4.4. Biopsy

Puncture biopsy is an excellent way to confirm a diagnosis of bone metastasis. CT-guided fine-needle aspiration and thick- or trephine-needle biopsies are very precise techniques, and they are easy to use. The orthopaedic surgeon must choose the exact location, taking into account the location of the lesion, viable access routes and, whenever possible, the final incision line of the operation, in case of resection surgery, excising the entire area of the biopsy, because it might be contaminated.

When finding certain locations (usually on the pelvis), a CT scan may be necessary in order to identify the best point and route of access that will reach the metastatic area and to avoid regions with reactive sclerotic bone, because these parts may not have tumor cells.

If colorectal carcinoma presents itself with a bone metastasis and the lesion is biopsied, the biopsy may not always provide a diagnosis for the primary tumor, because a tissue compatible with adenocarcinoma does not always tell the difference between primary tumors of the digestive system, prostate, breast and lung.

4.5. Supportive measures

4.5.1. Analgesic therapy

Around 70% of all patients with a bone metastasis report pain at some point along the course of the disease. The physiopathological pain may be due to medullary compression, distension of the periosteum or peripheral neurovascular involvement, as well as to pathological fractures, whenever they are present and mediated by substances such as histamine, substance P or other cytokines.

4.5.2. Bisphosphonates

Metastatic osteolysis is caused by the stimulation of osteoclast activity. For this reason, bisphosphonates can play an important role in this process, because they inhibit the osteoclast activity. They bind with the mineral bone matrix and they have a great physicochemical impact on the hydroxyapatite crystals.

Some authors have suggested that they are not only useful in the treatment of pain and the prevention of osteolytic complications, but that they can also modify the natural course of evolution of cancer in some cases, due to the effect they have on some intermediate products, such as growth factors.

Ross et al. carried out a systematic review of all randomized essays on patients with bone metastasis. It is a meta-analysis based on 18 randomized studies in which different bisphosphonates have been compared with a placebo or between themselves. Most of these studies were performed on patients with breast carcinoma (Ross et al, 2004). The review showed a decrease in the incidence and an increase in the time until the appearance of bone complications, with a better evolution of pain and functional capacity, with regard to the control group who received a placebo. Treatment with oral bisphosphonates (clodronate, etidronate) caused a decrease in the number of spinal and non-spinal fractures, but it had no effect on the indications of radiotherapy or in hypercalcaemia.

4.5.3. Treatment of hypercalcaemia

Hypercalcaemia affects 10-40% of cancer patients at some point, and it causes anorexia, nausea, vomiting, polydipsia, polyuria, dehydration, constipation, confusion and coma.

It is the result of PTHrP production, which activates bone metabolism and induces an excess of osteoclast activity. Osteoclasts are then stimulated by local factors produced by tumor cells, such as interleukin 6. Moreover, calcium levels are also increased due to lower levels of renal calcium elimination, because PTHrP acts on the renal receptors of the parathyroid hormone and it increases calcium resorption on the renal tubule. Polyuria and reduction of intravascular volume appear as a consequence, and for this reason, the initial treatment with these patients is rehydration with intravenous saline serum in order to balance the intravascular volume and to improve glomerular filtration and renal secretion of calcium.

Calcitonin inhibits osteoclasts and it has a rapid effect, although for a brief period of time. For this reason, it is mainly used in emergency treatments.

Plicamycin normalizes calcium levels in up to 50% of the cases, but its serious adverse effects make it unadvisable to use it.

4.6. Non-surgical treatment

4.6.1. Treatment of metastatic bone disease secondary to colorectal carcinoma

The treatment of bone metastases derived from colorectal tumors is the same as the treatment for other metastases caused by other tumors. Surgical resection of the primary tumor, together with chemotherapy and radiotherapy for the rectal cancer is the treatment of choice, depending on the cases.

4.6.2. Radiotherapy

Radiotherapy is the most widely used palliative treatment for bone metastasis. It is the treatment of choice for painful lytic bone metastases without short-term risk of fracture, and it is combined with surgery when there is an imminent fracture or when the fracture has already taken place. It leads to the necrosis of tumor cells, which makes it possible for the bone tissue to regenerate afterwards. The result is pain relief and, later on, a re-calcification of the destroyed areas of the bone, which is important for the functional recovery of the patient and the prevention of pathological fractures.

4.6.3 Surgical treatment

Surgery for bone metastases requires a previous complete general and local assessment. It presents its own indications, objectives, techniques and means, and it is associated to a program for postoperative radiotherapy that follows the lines that have been previously described.

5. Brain metastases

The increasing incidence of brain metastases in patients with metastatic colorectal cancer has been attributed to the longer survival rates seen with newer systemic therapies. Compared to the era when 5-fluorouracil was the primary agent for metastatic disease, median survival has increased markedly with the introduction of oxaliplatin, irinotecan, and biologic therapies (from 6 to 7 to approximately 24 months).

However, the incidence of brain metastases in metastatic colorectal cancer is still low, 2.3 percent in one of the series. Brain metastases are usually a late-stage phenomenon, and the vast majority of patients have metastases in other sites, particularly the lung. Outcomes are poor, despite aggressive treatment.

The most common mechanism of metastasis to the brain is by hematogenous spread. Metastases are usually located directly at the junction of the gray matter and white matter where blood vessels decrease in diameter and act as a trap for clumps of tumor cells. Brain metastases also tend to be more common at the terminal "watershed areas" of arterial circulation. The distribution of metastases roughly follows the relative weight and blood flow in each area:

- Cerebral hemispheres — approximately 80 percent
- Cerebellum — 15 percent
- Brainstem — 5 percent

Different primary tumors may have a predilection for metastasis to different areas within the brain. Gastrointestinal tumors more commonly metastasize to the posterior fossa.

5.1. Clinical presentation

Brain metastases have highly variable clinical features and should be suspected in any cancer patient who develops neurologic symptoms or behavioural abnormalities. However, multiple other causes can also be responsible. In the majority of patients, a gradually expanding tumor mass and its associated edema cause symptoms. Less commonly, intratumoral hemorrhage, obstructive hydrocephalus, or embolization by tumor cells result in symptoms.

Headache: Headaches occur in approximately 40 to 50 percent of patients with brain metastases. The frequency is higher when multiple lesions are present or a metastasis is located in the posterior fossa.

Focal neurologic dysfunction: Focal neurologic dysfunction is the presenting symptom of 20 to 40 percent of patients. Hemiparesis is the most common complaint but the manifestations depend upon the location of the metastases.

Cognitive dysfunction: Cognitive dysfunction, including memory problems and mood or personality changes, is the presenting problem in 30 to 35 percent of patients.

Seizures: New onset of seizures is the presenting symptom in 10 to 20 percent of patients. Seizures in patients with brain metastases are almost exclusively associated with supratentorial disease.

Stroke: Another 5 to 10 percent present acutely due to stroke caused by hemorrhage into a metastasis, hypercoagulability, invasion or compression of an artery by tumor, or embolization of tumor cells.

5.2. Diagnosis

Imaging studies provide useful information but brain biopsy is necessary in some cases for a definitive diagnosis.

Contrast-enhanced MRI is the preferred imaging study for the diagnosis of brain metastases.

Biopsy should be performed when the diagnosis of brain metastases is in doubt. This is particularly important in patients with a single lesion.

Positron emission tomography (PET) may also be useful in these patients by finding other sites of metastatic disease.

5.3. Treatment

Patients with BM from CRC have a poor prognosis, because they often have substantial extracranial metastatic disease.

Traditionally, the therapeutic goal in many of these patients has been to palliate debilitating neurologic symptoms, because most of these patients die of systemic disease. However, new advances in metastatic CRC management—including the incorporation of monoclonal antibody therapies bevacizumab, cetuximab, and panitumumab— are enhancing the outcomes of patients with systemic disease.

6. Ovarian metastases

Isolated ovarian metastases from primary CRC occur with a low frequency. The incidence of ovarian metastases (synchronous or metachronous) in patients with CRC is 1 to 14 percent. Bulky ovarian metastases are often symptomatic and less responsive to systemic chemotherapy than are other sites of disease. Resection is associated with fairly low morbidity and, in some cases, may improve quality of life and prolong survival, even in the setting of widespread extraovarian metastatic disease. There is a debate regarding prophylactic oophorectomy at the time of curative resection for primary CRC.

There is a rare variety of ovarian metastasis known as Krukenberg tumor (KT), which has been the focus of extensive research due to its poor prognosis. Although the age range of patients is highly variable, KT usually appears in premenopausal women, and for some authors, the diagnosis of primary tumor after KT is a factor for poor prognosis. They are usually large bilateral lesions, solid and bulbous, and they have a gastrointestinal origin in more than 90% of the cases. Although the form of presentation and the treatment are not different from the rest of metastatic ovarian lesions secondary to a primary tumor with a digestive origin, the prognosis is worse. It has been proven that a combined therapy of radical surgery and radiochemotherapy can achieve a slight improvement in long-term survival rates.

7. Peritoneum metastases

7.1. Definition and physiopathology

Colorectal cancer is a pathological process that spreads through the lymphatic channels through hematogenous ways and through the invasion of the intestine wall. These mechanisms result in metastases to the lymph nodes, liver and also peritoneal dissemination. Although the spread to the lymph and venous systems implies the existence of a local invasive process, peritoneal dissemination can appear in tumors with high as well as low malignancy. The dissemination of the cancer that leads to liver and lymph node metastases takes place before the surgical resection of the primary colorectal neoplasm. Peritoneal dissemination, as well as dissemination in the resection area (local recurrence) can also take place as a result of the surgical trauma associated to the resection of the primary neoplasm. The filtration of malignant cells through the severed lymph channels can also be a mechanism in this intraoperative phenomenon of cancer dissemination. Dissemination inside the peritoneal cavity is one of the most severe forms of carcinomatous dissemination from the colon, because it rapidly takes away —provisionally— all hope for a surgical resection of the lesion. Together with lymphatic and hematogenous dissemination, transcoelomic spread is one of the routes of tumor dissemination. In the early stages of peritoneal invasion, transcoelomic spread may be limited to the neighbouring structures just around the primary tumor, with a potential development of isolated carcinoid plaques in the adjacent peritoneum. It is of course a possibility that some of these nodes are not originated in a transperitoneal spread but in a dissemination of the subperitoneal lymph nodes, as Miles proposes (1926). In a later stage, peritoneal metastases spread until there is a diffuse peritoneal carcinomatosis in which there are tumor nodes that spread through the entire parietal peritoneum, greater omentum and adjacent viscera, and abundant ascites appears (Cirugía del ano, recto y colon. John Golligher 2ª edición). For Hara (Hara *et al.* Comparative analysis of intraperitoneal minimal free cancer cells between colorectal and gastric cancer patients using quantitative RT-PCR: possible reason for rare peritoneal recurrence in colorectal cancer. Clin Exp Metastasis 2007;24:179–89), peritoneal metastases take place in two stages: first of all, the tumor cells detach themselves from the serosal surface of the primary tumor and are transported in the peritoneal cavity, and in the second stage, malignant cells in the peritoneum adhere to places like the omentum and the mesenterium, and they grow and spread through the peritoneal cavity afterwards.

Four characteristics have been identified as risk factors for tumor cell exfoliation in the peritoneal cavity: 1. Depth of the invasion, 2. Involvement of lymph nodes, 3. Lymph node invasion, and 4. Venous invasion (Peritoneal cytology in colorectal cancer. Noura *et al*: Diseases of the Colon & Rectum. volume 52: 7 2009).

The identification of these tumor cells with preoperative peritoneal washing cytology can identify those patients at risk of presenting a peritoneal recurrence of the tumor process.

Peritoneal carcinomatosis is a common form of recurrence, and it is frequently the only one, after surgical curative treatment in digestive and gynecological tumors. It is logical to think that the dissemination of tumor cells by the tumor is a common previous mechanism for peritoneal carcinomatosis of abdominal tumors.

There are studies about the mechanisms and incidence of intraperitoneal dissemination of CRC that have contributed to a better comprehension and a different perception of the pathological basis of peritoneal carcinomatosis. Although the incidence rates for the presence of tumor cells during the resection of primary tumors widely vary, the presence of free tumor cells in the peritoneal cavity (similar to the micrometastases in the blood or the bone marrow) is not an independent prognostic factor, and it seems possible that these tumor cells can effectively contribute to the failure of the treatment at an intraperitoneal level. In fact, two studies found a correlation between the presence of free tumor cells in the peritoneal cavity and the recurrence of the tumor in the peritoneal cavity (Peritoneal Carcinomatosis of Colorectal Origin. M.J. Koppe. Ann Surg 2006 Febrero. 243("): 212-222).

Approximately 50% of the patients with CRC stage IV present peritoneal carcinomatosis, and approximately 25% of the patients present a recurrence of their tumor in the peritoneal cavity (peritoneal carcinomatosis), without a clear involvement of the liver or the lungs (Chu DZ, Lang NP, Thompson C, et al. Peritoneal carcinomatosis in nongynecologic malignancy: a prospective study of prognostic factors. *Cancer*. 1989;63:364–367. Sugarbaker PH, Cunliffe WJ, Belliveau J, et al. Rationale for integrating early postoperative intraperitoneal chemotherapy into the surgical treatment of gastrointestinal cancer. *Semin Oncol*. 1989;16:83–97).

Local or peritoneal metastases are factors that represent a poor prognosis for colorectal cancer (Graf et al, 1991; Mahteme et al, 1996; Shepherd et al, 1997; Assersohn et al, 1999) and their treatment is still an important challenge.

The EVOCAPE study shows an average survival of 5.2 months in patients with peritoneal carcinomatosis of colorectal origin. (Sadeghi B, Arvieux C, Glehen O, et al. Peritoneal carcinomatosis from non-gynecologic malignancies: results of the EVOCAPE Multicentric prospective study. *Cancer*. 2000;88:358–363.).

Patients with peritoneal metastases or locally advanced tumors without distance metastases can benefit from cytoreductive surgery with intraperitoneal chemotherapy (Mahteme et al. British Journal of Cancer (2004) 90 403-407).

The average survival rate for patients with carcinomatosis treated with chemotherapy is around 6-12 months (Gramont er al.2000), although this does not factor the modern therapeutic approaches that include immunomodulating agents, which have not yet been evaluated enough and appeared after the year 2000.

7.2. Peritoneal cytology

In this situation, peritoneal cytology before the resection of the primary tumor and, when needed, cytoreduction, is a useful tool to assess the prognosis of the patients (both with and without peritoneal carcinomatosis). And it can also be useful when deciding whether to choose systemic or intraperitoneal chemotherapy.

In a multivariate analysis, peritoneal cytology appears as an independent predictor for survival in patients with tumors pT3 or pT4 (Peritoneal cytology in colorectal cancer. Noura *et al*: Diseases of the Colon & Rectum. volume 52: 7 2009). Patients with negative cytology results show better five-year survival rates in cases in which at least the serosal layer is affected by the tumor than patients with positive results (68% vs. 20.6%). These results are also reflected in the fact that patients with positive cytology results present a higher rate of peritoneal dissemination than patients with negative cytology results. Some patients with macroscopic peritoneal dissemination and negative cytology have been proven to have survived for a long time (more than 10 years, in some cases); whereas patients with peritoneal dissemination and positive cytology results show five-year survival rates close to zero. When the peritoneal cytology results are positive, monitoring has to be particularly careful in order to obtain an early detection of recurrence (Peritoneal Cytology in Colorectal Cancer. Nishikawa et al. Disease of the Colon and Rectum. Volume 52:12 (2009). All these promising results with regard to peritoneal cytology must be included in the evaluation, prognosis and therapeutic approach, and this requires subsequent prospective studies that homogenize the way in which the cytology is performed (technique, staining, etc.) and its inclusion in the different studies, such as its inclusion in the selection protocols to perform Sugarbaker technique.

7.3. Treatment

Peritoneal carcinomatosis and ascites are usually signs of advanced colorectal cancer, and survival rates, as we have said, are low. However, a more aggressive approach for surgical cytoreduction of the peritoneal disease has been used as in the treatment for ovarian cancer, primary peritoneal cancer and appendicular mucinous tumors such as pseudomyxoma and cystadenocarcinoma, and it shows better results than palliative surgery and conventional chemotherapy by themselves. The extrapolation of these therapies to the treatment of CRC seems inappropriate, because these tumors are biologically different, and they are mainly of a low grade. The arrival of intraperitoneal chemotherapy combined with peritoneal debulking seems to offer an increased survival rate in selected patients with colorectal carcinomatosis. Sugarbaker described in 1995 the surgical techniques that lead, when this is not possible, to a complete resection of the peritoneal neoplastic disease. As in other scenarios of resectable metastatic disease, it is advisable to consolidate the results obtained thanks to surgery with a complementary treatment that eradicates the residual microscopic disease. The intraperitoneal administration of certain cytostatic drugs leads to a higher exposure of the peritoneal surface to the drugs than with the usual systemic administration. The perioperative administration (hypertermia-modulated intraoperative administration and/or early postoperative administration) avoids the difficulties that have been traditionally associated with the intraperitoneal administration of cytostatic drugs (difficulty of access, erratic distribution, pain...), which have been one of the main causes of its poor reception by specialists in medical oncology.

This way, and after decades of preclinical and clinical efforts, cytoreductive surgery combined with preoperative hyperthermic intraperitoneal chemotherapy (HIPEC) appear in this new century as an indissoluble and feasible multimodal strategy with proven effectiveness in the treatment of selected cases of peritoneal carcinomatosis in colorectal cancer, although, as we have said before, it can also be useful for other tumors (González-Moreno S. Cirugía citoreductora y quimioterapia intraperitoneal perioperatoria para las neoplasias con diseminación peritoneal: ha llegado el momento. Cir Esp. 2005;78(6):341-3)(Sugarbaker PH, Mora JT, Carmignani P, Stuart OA, Yoo D. Update on chemotherapeutic agents utilized for perioperative intraperitonealchemotherapy. Oncologist. 2005;10:112-22.)(Treatments and Outcomes of Peritoneal Surface Tumors Through a Centralized National Service (United Kingdom) S. Rout, Diseases Of The Colon & Rectum Volume 52: 10 (2009).

There are protocols for the selection of patients which, among other things, try to establish the mass of the tumor and its location by mapping the abdominal cavity in order to assess the size of the tumor and the possibility of achieving an adequate cytoreduction. Laparoscopy is a technique that is currently included in the treatment protocols when there is suspicion or preoperative evidence of peritoneal carcinomatosis. After obtaining a laparoscopic diagnosis of the affected areas (including images obtained during the process, if possible), the patient is sent to a health centre with experience in cytoreductive surgery and HIPEC in order to assess the procedure (commonly referred to as Sugarbaker technique).

The prognosis and results depend on the level of cytoreduction. It is necessary to take into account the fact that this cytoreduction goes through a peritonectomy and the resection of visceral metastases that sometimes involve several days of surgery, with the corresponding increase of morbidity and mortality. For this reason, it is essential to have specialized or experienced centres when assessing the results.

As we have said, the level of cytoreduction is directly related to the prognosis. The success rate of cytoreduction has been established according to different systems, although it is generally classified as CCR 0 (Completeness of Cancer Resection) when there is no microscopic tumor, CCR 1 when there are no nodes larger than 0.5 cm and CCR 2 when there are clearly visible tumors (more than 0.5 cm). Average survival is 33 months for CCR 0, 12.5 months for CCR 1 and 8.5 months for CCR 2 (Glehen O, Cotte E, Schreiber V, Sayag-Beaujard AC, Vignal J, Gilly FN. Intraperitoneal chemohyperthermia and attempted cytoreductive surgery in patients with peritoneal carcinomatosis of colorectal origin. *Br J Surg*. 2004;91:747–754).

The most commonly used chemotherapeutic agents are mitomycin C and cisplatin combined with 5-FU. These agents are heated to 47-59 ºC and inserted in the peritoneal cavity, which lets the surgeon spread it to all necessary spaces. They are left in the cavity for one hour and a half to two hours, and then they are drained. The catheters are left in place for postoperative drainage (Royal RE, Pingpank JF Jr. Diagnosis and management of peritoneal carcinomatosis arising from adenocarcinoma of the colon and rectum. *Semin Oncol*. 2008;35:183–191).

Morbidity rates in the procedure of cytoreduction and HIPEC are around 30% and 60%, and mortality is less than 2%. Logically, covering the logistic needs for intensive care, chemotherapy and trained surgeons with an established protocol allow for an adequate morbidity and mortality. This therapy must be applied to patients in whom a complete or almost complete cytoreduction can be achieved. With these conditions, the existing studies (although retrospective) show an important improvement of survival, with some results showing a five-year survival rate of 49% when cytoreduction is complete. (Yan TD, Black D, Savady R, Sugarbaker PH. Systematic review on the efficacy of cytoreductive surgery combined with perioperative intraperitoneal chemotherapy for peritoneal carcinomatosis from colorectal carcinoma. *J Clin Oncol.* 2006;24: 4011–409).

It is possible to apply delayed and repeated intraperitoneal systemic chemotherapy after the cytoreduction with acceptable morbidity rates. It is also possible to administer delayed intraperitoneal chemotherapy in up to 83% of the patients who had previously undergone cytoreduction (Delayed Repeated Intraperotoneal Chemotherapy. Fajardo et al. Diseases of Colon and Rectum. Volumen 55.: 10 (2012)).

On the other hand, there are reasons to be optimistic about the use of immunomodulating treatments (targeted monoclonal antibodies) which, when combined with other 'traditional' chemotherapeutic approaches, are showing some really promising results. We still need more studies that let us know what conditions lead to a successful outcome (such as the KRAS status of the primary tumor) and also whether they have a beneficial effect in peritoneal carcinomatosis.

Chemotherapy and targeted therapies: There are currently eight active and approved drugs for patients with metastatic colorectal cancer which are used separately or combined with other drugs:

5-FU, Capecitabine, Irinotecan., Oxaliplatin, Bevacizumab, Cetuximab, Aflibercept and Panitumumab.

These chemotherapeutic agents, some of which are monoclonal antibodies, can be combined in different ways and represent an encouraging future for patients with peritoneal metastases who were previously called 'terminally ill'.

7.4. Treatment of metastatic disease

Initial management of the primary site in patients who present with stage IV disease is controversial, and there are no data from prospective randomized studies to guide treatment. In general, the choice and sequence of treatment is guided by the presence or absence of symptoms from the primary tumor and whether or not the metastases are potentially resectable.

Surgery provides a potentially curative option for selected patients who present with limited metastatic colorectal cancer.

Management in patients with unresectable metastatic disease: systemic and hepatic arterial infusion chemotherapy may be useful treatment options in patients with unresectable disease.

Other established treatment is radiofrequency ablation.

Author details

C. Alberto Blanco[1*], R. Sánchez[2], F. Piniella[3], D. Pescador[3], G. Borobio[3], A. García[3] and C. Cano[3]

*Address all correspondence to: titoberto2002@hotmail.com

1 Hospital Santos Reyes, Aranda de Duero (Burgos), Spain

2 Health Care Centers of Aranda de Duero (Burgos), Ávila, Spain

3 Health Care Centers of Aranda de Duero (Burgos), Salamanca, Spain

References

[1] Hara et al. Comparative analysis of intraperitoneal minimal free cancer cells between colorectal and gastric cancer patients using quantitative RT-PCR: possible reason for rare peritoneal recurrence in colorectal cancer. Clin Exp Metastasis 2007;24:179–89.

[2] Noura et al. Peritoneal cytology in colorectal cancer.: Dis Colon Rectum. Vol 52: 7 (2009)

[3] Koppe et al. Peritoneal carcinomatosis of colorectal origin.. Ann Surg 2006 243: 212-222.

[4] Chu et al. Peritoneal carcinomatosis in nongynecologic malignancy: a prospective study of prognostic factors. *Cancer*. 1989;63:364–367.

[5] Sugarbaker et al. Rationale for integrating early postoperative intraperitoneal chemotherapy into the surgical treatment of gastrointestinal cancer. *Semin Oncol.* 1989;16:83–97.

[6] Sadeghi et al. Peritoneal carcinomatosis from non-gynecologic malignancies: results of the EVOCAPE Multicentric prospective study. *Cancer*. 2000;88: 358–363.

[7] Wagner et al. Eartly postoperative intraperitoneal chemotherapy folloeonng cytoreductive surgery for appendiceal mucinous neoplasms with isolated peritoneal metastasis. Dis Colon Rectum Vol 55: 4 (2012) 407-415.

[8] Mahteme et al. Improve survival in patients with peritoneal metastases from colorectal cancer: a preliminary study. British Journal of Cancer (2004) 90 403-407.

[9] Nishikawa et al. Peritoneal Cytology in Colorectal Cancer.. Dis Colon Rectum. Vol 52:12 (2009)

[10] González-Moreno S. Cirugía citoreductora y quimioterapia intraperitoneal perioperatoria para las neoplasias con diseminación peritoneal: ha llegado el momento. Cir Esp. 2005 ;78(6):341-343

[11] Sugarbaker et al.. Update on chemotherapeutic agents utilized for perioperative intraperitonealchemotherapy. Oncologist. 2005;10:112-22

[12] Rout et al. Treatments and Outcomes of Peritoneal Surface Tumors Through a Centralized National Service (United Kingdom) Dis Colon Rectum Volume 52: 10 (2009)1705-1715.

[13] Glehen et *al*. Intraperitoneal chemohyperthermia and attempted cytoreductive surgery in patients with peritoneal carcinomatosis of colorectal origin. *Br J Surg*. 2004;91:747–754.

[14] Royal et al.. Diagnosis and management of peritoneal carcinomatosis arising from adenocarcinoma of the colon and rectum. *Semin Oncol*. 2008;35:183–191

[15] Yan et al. Systematic review on the efficacy of cytoreductive surgery combined with perioperative intraperitoneal chemotherapy for peritoneal carcinomatosis from colorectal carcinoma. *J Clin Oncol*. 2006;24: 4011–409.

[16] Fajardo et al. Delayed repeated intraperotoneal chemotherapy.. Dis Colon Rectum. Vol 55.: 10 (2012);1044-1052

[17] Soumaoro et al. Coexpression of VEGF-C and Cox-2 in Human Colorectal Cancer and its Association With Lymph Node Metastasis Dis Colon Rectum, March 2006 vol 49, nº 3; 392-398.

[18] Óberg, A. e*t al*. Are lymph node micrometastases of any clinical significance in Dukes stages A and B colorectal cancer? Dis Colon Rectum, October 1998 Vol 41, No. 10 1244-1249.

[19] Edge SB, Byrd DR, Compton CC, et al., eds.: AJCC Cancer Staging Manual. 7th ed. New York, NY: Springer, 2010, pp 143-64.

[20] Wong et al. Staging accuracy in colorectal carcinoma. Journal of Clinical Oncology. Vol 17. nº 9 (1999) 2896-2900.

[21] Wang et al. Curative resection of T1 colorectal carcinoma: risk of lymph node metastasis and long-term prognosis. Dis Colon Rectum June 2005. Vol 48, No. 6, 1182-1192.

[22] Kelder et al. Impact of the number of histologically examined lymph nodes on prognosis in colon cancer: a population-based study in the Netherlands. Dis Colon Rectum. Vol. 52 (2009); 260-267.

[23] J. Gastroenterol Heptol 6:325-244. 1991

[24] Park et al. Comparative analisis of limph node metastasis in patients with ypT0-2 rectal cancers after neoadjuvant chemoradiotherapy. Dis Colon Rectum. Vol 56: 2 (2013).135-141.

[25] Sardon et al. Técnica del ganglio centinela en el cáncer de colon. Experiencia en 125 casos.CIR ESP. 2013; 91(6) 366-371

[26] Watanabe et *al*. Heterogeneity of KRAS status may explain the subset of discordant KRAS status between primary and metastatic colorectal cancer. Dis Colon Rectum Vol 54: 9(2011) 1170-1178.

[27] Faerden et al. Sentinel node mapping in colonic cancer Dis Colon Rectum. Vol 51: (2008) 891–896

[28] (2013). "Rectal Cancer." *National Comprehensive Cancer Network (NCCN) guidelines* Retrieved Jun 30, 2013, from www.nccn.org.

[29] Ambiru, S., M. Miyazaki, H. Ito, K. Nakagawa, H. Shimizu, A. Kato, S. Nakamura, H. Omoto and N. Nakajima (1998). "Resection of Hepatic and Pulmonary Metastases in Patients with Colorectal Carcinoma." *Cancer* 82(2): 274-278.

[30] Carballo, M., M. S. Maish, D. E. Jaroszewski and C. E. Holmes (2009). "Video-Assisted Thoracic Surgery (Vats) as a Safe Alternative for the Resection of Pulmonary Metastases: A Retrospective Cohort Study." *J Cardiothorac Surg* 4: 13.

[31] Collie, D. A., A. R. Wright, J. R. Williams, B. Hashemi-Malayeri, A. J. Stevenson and C. M. Turnbull (1994). "Comparison of Spiral-Acquisition Computed Tomography and Conventional Computed Tomography in the Assessment of Pulmonary Metastatic Disease." *Br J Radiol* 67(797): 436-444.

[32] Ehrenhaft, J. L., M. S. Lawrence and D. M. Sensenig (1958). "Pulmonary Resections for Metastatic Lesions." *A.M.A. archives of surgery* 77(4): 606-612.

[33] Fiorentino, F., I. Hunt, K. Teoh, T. Treasure and M. Utley (2010). "Pulmonary Metastasectomy in Colorectal Cancer: A Systematic Review and Quantitative Synthesis." *J R Soc Med* 103(2): 60-66.

[34] Gonzalez, M., A. Poncet, C. Combescure, J. Robert, H. B. Ris and P. Gervaz (2013). "Risk Factors for Survival after Lung Metastasectomy in Colorectal Cancer Patients: A Systematic Review and Meta-Analysis." *Ann Surg Oncol* 20(2): 572-579.

[35] Greelish, J. P. and J. S. Friedberg (2000). "Secondary Pulmonary Malignancy." *Surg Clin North Am* 80(2): 633-657.

[36] Hellman, S. and R. R. Weichselbaum (1995). "Oligometastases." *J Clin Oncol* 13(1): 8-10.

[37] 10. Hendriks, J. M., S. Romijn, B. Van Putte, E. Eyskens, J. B. Vermorken, E. Van Marck and P. E. Van Schil (2001). "Long-Term Results of Surgical Resection of Lung Metastases." *Acta Chir Belg* 101(6): 267-272.

[38] Inoue, M., Y. Kotake, K. Nakagawa, K. Fujiwara, K. Fukuhara and T. Yasumitsu (2000). "Surgery for Pulmonary Metastases from Colorectal Carcinoma." *Ann Thorac Surg* 70(2): 380-383.

[39] Irshad, K., F. Ahmad, J. E. Morin and D. S. Mulder (2001). "Pulmonary Metastases from Colorectal Cancer: 25 Years of Experience." *Can J Surg* 44(3): 217-221.

[40] Jaklitsch, M. T., C. M. Mery, J. M. Lukanich, W. G. Richards, R. Bueno, S. J. Swanson, S. J. Mentzer, B. D. Davis, E. N. Allred and D. J. Sugarbaker (2001). "Sequential Thoracic Metastasectomy Prolongs Survival by Re-Establishing Local Control within the Chest." *J Thorac Cardiovasc Surg* 121(4): 657-667.

[41] Kondo, H., T. Okumura, Y. Ohde and K. Nakagawa (2005). "Surgical Treatment for Metastatic Malignancies. Pulmonary Metastasis: Indications and Outcomes." *Int J Clin Oncol* 10(2): 81-85.

[42] Martini, N. and P. M. McCormack (1998). "Evolution of the Surgical Management of Pulmonary Metastases." *Chest Surg Clin N Am* 8(1): 13-27.

[43] McAfee, M. K., M. S. Allen, V. F. Trastek, D. M. Ilstrup, C. Deschamps and P. C. Pairolero (1992). "Colorectal Lung Metastases: Results of Surgical Excision." *Ann Thorac Surg* 53(5): 780-785; discussion 785-786.

[44] Mery, C. M., A. N. Pappas, R. Bueno, S. J. Mentzer, J. M. Lukanich, D. J. Sugarbaker and M. T. Jaklitsch (2004). "Relationship between a History of Antecedent Cancer and the Probability of Malignancy for a Solitary Pulmonary Nodule." *Chest* 125(6): 2175-2181.

[45] Pfannschmidt, J., H. Dienemann and H. Hoffmann (2007). "Surgical Resection of Pulmonary Metastases from Colorectal Cancer: A Systematic Review of Published Series." *Ann Thorac Surg* 84(1): 324-338.

[46] Pfannschmidt, J., H. Hoffmann and H. Dienemann (2010). "Reported Outcome Factors for Pulmonary Resection in Metastatic Colorectal Cancer." *J Thorac Oncol* 5(6 Suppl 2): S172-178.

[47] Pfannschmidt, J., T. Muley, H. Hoffmann and H. Dienemann (2003). "Prognostic Factors and Survival after Complete Resection of Pulmonary Metastases from Colorectal Carcinoma: Experiences in 167 Patients." *J Thorac Cardiovasc Surg* 126(3): 732-739.

[48] Poston, G. J., D. Tait, S. O'Connell, A. Bennett and S. Berendse (2011). "Diagnosis and Management of Colorectal Cancer: Summary of Nice Guidance." *BMJ* 343: d6751.

[49] Quiros, R. M. and W. J. Scott (2008). "Surgical Treatment of Metastatic Disease to the Lung." *Semin Oncol* 35(2): 134-146.

[50] Regnard, J. F., D. Grunenwald, L. Spaggiari, P. Girard, D. Elias, M. Ducreux, P. Baldeyrou and P. Levasseur (1998). "Surgical Treatment of Hepatic and Pulmonary

Metastases from Colorectal Cancers." *Ann Thorac Surg* 66(1): 214-218; discussion 218-219.

[51] Reinhardt, M. J., N. Wiethoelter, A. Matthies, A. Y. Joe, H. Strunk, U. Jaeger and H. J. Biersack (2006). "Pet Recognition of Pulmonary Metastases on Pet/Ct Imaging: Impact of Attenuation-Corrected and Non-Attenuation-Corrected Pet Images." *Eur J Nucl Med Mol Imaging* 33(2): 134-139.

[52] Remy-Jardin, M., J. Remy, F. Giraud and C. H. Marquette (1993). "Pulmonary Nodules: Detection with Thick-Section Spiral Ct Versus Conventional Ct." *Radiology* 187(2): 513-520.

[53] Rena, O., C. Casadio, F. Viano, R. Cristofori, E. Ruffini, P. L. Filosso and G. Maggi (2002). "Pulmonary Resection for Metastases from Colorectal Cancer: Factors Influencing Prognosis. Twenty-Year Experience." *Eur J Cardiothorac Surg* 21(5): 906-912.

[54] Saisho, S., M. Nakata, S. Sawada, M. Yamashita, H. Saeki, A. Kurita and S. Takashima (2009). "Evaluation of Video-Assisted Thoracoscopic Surgery for Pulmonary Metastases: 11-Years of Experience." *Surg Endosc* 23(1): 55-61.

[55] Sakamoto, T., N. Tsubota, K. Iwanaga, T. Yuki, H. Matsuoka and M. Yoshimura (2001). "Pulmonary Resection for Metastases from Colorectal Cancer." *Chest* 119(4): 1069-1072.

[56] Salah, S., K. Watanabe, J. S. Park, A. Addasi, J. W. Park, J. Zabaleta, F. Ardissone, J. Kim, M. Riquet, K. Nojiri, M. Gisabella, S. Y. Kim and K. Tanaka (2013). "Repeated Resection of Colorectal Cancer Pulmonary Oligometastases: Pooled Analysis and Prognostic Assessment." *Ann Surg Oncol* 20(6): 1955-1961.

[57] Salah, S., K. Watanabe, S. Welter, J. S. Park, J. W. Park, J. Zabaleta, F. Ardissone, J. Kim, M. Riquet, K. Nojiri, M. Gisabella, S. Y. Kim, K. Tanaka and B. Al-Haj Ali (2012). "Colorectal Cancer Pulmonary Oligometastases: Pooled Analysis and Construction of a Clinical Lung Metastasectomy Prognostic Model." *Ann Oncol* 23(10): 2649-2655.

[58] Villeneuve, P. J. and R. S. Sundaresan (2009). "Surgical Management of Colorectal Lung Metastasis." *Clin Colon Rectal Surg* 22(4): 233-241.

[59] Weichselbaum, R. R. and S. Hellman (2011). "Oligometastases Revisited." *Nature reviews. Clinical oncology* 8(6): 378-382.

[60] Yano, T., N. Hara, Y. Ichinose, H. Yokoyama, T. Miura and M. Ohta (1993). "Results of Pulmonary Resection of Metastatic Colorectal Cancer and Its Application." *J Thorac Cardiovasc Surg* 106(5): 875-879.

[61] Igor T. Gavrilovic and Jerome B. PosnerJournal of Neuro-Oncology (2005) 75: 5–14 _ Springer 2005

[62] Tim J. Kruser, Samuel T. Chao,Paul Elson, Gene H. Barnett,Michael A. Vogelbaum, Lilyana Angelov, Robert J. Weil, Robert Pelley, John H. Su CANCER July 1, 2008 / Volume 113 / Number 1

[63] Germán Borobio León, Asunción García Plaza, Roberto González Alconada, Ignacio García Cepeda, Jorge López Olmedo, Alberto Moreno Regidor and David Pescador Hernández A Multidisciplinary Approach to Management, Dr. Giulio A. Santoro

[64] Borobio León, G; García Plaza, A; García Cepeda, I; González Alconada, R.; Hernández Cosido, L. (2010). Metástasis en mano de adenocarcinoma de recto. Un caso excepcional. *Cirugía Española 2010;88:195-7.-vol. 88 núm. 03*

[65] Bonnheim, D.C; Petrelli, N.J; Herrera, L.; Walsh, D; Mittelman, A.(1986). Osseous metastases from colorectal carcinoma. *Am J Surg*, vol. 151(4), (April 1986), 457-459.

[66] Chang, H.C; Lew, K.H; Low, C.O .(2001). Metastasis of an adenocarcinoma of the stomach to the 4th metacarpal bone. *Hand Surgery 2001 December; 6(2): 239-242.*

[67] Clohisy, DR; Perkins, SL; Ramnaraine ML. Review of cellular mechanisms of tumor osteolysis (2000). *Clin Orthop 2000;3743:104-114*

[68] Desmanet, E; Amrani, M; Fievez, R; Six Ch. Les acrométastases. A propos de deux cas.(1991). *Revue de la littérature. Ann Chir Main 1991; 10, nº2: 154-157.*

[69] Flynn, CJ; Danjoux, C; Wong, J; Christakis, M; Rubenstein, J; Yee, A; et al.(2008). Two cases of acrometastasis to the hands and review of the literature. *Curr Oncol 2008 October; 15 (5): 51-58.*

[70] Galasko, CS. Diagnosis of skeletal metastases and assessment of response to treatment.(1995). *Clin Orthop 1995;312:64-75*

[71] García Plaza, A. (2003). *Aspectos terapéuticos y pronósticos del carcinoma colorrectal.* Ediciones Universidad de Salamanca. (Marzo 2003). Colección Vitor 105.

[72] Healey, J.H; Turnbull, A.D; Miedema, M; Lane, J.M.(1986). Acrometastases. A study of twenty-nine patients with osseous involvement of the hands and feet. *.J Bone Joint Surg Am. 1986; 68:743-746.*

[73] Kose, F; Sakalli, H ; Sezer, A; Mertsoylu, H; Pourbagher, A; Reyhan, M; Ozyilkan, O. (2008). Colon adenocarcinoma and solitary tibia metastasis: Rare entity. *J Gastrointest Canc*, vol.39, (February 2008), 146-148.

[74] Méndez López, JM; García Mas, R; Salvà Coll, G. (1997). Metastasis of an adenocarcinoma of the colon to the 1st metacarpal bone. *Ann Chir Main Memb Super 1997; 16(2): 134-7.*

[75] Mundy, JR & Yoneda, T. Facilitation and supresion of bone metastasis (1995). *Clin Orthop 1995;312:34-44*

[76] Nozue, M; Oshiro, Y; Kurata, M; Seino, K; Koike, N; Kawamoto, T et al (2002). Treatment and prognosis in colorectal cancer patients with bone metastasis. *Oncol Rep 2002 Jan-Feb; 9(1): 109-112.*

[77] Ross, J.R; Saunders ,Y; Edmonds, P.M; Patel, S; Wonderling, D; Normand, C. (2004). A systematic review of the role of bisphosphonates in metastatic disease. *Health Technol Assess*. vol 8. (August 2004). 1-176.

[78] Roth, E.S; Fetzer, D.T; Barron,B.J; Usha, A; Joseph, U. A; Isis, W; Gayed, I. W; Wan, D.Q. (2009). Does colon cancer ever metastasize to bone first? a temporal analysis of colorectal cancer progression. *BMC Cancer*. vol. 9, (August 2009), 274.

[79] Schlüter, K; Gassmann, P; Enns, A.(2006) Organ-Specific Metastatic Tumor Cell Adhesion and Extravasation of Colon Carcinoma Cells with Different Metastatic Potential. *The American Journal of Pathology. vol.169,* (September 2006),1064–1073.

[80] Schlüter, K; Gassmann, P; Enns, A; Korb, T; Hemping-Bovenkerk, A; Hölzen, J; Haier,J. (2006). Organ-Specific Metastatic Tumor Cell Adhesion and Extravasation of Colon Carcinoma Cells with Different Metastatic Potential. *American Journal of Pathology.* Vol 169, (September 2006), 1064-1073.

[81] Spiteri, V; Bibra, A; Ashwood, N; Cobb, J. Managing acrometastases treatment strategy with a case illustration (2008). *Ann R Coll Surg Engl 2008 October; 90(7): 8-11.*

[82] Sundermeyer, M. L; Meropol, N.J; Rogatko, A; Wang, H; Cohen, S.J. (2004). Changing patterns of colorectal cancer metastases: A 10-year retrospective review. *Journal of Clinical Oncology,* vol 22, nº 14S ,(July 15 Supplement 2004), 3548.

[83] Sundermeyer, M. L; Meropol, N.J; Rogatko, A; Wang, H; Cohen, S.J. (2005).Changing Patterns of Bone and Brain Metastases in Patients with Colorectal Cancer. Clinical Colorrectal Cancer. vol 5, nº 2 (July 2005). 108-113. www.intechopen.

3

New Strategies to Enhance the Efficacy of Surgical Treatment for Colorectal Liver Metastasis

Teodoro Palomares, Ana Alonso-Varona,
Ignacio García-Alonso and Vicente Portugal

1. Introduction

Colorectal cancer (CRC) is the second most common cause of cancer death worldwide [1]. The liver is the most frequent site of metastasis in CRC, both at the time of diagnosis (15-20% of cases) and after apparently radical surgery on the primary tumour (nearly 40% of cases). If patients with colorectal liver metastasis (CRC-LM) are not treated, prognosis is very poor, with a near zero five-year survival rate. At present, liver resection is the only treatment modality that has the potential to achieve long-term survival and to offer the possibility of a cure. Patients who undergo complete (R0) resection of liver metastases have a five-year survival rate of approximately 40-50% [2]. Unfortunately, however, 50% to 70% of patients develop secondary metastatic disease after R0-resection of CRC-LM [3].

In order to obtain the best results in a systemic disease such as metastatic CRC (mCRC), the optimal integration of medical treatment and surgery is essential. The introduction of several effective cytotoxic and targeting agents, in combination with surgical treatment, has extended survival [4]. In addition, promising emerging therapies –cancer stem cell (CSC)-targeted therapies, pathway inhibitors for CRC, induction of tumour cell differentiation, improving liver regeneration, and nanoparticle (NP)-guided tumour ablation, among others– may be found to be effective in achieving better control and even complete eradication of CRC-LM. If confirmed, these strategies will bring significant benefits to patients, particularly in terms of long-term survival. Further, in this era of multimodality treatment of CRC, it is critically important to identify effective biomarkers for prognosis and prediction of individual treatment responses, and these are expected to become useful tools for improving therapeutic approaches.

The present chapter aims i, to present the state of the art related to criteria for appropriate decision making for CRC-LM treatment; ii, to review the current data on the role of biomarkers used for the prediction of response to CRC-LM therapies; and iii, to outline emerging targeting agents and new therapeutic techniques to improve life expectancy and quality of life in CRC-LM patients.

2. Therapeutic approaches to colorectal liver metastases: The state of the art

More than half of patients with CRC will develop liver metastases, and nearly 80% of them are initially unresectable. Hence, optimal management of hepatic metastases often requires a multidisciplinary approach. The availability of new medical therapies, including neoadjuvant chemotherapy and targeted therapies, render a considerable percentage (up to 40%) of initially unresectable patients potentially resectable, improving the overall outcomes of patients with mCRC.

Nowadays, to optimise the integration between surgery and medical approaches in the treatment of mCRC it is necessary to consider different groups, based on current guidelines for stratification of patients according to clinical goals and treatment. In this section, we summarise the recommended therapeutic approaches for CRC-LM according to the aforementioned patient stratification.

2.1. Selection criteria for resection of colorectal liver metastases: Definition of resectability

Patients diagnosed with mCRC should undergo an upfront evaluation by a multidisciplinary team, including medical oncologists, surgeons, radiotherapists and radiologists, in order to assess resectability status and to achieve the best therapeutic results [5]. The target end point for assessing resectability is the potential of surgery to cure the disease when achieving RO resection of all evident disease. Incomplete resection (macroscopic or microscopic), so-called debulking surgery, has not been found to help achieve this end point [6].

Classically, surgical criteria have determined resectability [7], but over recent years several authors have questioned the relevance of many of them. Nowadays, the only surgical criteria that continue to be widely used are complete tumour resection with the preservation of two contiguous liver segments (with adequate vascular inflow and outflow) and an adequate liver remnant (at least 25% of the total liver volume considering the healthy organ) [8]. If, however, we seek a more comprehensive definition of resectability, we should also take into account prognostic evaluation and predicted response to different treatments, by including multiple clinical and molecular factors, which influence patient outcome. Some validated clinical scores are already available, while molecular factors are still under investigation (discussed in more detail below in the section entitled *Predictive biomarkers for response to treatment in colorectal cancer*. In relation to this, the study conducted by Fong *et al.* [9]at the Memorial-Sloan Kettering Cancer Center has been one of the most useful attempts to define prognosis after surgical management of CRC-LM. The score proposed integrates a range of risk factors which influence the risk of death after surgery: preoperative carcinoembryonic antigen (CEA) level > 200 ng/ml, synchronous metastases or metachronous metastases with a disease-free interval of less than twelve months, more than one metastasis, extrahepatic disease, a tumour > 5 cm in diameter and lymph node involvement associated with the primary tumour.

Over recent years, several studies, well summarised in the systematic review of Quan *et al.* [10], have investigated the validity of these various criteria. Notably, the value of the following indicators have been questioned: the number of lesions, maximum lesion dimensions, timing of metastases, absence of metastatic spread outside the liver, and margin of healthy liver tissue, as has the definition of an adequate liver remnant after resection [11].

In summary, the criteria listed in this section can be regarded as an invaluable tool for patient stratification before liver resection, but failure to meet them should not constitute an absolute contraindication to surgery.

2.2. Optimal chemotherapy timing and regimes

In the case of resectable CRC-LM, current guidelines recommend the administration of a course of an active systemic chemotherapy regimen for a total perioperative treatment time of approximately six months [12]. The preferred regimens are combination chemotherapy based on fluoropyrimidines XELOX (capecitabine plus oxaliplatin), FOLFOX (5-fluorouracil, leucovorin and oxaliplatin) and FOLFIRI (5-fluorouracil, leucovorin and irinotecan), optionally together with antiangiogenic biological agents (bevacizumab, cetuximab or panitumumab). In order to improve the selection of the regimen to be used, KRAS mutation status should be determined in all patients at the time of diagnosis of metastatic disease. If no KRAS mutations are identified, BRAF testing should be considered [13]. New targeting biological agents are emerging and they can be expected to lead to improvements in clinical effectiveness. Their effects, pathways and theoretical and practical applications will be discussed in more detail below in the section entitled *Emerging targeting agents for colorectal liver metastases.*

In patients with few metastases that are easy to surgically resect and no poor prognostic indicators, postoperative chemotherapy is usually preferred [14]. On the other hand, in other clinical situations, perioperative (neoadjuvant plus postoperative) chemotherapy can be used [15]. The optimal sequencing of chemotherapy is not clear, however, and recent studies have assessed the pros and cons of different possible timings of administration [16-17]. Potential advantages of administering chemotherapy preoperatively include earlier treatment of micrometastatic disease, evaluation of responsiveness to chemotherapy (which can be prognostic and help decision making) and avoidance of surgery in patients who progress early. On the other hand, several disadvantages have also been highlighted: the risk of missing the window of opportunity for resection, which may be due to disease progression or due to a complete response making it difficult to identify areas for resection; radiological complete response does not always mean pathological response, as viable cancer cells can remain at the original sites of metastases [18]; hepatotoxicity develops with some regimens with serious clinical implications both before and after surgery [19]; and finally, frequent radiological examinations must be undertaken to determine the appropriate timing for surgery [20]. There is now a general trend towards the use of perioperative chemotherapy for patients with resectable CRC-LM, but more studies are necessary to provide stronger evidence regarding the benefit of this approach.

It is important to note that patients diagnosed with rectal cancer and resectable synchronous liver metastases usually need a specific approach due to the risk of locoregional failure. Preoperative chemoradiotherapy in locally advanced rectal tumours (cT3/4, cN+) decreases the risk of pelvic recurrence after surgery, and postoperative chemotherapy is also mandatory [21]. Some studies suggest that pelvic radiotherapy diminishes tolerance to biological agents, but there is not enough data to guide decisions on when this approach may be suitable. After surgical resection of metastases and rectal lesions, pathological rectal disease determines adjuvant therapy. Specifically, postoperative chemoradiotherapy is advised for patients who have not received prior chemoradiation and have a higher risk of pelvic recurrence (pT3/4 or pN1/2) [22]. Patients with pT1-2pN0 tumours should receive six months of adjuvant chemotherapy without pelvic radiation.

In brief, the choices of type of chemotherapy/chemoradiotherapy regimen and its timing depend on a number of factors, namely a patient's disease history and pathological status, tumour gene expression, and previous treatment (including chemotherapy and associated drug toxicity/safety), as well as institutional preferences.

2.3. Conversion or downsizing chemotherapy

When patients present initially unresectable disease, owing to technical difficulties and/or the presence of poor prognostic factors, treatment decisions are difficult. In this clinical situation, preoperative chemotherapy is being considered in highly selected cases in an attempt to downsize CRC-LM and convert them to a resectable status. In these cases, any active metastatic chemotherapy regimen can be used, the goal being to reduce the size of the visible metastases as much as possible. Several trials have been conducted using different combinations of chemotherapy and biological agents, but they have not provided compelling evidence to favour one regimen over another [23-24].

Further, there are other factors we must keep in mind when considering this kind of treatment. Some chemotherapy regimens may cause hepatotoxicity (steatohepatitis and sinusoidal liver injury, among others) [25]with clinical implications for liver surgery, and we must measure responsiveness, so radiological and clinical reassessment should be scheduled approximately every two months after the initiation of chemotherapy. If the disease becomes resectable, surgery should be performed as soon as possible, in order to limit toxicity.

In addition, we must optimise imaging of CRC-LM choosing the most accurate methods. Radiological imaging techniques, namely computed tomography (CT), magnetic resonance imaging (MRI), and positron emission tomography-PET/CT in selected cases, are the essential tools to measure patient tumour response and resectability, while intraoperative ultrasonography (IOUS) remains mandatory in all patients undergoing surgical resection of CRC-LM. Indeed, several authors have demonstrated that IOUS can change the surgical management in up to 35% of patients [26-27].

Furthermore, it must be taken into account that sometimes a radiological complete response can be achieved in patients with one or more metastases. However, a systematic review of the literature suggests that between 17 and 51% of such patients will have residual microscopic disease [28-29]. Accordingly, all liver metastases, including those with radiological complete response after chemotherapy, should be resected when technically feasible. In addition, almost all authors recommend postoperative chemotherapy in these cases.

Overall, recent studies have reported that resectability is achieved in 10 to 40% of selected patients after chemotherapy. It remains difficult, however, to draw firm conclusions as the definition of unresectable disease, patient selection criteria, drug regimens, and outcome measures vary, and there is insufficient data from randomised controlled trials [10].

2.4. Surgical strategy

Liver resection remains the only treatment modality that can achieve long-term survival and offers a possibility of a cure [2]. Selection criteria for resection of CRC-LM are continually being refined (see the aforementioned *Definition of resectability*). In this field, advances in surgical strategy (timing, techniques, etc.) have improved results, but patient management is complex and tends to require a combination of different approaches (colorectal resection, liver resection, chemotherapy, and radiotherapy, among others).

At present, when oncology committees evaluate CRC-LM for surgical treatment, several clinical scenarios are considered: resectable synchronous metastases, resectable metachronous metastases and unresectable disease amenable to conversion chemotherapy.

2.4.1. Resectable synchronous metastases

Close to a third (15-34%) of patients have liver metastases at the time of diagnosis (synchronous metastases). Evidence-based protocols for the management of synchronous metastases are, however, poor, and few prospective studies have been published recently, such results as are available being difficult to generalise [30]. In any case, some suggestions can be made.

One of the open questions is the timing of colorectal and liver surgery (simultaneous versus staged). The traditional approach has been to perform surgery on the primary lesions (colorectal resection), followed by chemotherapy and subsequent liver surgery. Nowadays, simultaneous colorectal and liver resections are preferred when feasible [31]. This combined surgery can be safely performed whenever minor hepatectomies are planned, but there is no consensus on the best approach in cases requiring major hepatectomies. Considering the largest series, some show similar rates in simultaneous and staged resections [32], but a multicentre database analysis in the USA found increased morbidity and mortality after simultaneous major hepatectomy and colorectal resection [33]. Thus, in the absence of clear evidence, the decision to undertake more complex procedures must be made on a case-by-case basis. Even though surgery is the key treatment in patients with CRC-LM, chemotherapy (and sometimes radiotherapy) must also be administered. The sequencing of chemotherapy has been discussed above, and often influences surgical timing.

On the other hand, we should not forget that patients with synchronous metastases have a poorer prognosis [34]. Various strategies have been proposed in an attempt to improve results. One possibility, suggested by Mentha *et al.* [35], is a change in the treatment sequence, the so-called reverse approach, which consists of treatment with systemic chemotherapy followed by liver resection and subsequent primary tumour treatment (with the option of radiotherapy of the rectal tumour prior to resection). More recently, Bruquet *et al.* [36], have reported their experience at the MD Anderson Cancer Center comparing the traditional approach, combined or simultaneous resection, and a "reverse" strategy. These authors found similar oncological outcomes, morbidity and mortality with the three options. This lack of strong evidence makes us cautious, but we believe that the reverse strategy can be considered a reasonable option in patients with asymptomatic primary CRC but advanced CRC-LM.

2.4.2. Resectable metachronous metastases

Most patients with CRC-LM (2/3 of cases) develop liver metastases after initial treatment, during the course of the disease (metachronous metastases). The management of resectable metachronous disease is distinct from that of synchronous disease, though it should also include diagnostic imaging of CRC-LM, as well as evaluation of the chemotherapy and surgical history.

In this group of patients, PET/CT should be considered preoperatively to characterise the extent of metastatic disease and to identify possible sites of extrahepatic disease that could preclude surgery [37]. In addition, it is important to evaluate previous chemotherapy to guide the choice of regimen. In general, six months of perioperative (pre- and/or postoperative) chemotherapy is recommended, but in selected cases observation is also considered appropriate. In addition, previous hepatotoxicity and other side effects should be taken into account [12].

In relation to the type of surgery to be performed, previous surgery can preclude surgical treatment of metachronous metastases, especially if upfront liver resection was performed, it being necessary to assess the remnant liver and technical difficulties. Finally, recent data suggest that it is safe to adopt a surgical approach to the treatment of recurrent hepatic disease isolated to the liver, but that survival decreases with each subsequent curative surgical approach [38].

2.4.3. Unresectable disease amenable to conversion chemotherapy

In this clinical situation, preoperative chemotherapy is considered in highly selected cases, with the aim of downsizing CRC-LM [39]. After disease becomes resectable, surgery should be performed as soon as possible and all liver metastases, including those with radiographic complete response after chemotherapy, should be resected when technically feasible [10]. The treatment of the primary tumour can be postponed until the completion of adjuvant therapy [36].

2.4.4. New surgical techniques

A feasible approach has emerged for patients who would be left with an inadequate future liver remnant (FLR) if complete disease clearance were to be attempted with a single hepatectomy: this is a two-stage hepatectomy for bilobular liver metastases in combination with selected use of portal venous embolization. It offers the best chance of achieving an adequate degree of liver remnant hypertrophy, being more effective than portal venous embolization before a single hepatectomy [40].

Although the standard of care for resectable liver metastases is surgical resection, in selected patients other liver-directed therapies can be used in addition to or instead of surgical resection. These include intrahepatic arterial chemotherapy [41], radiofrequency tumour ablation [42], radioembolization [43]and stereotactic external beam radiation [44]. Some of these innovative techniques will be discussed in more depth below in the section entitled *New therapeutic techniques for colorectal liver metastases*.

3. Predictive biomarkers for response to treatment in colorectal cancer

Over the past decade, developments in CRC-LM therapy have improved the prognosis of patients. Combination chemotherapy, such as FOLFOX or FOLFIRI, has become the standard regimen for unresectable advanced or recurrent CRC, and high response rates have been reported. On the other hand, not all patients respond well to these therapies, and it has been suggested that differential responses are due to the specific molecular profile of each patient and/or tumour. To facilitate the design of personalised therapeutic strategies for CRC patients, it is therefore important to identify biomarkers which are able to accurately predict the sensitivity of patients to the potential therapies and to estimate the likely course of the illness.

Recent advances in the fields of genomics and proteomics have contributed to our understanding of CRC at the molecular level by evaluating the expression profiles of genes and proteins in tissues and body fluids. To date, some of the candidate biomarkers have yielded somewhat contradictory results. On the other hand, several studies have identified candidate molecular biomarkers that may help to predict the response to cytotoxic chemotherapy and guide treatment selection.

3.1. Molecular predictors of response to chemotherapy

5-Flurouracil (5-FU) is the main stay of all current standard CRC chemotherapy regimens, despite the fact that it causes serious side effects (grade 3 or 4) in up to 30% of patients. Several enzymes involved in 5-FU metabolism have been proposed as predictors of response to fluopyrimidine treatment: 5-FU exerts its activity by inhibiting thymidylate synthase (TS), a key enzyme of nucleotide pyrimidine metabolism that is essential for DNA synthesis and cellular proliferation. Thymidine phosphorylase (TP) is another enzyme involved in thymidine metabolism, which regulates the conversion of thymine to thymidine; this is why it is thought to limit the toxicity of high levels of thymidine and prevent replication errors during DNA synthesis. In this role, TP degrades 5-FU, limiting the activity of this chemotherapeutic agent. Dihydropyridimine dehydrogenase (DPD) is a rate-limiting hepatic enzyme involved in the catabolism of 5-FU [45]. It was found that low levels of expression of TP, DPD and TS were independently associated with improved overall survival [46]. Specifically, deficiency in DPD activity caused by mutations in the gene encoding DPD (the *DYPD* gene) can lead to severe 5-FU-related toxicities, which can be fatal. However, as mutations in the *DPYD* gene are responsible for only some of the adverse reactions to 5-FU and the association between genotype and phenotype is not clear [47], further assay development and prospective trials are needed to evaluate the clinical usefulness of these enzymes in predicting which patients are likely to develop serious, life-threatening toxicity to 5-FU [48].*Irinotecan (CPT-11),* a topoisomerase inhibitor, shows efficacy in the treatment of mCRC when used either as a single agent or in combination with radiotherapy and/or other chemotherapeutic drugs. Irinotecan acts as an inhibitor of DNA topoisomerase I (Topo I) and exerts a cytotoxic effect in replicating cells by inducing DNA strand breaks [49]. The active metabolite of irinotecan is SN-38, which is metabolised *in vivo* through conjugation by the liver enzyme uridine diphosphate glucuronosyltransferase (UGT1A1). A variant of the gene encoding this enzyme (UGTA1*28) has come to be considered the main pharmacogenetic marker for severe haematological toxicity (neutropaenia) of the drug. Nevertheless, UGT1A1*28 testing as a predictive marker of adverse effects needs to be further investigated before translation to clinical practice and the available data are not conclusive in defining a precise genotype-based dosage [50-51]. In addition, tumour expression of Topo-I has been explored as a biomarker of the efficacy of irinotecan-based therapies [52]. Although further studies are needed, it has been shown that high levels of Topo-I in tumour tissue are associated with a good response to irinotecan [53-54]; these data are consistent with the hypothesis that a larger amount of Topo I would facilitate the activity of a Topo I inhibitor [55].*Oxaliplatin* is a platinum analogue that improves response rate and survival in patients with advanced CRC. DNA kinking is the major feature of platinum-DNA adducts that block DNA replication and lead to cancer cell death. These DNA strand breaks are recognised and repaired by the nucleotide excision repair (NER) pathway, whose major components are excision repair cross-complementation group (ERCC1 and ERCC2) proteins, acting as the rate-limiting enzymes of oxaliplatin efficacy. Several studies have demonstrated that low levels of ERCC1 and/or ERCC2 gene expression correlate well with better response rates following oxaliplatin-based therapy in advanced CRC patients, leading to improved survival [56-58]. Despite these promising findings, most of the studies have been retrospective and differed significantly in design, and results have not been consistent. Further prospective trials are needed to assess the correlation between decreased expression of *ERCC1* and *ERCC2* and platinum toxicities.

3.2. Molecular predictors of response to anti-EGFR therapy

We should also consider other markers which it has been suggested may be useful for predicting patient responses to biological agents, in particular anti-epidermal growth factor receptor (EGFR) monoclonal therapy. EGFR is a member of the transmembrane tyrosine kinase receptor family ErbB, involved in tumour cell proliferation, inhibition of apoptosis, invasion, migration and angiogenesis [59-60]. When a ligand binds the EGFR homo or hetero-dimers are formed with other ErbB family members, initiating two main intracellular cascades, which are important for cell survival, proliferation and migration. On the one hand, membrane localization of the lipid kinase PIK3CA counteracts PTEN and promotes AKT1 phosphorylation and, on the other, KRAS activates BRAF, which in turn triggers the mitogen-activated protein kinases [61]. Abnormal expression of EGFR has been demonstrated in many advanced tumours, including in breast cancers, gliomas and lung cancer. In the case of mCRC, EGFR overexpression has been detected in 60-80% of cases [59]and a correlation has been reported with early tumour recurrence and extra-hepatic metastasis [62]. For these reasons, researchers started to explore therapeutic strategies to disrupt EGFR function.

Cetuximab, a chimeric IgG1 monoclonal antibody (mAb), and panitumumab, a humanised IgG2 mAb, target the EGFR and have small, but nonetheless clinically important response rates of around 10% in unselected patients with chemotherapy-refractory metastatic CRCs. However, its exact role in the CRC metastatic cascade has not yet been characterised due to controversial results obtained with anti-EGFR antibody therapy. In fact, it has been shown that the response to this therapy is independent of EGFR expression in tumour tissue [63]. In relation to this, some studies suggest that EGFR expression in the primary tumour does not necessarily correspond with the level of expression in metastatic tissue, while other studies have reported 78-100% concordance in EGFR expression in the two tissue compartments [64]. These findings prompted an effort to identify alternative predictive molecular biomarkers that could help to select patients more likely to benefit from anti-EGFR agents. Candidates that have been investigated so far include not only molecular alterations affecting the EGFR, but also molecular events downstream in the pathway, such as aberrations in the interlinked RAS-RAF-mitogen-activated protein kinase and PI3K-AKT-mTOR intracellular signalling transducers.

KRAS encodes for a cytoplasmic GTP-binding protein with low inherent GTPase activity. When the KRAS protein is bound to GTP, it relays signals of cellular proliferation and inhibition of apoptosis, acting as a typical oncogene. Activating mutations in KRAS lead to a gain in function of this gene, and hence over-expression of RAS/RAF-dependent proteins. Specifically, mutations in codons 12 and 13 of exon 2 have been demonstrated to predict low response rate to EGFR monoclonal antibodies-targeted therapy [65]. A lack of efficacy and also a possible detrimental effect on anti-EGFR–based chemotherapy in KRAS-mutated patients have been suggested by some trials using cetuximab in first-line therapy for mCRC, such as OPUS (oxaliplatin plus cetuximab) [66] and CRYSTAL (irinotecan plus cetuximab) [67]. These data indicate that KRAS mutations can be considered a highly specific biomarker to predict poor response to treatment with anti-EGFR mAbs. In addition, due to the fact that anti-EGFR agents fail to achieve either objective responses or disease stabilization in a substantial proportion of patients with wild-type KRAS tumours also, it seems necessary to investigate mutations in other genes involved in signalling pathways downstream of EGFR, including NRAS, BRAF, PIK3CA and PTEN.

Activating mutations in other members of the RAS family are less common than those found in KRAS. For instance, the reported frequency of *NRAS* mutations is 2.2 to 2.6%. Patients with tumours with these mutations had a significantly poorer response rate to anti-EGFR therapy [68], although no significant differences were seen in overall survival between patients with wild-type and mutant *NRAS*.

Mutations in *BRAF*, the major effector of *KRAS*, have also been associated with reduced sensitivity to EGFR-directed therapy. In a retrospective study, Di Nicolantino *et al.*

[69]examined tumours from patients who had received anti-EGFR therapy. They found that none of the patients carrying the BRAF V600E mutation responded and that none of the responders had a BRAF mutation. Moreover, De Roock *et al.* [68]recently conducted a large trial in which they analysed tumour specimens from CRC patients treated with the anti-EGFR agent cetuximab. They found that KRAS and BRAF mutations were mutually exclusive; the *BRAF* mutation was identified in 4.7% of cases and those carrying the mutation had a significantly lower response to anti-EGFR therapy, than those with BRAF wild-type tumours.

The phosphatidylinositol 3-kinase/Akt/mammalian target of rapamycin, *PI3K/AKT/mTOR,* pathway is another major intracellular signalling effector pathway activated by EGFR stimulation. Mutations in this pathway are present in as many as 30-40% of CRC patients. In particular, mutations in PI3KCA have been described in 15% of colon carcinomas, 20% of these being found in exon 20. Patients carrying these mutations and treated with anti-EGFR therapy have poorer clinical outcomes than wild-type PIK3CA carriers. However, because the number of patients with these mutations is very low in most studies, there is a need for controlled trials to assess whether the use of BRAF and PIK3CA mutation analysis as predictors of anti-EGFR therapy efficacy improves clinical outcomes [70].

PTEN is the only tumour suppressor gene involved in the PI3K/AKT-mTOR pathway. Loss of PTEN function, due to mutations, deletions or epigenetic silencing, leads to activation of this pathway. On the other hand, intact PTEN expression in metastatic tissue was found to be predictive of response to cetuximab, while this was not observed in patients with intact PTEN expression in primary tumour tissue [71]. These data are, however, limited and the findings need to be explored in larger confirmatory studies.

3.3. Molecular predictors of response to anti-VEGFR therapy

VEGF is overexpressed in CRC and the level of expression is directly correlated with the development of metastasis [72]. The VEGF family is made up of six growth factors (GFs) which exert their effects via binding to one of the three VEGFRs which belong to the tyrosine kinase receptor (TKR) family, mostly found in endothelial cells and angioblasts [64]. Bevacizumab is a humanised mAb which binds to VEGFA blocking the binding of this GF to VEGFR, thereby avoiding the corresponding intracellular signal transduction. Although several groups have focused their research efforts on finding a biomarker to accurately predict the clinical benefit of adding bevacizumab to therapy, no predictive molecules have yet been identified.

Several candidate predictive biomarkers similar to the KRAS mutation for cetuximab, have been proposed for bevacizumab, but they have remained elusive [73]. Specifically, it has been shown that the efficacy of bevacizumab therapy is independent of KRAS, BRAF and p53 status [74-75].

Another candidate is Ang-2, a regulator of angiogenesis that exerts context-dependent effects on endothelial cells. Although this ligand binds the endothelial-specific receptor tyrosine kinase 2 (TIE2) and acts as a negative regulator of angiogenesis, recent data from analysis of tumours indicate that, under certain conditions, Ang-2 can stimulate endothelial cells, acting as an anti-apoptotic agent in these cells [76]. In this context, serum Ang-2 has been proposed as a candidate biomarker due to the fact that patients having low pre-therapeutic Ang-2 serum levels was significantly associated with response rate after receiving bevacizumab-containing treatment, though results should be further validated [77].

Recently, the development of quantitative predictive biomarkers has led to the increased use of imaging in the evaluation of tumour angiogenesis. Dynamic contrast enhanced-MRI (DCE-MRI) is a technique that can assess tumour perfusion and microvascular vessel wall permeability. Although it is difficult to evaluate the subtle changes occurring during bevacizumab treatment, correlations between tumour grade, microvessel density and VEGF expression in clinical trials of angiogenesis inhibitors have led to DCE-MRI parameters being proposed as biomarkers of drug efficacy [73]. Lastly, some authors have investigated changes in plasma cytokines and angiogenic factors during treatment as potential markers of therapeutic response and resistance [78].

3.4. DNA microarray-based gene expression profiling

Due to the genetic heterogeneity of CRC, many authors agree that it is likely to be necessary to assemble a panel of biomarkers to obtain high enough sensitivity to use these types of biomarkers as a screening test in clinical practice [48, 52]. To date, however, a limited number of markers have been identified in CRC, and their individual use has led to conflicting results.

In this context, advances in genomic techniques, such as DNA microarrays (allowing high-throughput analysis of genes), are very important as they provide large volumes of data which increases the probability of uncovering potential biomarkers. Recently, a total of 66 genes associated with benefit from adjuvant 5-FU/leucovorin treatment were identified. Six of the so-called "chemotherapy benefit genes" were selected to create treatment score algorithms. If validated, these signatures will quantify the likelihood of differential treatment benefit from 5-FU-based therapy [79]. Further, DNA microarray-based gene expression profiling provides a strategy to search systematically for molecular markers of colon cancer. Gene expression analysis studies have already resulted in many new insights into cancer biology and mRNA expression analysis is turning out to be a very useful tool for disease outcome prediction [80-81].

4. Emerging targeting agents for colorectal liver metastasis

The current treatment recommendations for mCRC indicate that therapeutic approach should be multidisciplinary [82], as surgery plus perioperative treatment offers better survival than surgery alone in patients with resectable or potentially resectable disease. Thus, whereas primary surgery is the gold standard for individuals with a single mestatasis, it seems that for multinodular disease, neoadyuvant chemotherapy followed by surgery may be more appropriate [83]. Though in cases of unresectable aggressive disease, treatment should be decided on a case-by-case basis (adapting the strategy to the characteristics of the patient), a multidisciplinary approach should be taken to planning treatment from the outset. In fact, in select unresectable patients chemotherapy allows subsequent rescue surgery and achieves a significant increase in five-year survival rates [39]. An essential aspect of the treatment strategy for advanced CRC is the consideration of treatment as a continuum. Thus, sequential administration of conventional drug combinations based on fluoropyrimidines plus oxaliplatin or irinotecan, results in longer survival. While XELOX, FOLFOX and FOLFIRI are the schemes most commonly used, the trend has been for the standard of care chemotherapy for first-line mCRC to change from FOLFIRI to FOLFOX [84]. In order to improve the poor prognosis of patients with mCRC, treatment intensification has been also tested using the combination of the three active agents 5-FU/leucovorin, oxaliplatin and irinotecan (FOLFOXIRI), and this has achieved increase in R0 secondary resection rate and in overall survival [85]. Other schemes are currently being evaluated in randomised phase II trials as first-line chemotherapy for advanced CRC; these include TOMOX (oxaliplatin plus raltitrexed) which has been found to have a similar efficacy to FOLFOX [86].

The development of new drugs that selectively target specific molecular pathways involved in tumour progression (targeted therapy) has resulted in one of the most important advances in mCRC in the last decade, with biological agents today being a commonly used weapon in the armamentarium against mCRC, particularly in chemorefractory patients and those who are not initially suitable liver resection candidates [87]. In recent years, intense efforts have been focused on developing new molecules to inhibit targets that are critical for CRC, including new anti-angiogenesis agents, novel tyrosine kinase inhibitors (TKIs), agents to act on the PI3K/Akt signalling pathway, modulators of autophagy, and proteasome inhibitors, as well as targeted therapies against cancer stem cells, among others.

4.1. Targeting angiogenesis

GFs have been identified as important targets [88]and the development of targeting biological agents, directed to block effects of GFs on tumour cells, and their integration with cytotoxic chemotherapy regimens has resulted in significant improvements in efficacy outcomes.

One of the most important effects of some GFs is the promotion of angiogenesis, an essential mechanism for both primary tumour growth and metastasis. Due to this, novel therapeutic approaches have focused on the role of angiogenesis-targeting inhibitors. So far, three antiangiogenic biological agents have been approved for the treatment of patients with mCRC: bevacizumab, cetuximab and panitumab. The first successful targeting agent was bevacizumab: today, there is clear evidence to recommend addition of this anti-VEGF antibody to cytotoxic therapy (irrespective of the selected chemotherapy regimen) in both the first- and second-line treatment, this significantly increasing overall survival [75]. Moreover, it has been shown that bevacizumab, combined with FOLFOX or FOLFIRI, may also be active in chemorefractory and selected mCRC patients [89]. Currently, new trials (CHARTA and PERIMAX) are being conducted with bevacizumab plus FOLFIRI, designed to assess the benefits and limitations of a highly active four-drug regimen in mCRC [4]. In addition, it is also important to note that in patients with mCRC on a bevacizumab-containing regimen who show disease progression and hence need a change in the chemotherapy regimen, maintenance therapy with bevacizumab appears to be associated with significantly longer overall survival than the same regimen without bevacizumab [90]; this fact highlights the importance of bevacizumab therapy beyond disease progression in patients with mCRC, although this use is not currently recommended outside clinical trials.

The other two antiangiogenenic biological agents, cetuximab and panitumumab target the ligand-binding domain of EGFR. Signalling of this receptor appears to modulate angiogenesis via the upregulation of VEGF and other angiogenic factors [60]. The use of these EGFR inhibitors was approved for mCRC in patients with wild-type KRAS, whose tumours express EGFR. In fact, as described previously, BRAF and codon 12 KRAS mutations are predictive of adverse outcome in CRC patients receiving cetuximab, being associated with a shorter time to progression and poor survival [91]. In contrast, it has been demonstrated that the combination of chemotherapy, such as irinotecan or FOLFIRI, and cetuximab as a first line in patients with wild-type KRAS significantly improves survival [67, 92]. Cetuximab is also indicated as a monotherapy in such patients following failure of both irinotecan- and oxaliplatin-based chemotherapy [93], while panitumumab is also a valid second-line option for wild-type KRAS patients, as a monotherapy or combined with FOLFIRI [94], though the addition of this EGFR inhibitor to oxaliplatin-based chemotherapy in first-line treatment of mCRC did not improve survival or response rate [95]. In an attempt to increase anti-tumour activity by simultaneously blocking both VEGF and EGFR pathways, some randomised studies have explored the combination of cetuximab or panitumumab with bevacizumab plus chemotherapy, but no benefits were observed, and in some cases the outcome was actually poorer with a greater toxicity, so this type of combination is not recommended for mCRC [64].

In relation to toxicity, treatment with these biological agents is associated with a wide range of adverse events that sometimes require discontinuation of treatment; these include severe hypersensitivity and skin toxicities, in the case of EGFR mAbs, and hypertension, thromboembolic events, bleeding and proteinuria, with bevacizumab treatment [93].

Despite the aforementioned advances, the targeted biological agents currently available are only effective in a small subset of patients (for example, less than half of the KRAS-wild type patient population benefits from anti-EGFR strategies) [96]and their overall impact on the treatment of mCRC has been relatively modest (beneficial effects only lasting on the order of weeks to a few months). These limited results, coupled with the undesirable effects, has led to intensification of the search for novel antiangiogenic therapies to increase the anti-tumour activity in advanced CRC. There are currently several molecules in phase II and III trials for treatment of mCRC that target various members of the VEGF family (aflibercept), signalling by VEGFRs (ramucirumab and IMC-18F1) or the tyrosine kinase components of these receptors (regorafenib, brivanib alaninate, cediranib and linifanib) [93, 97].

Aflibercept is a multiple angiogenic factor trap designed to block the angiogenesis network by binding VEGF-A, VEGF-B and placental growth factor (PLGF) [98]. The recent results of a multinational phase III study (VELOUR trial: aflibercept/FOLFIRI *vs.* placebo/FOLFIRI) demonstrated significant improvements in median overall survival, supporting the use of this VEGF Trap as a second-line option for patients with prior oxaliplatin treatment [99]. Ramucirumab is a fully humanised mAb directed against the extracellular domain of VEGFR-2, which binds VEGF-A and is believed to be the key VEGFR involved in tumour angiogenesis. Like aflibercept, ramucirumab is currently being evaluated in combination with FOLFIRI in a phase III trial for the second-line treatment of mCRC patients for whom prior oxaliplatin- and bevacizumab-containing initial therapy has failed [100]. In addition, a phase II study of ramucirumab in the first-line setting in combination with FOLFOX6 therapy is also in progress [101]. Another anti-VEGFR mAb, IMC-18F1, which targets VEGFR-1 has been developed recently [102], and is also being studied in a phase II trial in mCRC.

Other candidate molecules represent new approaches to intracellular signal blockade of the VEGF and fibroblast growth factor (FGF) signalling pathways, via TKIs. In a recent phase III study (CORRECT trial), regorafenib has been found to improve survival in mCRC patients who progressed after all standard therapies, making it the first small-molecule multikinase inhibitor to have demonstrated survival benefits in such patients [103]. Brivanib alaninate is an oral TKI that specifically inhibits the VEGFR-1 and FGFR. This FGF signalling blockade may represent an important advantage, since it has been suggested that resistance to bevacizumab is associated with increased expression of FGF [78], and hence brivanib could have antiangiogenic activity in bevacizumab-resistant patients. In addition, a phase III trial combining brivanib and cetuximab in second/third line therapy in patients with advanced wild-type *KRAS* mCRC found improved progression free survival with no impact in overall survival [97]. Cediranib is an inhibitor of VEGFRs, platelet-derived growth factor-(PDGF) receptor beta and FGF receptor, whose activity has been compared with that of bevacizumab as a first-line treatment in combination with FOLFOX (HORIZON phase III trial) for mCRC patients; although cediranib activity was comparable to that of bevacizumab, the patient-reported outcomes were significantly less favourable [104]. Similarly, linifanib (a TKI that targets both VEGFRs and PDGFRs), in combination with FOLFOX, did not offer any advantages (over bevacizumab) in a randomised phase II trial as a second-line treatment for mCRC [105].

4.2. Targeting PI3K/Akt/mTOR pathway

The PI3K/Akt/mTOR pathway, an essential regulator of protein translation and cell proliferation, is another important target being investigated for mCRC in phase II and III trials. The PI3K/AKT/mTOR signalling cascade is constitutively active in many types of cancer and, in particular, it plays a critical role in the growth and progression of CRC. In addition, it has been demonstrated that this pathway may be upregulated after blockade of both VEGF- and EGFR-mediated signalling [101].

These aforementioned data provide the rationale for targeting this pathway therapeutically in CRC patients. Perifosine is an oral alkylphospholipid that targets both AKT and nuclear transcription factor-kappa B (NF-κB) pathways. This novel molecule appears to enhance the cytotoxic effects of 5-FU: it has produced promising results in a phase II randomised trial of capecitabine ± perifosine in previously treated patients with mCRC and, hence, is currently in phase III clinical development in combination with this 5-FU prodrug [106].

Activation of the PI3K/AKT cascade promotes mTOR, a serine-threonine kinase whose activation results in cell cycle progression and protein synthesis, and is involved in the CRC metastatic process. The mTOR inhibitors are analogues of rapamycin, including everolimus and temsirolimus, which are being investigated in clinical trials in combination with irinotecan, cetuximab, FOLFOX, bevacizumab or panatimumab in patients with mCRC progressing on prior chemotherapy [101]. Current expert opinion suggests that mTOR inhibitors may represent an attractive anti-tumour target in combination with strategies to target other pathways that may overcome resistance [107]. In relation to this, it has been demonstrated that addition of the multikinase inhibitor, sorafenib, enhances the therapeutic effect of rapamycin on induction of apoptosis and inhibition of cell-cycle progression, migration and invasion of CRCs [108]. In addition, it has been suggested that mTOR inhibition by metformin (an antidiabetic drug), via activation of the AMP-activated protein kinase (AMPK) pathway, which functions as a sensor for cellular nutrient and energy levels, could be a new option for CRC [109].

4.3. Autophagy modulators and proteasome inhibitors

Autophagy is a multistep process of sequestration and subsequent elimination of cytosolic proteins, damaged organelles and protein aggregates in autophagosomes [110]. This self-degradation, via the lysosome, is responsible for the maintenance of intracellular homeostasis and enables cell survival under stress conditions. In the cancer cell, autophagy can be used as a strategy of self-adaption to generate nutrients and energy during tumour progression and in periods of hypoxia and stress, such as induced by chemotherapy, leading to development of drug resistance. The role of autophagy after chemotherapy remains controversial, it having been suggested that autophagy induction may increase efficacy of other anti-tumour agents, while most evidence suggests that the inhibition of autophagy is what can increase the effectiveness of these agents. As autophagy inhibitor, an analogue of chloroquine, hydroxy-chloroquine (HCQ), is currently involved in two different phase II studies for advanced CRC in combination with FOLFOX/bevacizumab or capecitabine/oxaliplatin/bevacizumab [111]. Given that HCQ induces ocular toxicities, such as retinopathy, novel autophagy inducers, such as Lys05, are currently being investigated in CRC [112].

In relation to autophagy inducers, since the PI3K/Akt/mTOR pathway is a key regulator of autophagy [113], mTOR inhibitors have been also used to modulate this mechanism, proving to be effective in many models for CRCs, but their clinical use has been less successful [114]. Proteasome inhibitors have also been described as autophagy inducers. It has been shown that proteasome inhibition generates a stress response through alteration of the protein milieu, which, in turn, induces endoplasmic reticulum stress; this causes an accumulation of misfolded proteins in the endoplasmic reticulum lumen and, consequently, induction of cellular stress responses, such as the unfolded protein response and autophagy to maintain endoplasmic reticulum homeostasis [110]. Bortezomib, the main proteasome inhibitor, was shown to induce autophagy in CRC cells [115]. However, in a randomised phase II study in relapsed or refractory CRC, bortezomib alone or in combination with irinotecan was not effective [116]. There are current trials examining combinations of bortezomib with other chemotherapies, such as oxaliplatin, 5-FU and leucovorin, in patients with advanced CRC [117]. In view of the limited results with autophagy inducers, some authors have suggested that optimal anti-tumour efficacy might be achieved by the combination of proteasome inhibitors and autophagy inhibitors [118].

4.4. Targeting cancer stem cells, Wnt pathway inhibitors, and tumour cell differentiation inducers

Cancer stem cells (CSCs) are a subpopulation of tumour cells that possess the capacity to self-renew and to give rise to the heterogeneous lineages of cancer cells that comprise the tumour, and it is believed that they could be crucial in controlling and curing cancer [119]. Specifically, there is increasing evidence that CSCs play an important role in the occurrence, growth, and progression of tumours, as well as possibly in the initiation of distant metastases. In addition, CSCs are also involved in resistance to conventional chemotherapeutic drugs, novel tumour-targeted drugs, and radiation therapy [120].

CSCs have been identified not only in leukaemias, but also in solid tumours, including CRC. In fact, it has been suggested that CRC stem cells are responsible for tumour relapse, because conventional drugs fail to eliminate the CSC reservoir [121]. Due to this important clinical feature, CRC stem cells have recently been identified as a rational therapeutic target. Several CSC-targeted therapies have been proposed, including microbial- and plant-derived biomolecules; therapies directed at CSC-specific surface markers; some classical drugs, such as tranilast, curcumin and thioridazine; and reversal of their resistance to anti-tumour agents; so far, however, the toxicity of some of these approaches in normal stem cells and treatment resistance remain important limitations [122].

Various signalling pathways, such as Wingless/Int (Wnt), Hedgehog and Notch, are involved in maintaining the stemness of CSCs. Among these, Wnt, stands out for being particularly active in the majority of CRCs, and hence is the first being investigated for therapeutic targeting in CRC. A primary consequence of Wnt signalling activation is the stabilization of β-catenin in the cytoplasm, resulting in an increased translocation of β-catenin to the nucleus and, in turn, activation of Wnt target gene expression. Misregulation of the canonical Wnt/β-catenin pathway and aberrant activation of Wnt signalling target genes are common in CRC and contribute to cancer progression [123]. Despite the importance of this pathway, few compounds have progressed beyond preclinical development. Efforts have been made to investigate the inhibition of a number Wnt genes, including the matrix metalloproteinases (MMPs), which play an important role in the degradation of extracellular matrix component, crucial for invasion and metastasis. Some studies have shown that increased expression of various MMPs (MMP-1, MMP-2 and MMP-9) favours CRC progression and could predict liver metastasis. Further, several therapeutic MMP inhibitors have been developed, but so far they have failed to produce a survival benefit and, in addition, they have been associated with adverse effects, such as musculoskeletal syndrome. The development of more selective MMP inhibitors is seen as a possible way forward [124].

Another novel compound is salinomycin, a polyether ionophore antibiotic that has been shown to kill CSCs in various types of human cancer, including CRC cells, mostly by interfering with ABC drug transporters and the Wnt/β-catenin signalling pathway. Salinomycin inhibits the migratory and invasive capacity, and reduces the proportion of CD133 CSCs in HT29 and SW480 CRC cells [125]. The results from preclinical trials and its ability to kill therapy-resistant cancer cells make salinomycin a promising anticancer drug [126].

In recent years, other agents have been shown to suppress the self-renewal of CSCs *in vitro* and *in vivo*; these include metformin, DECA-14, rapamycin, oncostatin M, some natural compounds, oncolytic viruses, microRNAs, TNF-related apoptosis inducing ligand, telomerase inhibitors, mAbs and all-*trans* retinoic acid (ATRA). It has been suggested that combinations of these agents and conventional therapy could significantly reduce tumour growth, metastasis and recurrence [127].

CSCs are characterised by two main properties of normal stem cells, self-renewal and differentiation. Given this, the induction of differentiation using retinoids would be a plausible therapeutic strategy. ATRA, a potent differentiating agent, has been demonstrated to induce CSC growth inhibition, and this has been associated with down-regulation of Wnt/β-catenin signalling [128]. In a CRC tumour model of liver metastasis, we have demonstrated the anti-tumour effects of ATRA. This pro-differentiating agent hindered or completely abolished the pro-tumour stimulus produced by serum obtained from hepatectomised rats, and by a wide variety of GFs (HGF, VEGF, PDGF, EGF, and bFGF). In addition, in combination with 5-FU, an additive effect was observed in *in vitro* studies [129]. In *in vivo* experiments, ATRA also reduced tumour progression, though it failed to increase survival, both alone and in combination with 5-FU (unpublished data).

5. New therapeutic techniques for colorectal liver metastasis

Although surgical excision of tumour tissue remains the only potentially curative treatment for CRC-LM, several other techniques are now being developed to be used when surgery is not feasible or to improve surgical results.

The list of possible new therapeutic techniques for CRC-LM seems likely to increase over the next five years, including:

- Surgical approaches focused on increasing the size of the liver lobes (staged surgery or portal branch ligatures), as the percentage of remnant liver after hepatectomy is a limiting factor in many patients
- Techniques for percutaneous tumour ablation, which can reduce CRC-LM volume and allow surgery or at least delay the progression of the illness
- Nanoparticles (NPs) to selectively deliver drugs to tumour cells or induce local hyperthermia.

First, let us consider patients who could benefit from surgical excision of their liver metastases, but in whom the FLR would be less than 25%, which is currently considered the threshold of what can be tolerated. Initially, strategies for such cases were focused on selectively increasing the liver mass of liver lobes free of tumour. Some clinical trials have found that portal vein embolization (PVE) of the lobes bearing metastases induces regeneration of the other lobes, and this has been found to result in a 20-45% increase in their relative volume in two to eight weeks [130]. However, the clinical benefit of this procedure is not clear and, as there were also reports of tumour progression due to hepatectomy, it has not been widely adopted.

In patients who have inadequate FLR to undergo disease clearance with a single hepatectomy, two-stage hepatectomy for bilobar liver metastases in combination with selected use of portal venous embolization is feasible. It offers the best chance of achieving adequate FLR hypertrophy, better than a strategy involving PVE before a single hepatectomy. In addition, rates of macroscopic surgical clearance greater than 65% have been reported [131].

Surgical strategies must be individualised after careful assessment of disease distribution and its relationship to key underlying vascular and biliary structures. Thus, the majority of authors perform the first surgical stage focused on the minor hepatectomy and concurrent procedures as required. When necessary, ligature or embolization of the portal vein is carried out, to enhance the hepatic regeneration response induced by hepatectomy [132]. Nowadays, embolization is preferred to avoid surgical manipulation of the porta hepatis prior to major hepatectomies, and to achieve segment IV total portal inflow occlusion if a right hepatectomy is planned. Hypertrophy after PVE is maximal in the first three weeks, and tends to plateau after this period [133]. The time interval between hepatectomies must be long enough for adequate recovery from the first hepatectomy and liver hypertrophy, but not so long as to enable disease progression, since tumour volume may still increase within the occluded liver [134]. This interval is not well defined but is believed to be around eight to sixteen weeks. In the second-stage operation, the liver surgery usually is complex, often involving other procedures such as radiofrequency ablation. Consequently, postoperative morbidity is significant (50-60%) after this second surgery, particularly due to transient or permanent liver insufficiency. Nevertheless, when performed in referral centres for hepatic surgery the mortality rate is low (2.6-5%). Further, reported three-year survival rates after two-staged hepatectomy range from 30 to 58% [135], and in all series were significantly higher than in those patients treated with best palliative chemotherapy. Given this survival benefit and the feasibility of the surgery, this two-stage approach can be justified in suitably selected patients.

More recently, *in situ* liver transection with portal vein ligation has been proposed as a useful alternative for patients who have some segments of the left liver free of tumour, but an FLR that is too small [136]. In a first surgical intervention, arterial vessels and veins draining the lobes containing metastases are dissected and marked with vessel loops; then, the portal branches to those lobes are severed (most commonly, all right portal branches and segment I and IV branches). Some clinical trials have found that a 40-80% increase in FLR is achieved after three to eight days, and the patient can be re-operated on to remove the previously prepared lobes [137]. The results so far reported (daily increases of FRL up to 22%) are promising, but further clinical trials need to be carried out before this procedure can be generally recommended.

A quite different approach is percutaneous tumour ablation, an old design that is continuously being refined and improved with new technical developments. Initially, ablation of liver metastases was achieved by alcoholisation (ethanol injection), this being used as a downstaging procedure prior to surgery, then came radiofrequency thermoablation [42], and this was soon followed by microwave thermoablation. These procedures proved to be useful tools to reduce tumour volume, but only provided a transient effect when applied to CRC-LM. More recently, laser tumour ablation and cryoablation have gone through experimental trials in animals and are now being tested in patients, but still limited to primary liver tumours. As with previous treatments, if and when they prove to be useful in hepatocarcinomas, they will be tried in CRC-LM [138]

A different, perhaps more subtle, approach is embolization of the arterial vessels supplying the tumour. Transarterial embolisation with 300- to 500-μm microspheres has been widely used either as a downstaging procedure or as a palliative treatment. This classic technique was improved by adding selective transarterial chemotherapy prior to embolisation, which allowed higher doses of chemotherapy with fewer side effects [139].

One of the problems in treating CRC-LM is the low tolerance of the liver parenchyma to radiation [140]. An elegant solution to overcome this limitation is known as *selective internal radiation therapy* and consists in the administration of ^{90}Y-resin microspheres through the arterial branches supplying the tumour. First applied to non-resectable hepatocarcinoma patients, achieving a reduction in tumour burden, relief of symptoms and increase in survival, it is now being tested in CLR-LM with promising results. However, the type of radiolabelled microspheres, indications and dosing schedules have to be better defined [141].

A novel approach has been the use of precharged particles to chemoembolise liver tumours. Smaller (50- to 100-μm) electrically-activated microspheres are exposed to a chemotherapeutic agent which binds to them by electrostatic forces. These spheres are delivered to the vascular tumour bed where they are widely and uniformly seeded; then the drug is released and exerts its effect specifically on the tumour tissue, while the spheres block further blood supply. Preliminary reports have been quite promising, and may lead to the procedure being applied in CRC-LM [142].

All these techniques can, however, only be applied to selected macroscopic liver metastases, leaving untreated residual microfoci responsible for tumour recurrence. We need therapeutic tools to attack individual cancer cells seeded throughout the whole liver parenchyma from the primary colorectal tumour. Currently, one of the most promising avenues is radioimmunotherapy, with ongoing preclinical and clinical studies in CRC. This type of therapy involves the administration of radiolabeled mAbs that are directed specifically against tumour-associated antigens or against the tumour microenvironment. Some phase II trials have suggested that radioiodinated antibodies against CEA, as an adjuvant treatment after R0-resection of CRC-LM, improve overall survival [143]. More recently, new studies are being undertaken to assess the safety and efficacy of combining anti-CEA-RIT and kinase inhibitors, such as imatinib, to increase antibody distribution in CRC tumours [144].

On the other hand, the new field of nanosystems for cancer diagnostics and treatment is highly promising [145]. NPs, which easily escape detection and destruction by our immune system, are being used to deliver drugs directly to the tumour bed and selectively destroy cancer cells. It has been suggested that this strategy may be able to overcome tumour resistance and reduce toxicity in healthy organs. Tumour tissue tends to retain NPs, probably due to its particular characteristics (abnormally leaky endothelium and underdeveloped lymphatic drainage) [146], and this could explain the tendency of NPs to accumulate in liver metastases more than in normal liver parenchyma when administered through the hepatic artery, as we have recently shown [147]. Further, in order to decrease the severe dose-limiting toxicity of 5-FU and to enhance the concentration of this agent in the tumour mass, some researchers are investigating the use of 5-FU-loaded biodegradable NPs, and have already shown a significant improvement in the anticancer activity of the drug in an *in vitro* CRC model [148]. Finally, magnetic NPs are being investigated in combination with high-frequency magnetic fields to induce local hyperthermia in the tumour, promising results having been obtained in experimental settings (CRC-LM in rats) [149].

6. Conclusion

Liver metastases are a common undesirable development in CRC and represent the leading cause of death in this high-prevalence disease. The management of CRC-LM has significantly changed over the past two decades, with dramatic improvements in patient outcomes. This has been made possible by the application of several key concepts when implementing different therapeutic approaches for subsets of patients with mCRC. Firstly, there is a clear consensus that the best management is achieved with a multimodality approach, including surgery, perioperative chemotherapy, biological agents and/or radiotherapy. Secondly, the therapeutic option with the best potential for cure in patients with CRC-LM remains complete resection of the metastases. Strategies to facilitate liver resection are allowing significantly increases in overall survival in this complex disease. In relation to this, the use of optimal first-line chemotherapy doublet (FOLFOX, FOLFIRI, XELOX) or triplet regimens (FOLFOXIRI) in combination with targeted therapy is now recognised as a good therapeutic approach in potentially resectable patients. In particular, the development of new biological molecules for targeted therapy (bevacizumab, cetuximab, and panatimumab) has been a key factor in the most important advances in mCRC treatment.

Nevertheless, much remains to be done. The fact that these current targeted biological agents are only effective in small subsets of patients with mCRC, and that their overall impact in the management of the disease is still relatively modest, has encouraged researchers to search for novel molecules that selectively target specific molecular pathways. This has resulted in a plethora of new antiangiogenic agents (aflibercept, ramucirumab, regorafenib, etc.) and novel molecules directed against new biological targets (such as, autophagy or CSCs) or various different signalling pathways (Wnt and PI3K/AKT/mTOR, among others); these are currently being tested in preclinical studies or in phase II and III trials.

Additionally, new therapeutic techniques, such as surgical approaches focused on increasing the size of the liver lobes, SIRT, radiofrequency ablations and, more recently, NPs to selectively deliver drugs or to induce local hyperthermia in the tumour bed, promise to increase overall outcome in patients with advanced mCRC, in particular, in those with special characteristics that complicate treatment of their disease (inadequate FLR and others).

Finally, it is important not to forget the need to continue the search for new biomarkers to enable better patient stratification for each treatment option. Based on a better understanding of the process involved in the development and progression of CRC, biomarker panels will be developed and this will greatly facilitate the design of personalized medicine for CRC patients.

Acknowledgements

Our ongoing research effort in this field is supported by research grants from the University of the Basque Country (Project GIU 10/16) and the Gangoiti Barrera Foundation.

Author details

Teodoro Palomares[1*], Ana Alonso-Varona[2], Ignacio García-Alonso[1] and Vicente Portugal[3]

*Address all correspondence to: teodoro.palomares@ehu.es

1 Dpt. of Surgery and Radiology and Physical Medicine, Faculty of Medicine and Dentistry, University of the Basque Country, Leioa, Spain

2 Dpt. of Biology and Histology, Faculty of Medicine and Dentistry, University of the Basque Country, Leioa, Spain

3 Unit of Colorectal Surgery, Hospital Galdakao-Usansolo, Galdakao, Spain

References

[1] Jemal A, Bray F, Center MM, Ferlay J, Ward E, Forman D. Global cancer statistics. CA Cancer J Clin 2011;61(2): 69-90.

[2] Kanas GP, Taylor A, Primrose JN, Langeberg WJ, Kelsh MA, Mowat FS, et al. Survival after liver resection in metastatic colorectal cancer: review and meta-analysis of prognostic factors. Clin Epidemiol 2012;4: 283-301.

[3] Lopez P, Marzano E, Piardi T, Pessaux P. Repeat hepatectomy for liver metastases from colorectal primary cancer: a review of the literature. J Visc Surg 2012;149(2): e97-e103.

[4] Stein A, Glockzin G, Wienke A, Arnold D, Edelmann T, Hildebrandt B, et al. Treatment with bevacizumab and FOLFOXIRI in patients with advanced colorectal cancer: presentation of two novel trials (CHARTA and PERIMAX) and review of the literature. BioMed Central Cancer 2012;12: 356. doi: 10.1186/1471-2407-12-356.

[5] Masi G, Fornaro L, Caparello C, Falcone A. Liver Metastases from Colorectal Cancer. How to Best Complement Medical Treatment With Surgical Approaches. Future Oncol 2011;7(11): 1299-1323.

[6] Yoo PS, Lopez-Soler RI, Longo WE, Cha CH. Liver resection for metastatic colorectal cancer in the age of neoadjuvant chemotherapy and bevacizumab. Clin Colorectal Canc 2006;6(3): 202-207

[7] Steele G Jr, Ravikumar TS. Resection of hepatic metastases from colorectal cancer. Biologic perspective. Ann Surg 1989;210: 127–138.

[8] Pawlik TM, Schulick RD, Choti MA. Expanding criteria for resectability of colorectal liver metastases. The Oncologist. 2008;13(1): 51-64.

[9] Fong Y, Fortner JG, Sun RL, Brennan MF, Blumgart LH. Clinical score for predicting recurrence after hepatic resection for metastatic colorectal cancer: analysis of 1001 consecutive cases. Ann Surg 1999;230(3): 309-18.

[10] Quan D, Gallinger S, Nhan C, Auer RA, Biagi JJ, Fletcher GG, et al. The role of liver resection for colorectal cancer metastases in an era of multimodality treatment: a systematic review. Surgery 2012;151(6): 860-870.

[11] Pulitanò C, Bodingbauer M, Aldrighetti L, de Jong MC, Castillo F, Schulick RD, et al. Liver resection for colorectal metastases in presence of extrahepatic disease: results from an international multi-institutional analysis. Ann Surg Oncol 2011;18(5): 1380-1388.

[12] Ciliberto D, Prati U, Roveda L, Barbieri V, Staropoli N, Abbruzzese A, et al. Role of systemic chemotherapy in the management of resected or resectable colorectal liver metastases: a systematic review and meta-analysis of randomized controlled trials. Oncol Rep 2012;27(6):1849-1856.

[13] Santini D, Spoto C, Loupakis F, Vincenzi B, Silvestris N, Cremolini C, et al. High concordance of BRAF status between primary colorectal tumours and related metastatic sites: implications for clinical practice. Ann Oncol 2010;21(7): 1565.

[14] Simmonds PC, Primrose JN, Colquitt JL, Garden OJ, Poston GJ, Rees M. Surgical resection of hepatic metastases from colorectal cancer: a systematic review of published studies. Brit J Cancer 2006;94(7): 982-999.

[15] Neumann UP, Thelen A, Rocken C, Seehofer D, Bahra M, Riess H, et al. Non-response to pre-operative chemotherapy does not preclude long-term survival after liver resection in patients with colorectal liver metastases. Surgery 2009;146(1): 52-59.

[16] Nordlinger B, Sorbye H, Glimelius B, et al. Perioperative chemotherapy with FOLFOX4 and surgery versus surgery alone for resectable liver metastases from colorectal cancer (EORTC Intergroup trial 40983): a randomised controlled trial. Lancet 2008;371(9617): 1007-1016.

[17] Nordlinger B, Sorbye H, Glimelius B, Poston GJ, Schlag PM, Rougier P, et al. EORTC liver metastases intergroup randomized phase III study 40983: Long-term survival results. J Clin Oncol 2012;30(15s): 3508.

[18] van Vledder MG, de Jong MC, Pawlik TM, Schulick RD, Diaz LA, Choti MA. Disappearing colorectal liver metastases after chemotherapy: should we be concerned? J Gastrointest Surg 2010;14(11): 1691-1700.

[19] Brouquet A, Benoist S, Julie C, Penna C, Beauchet A, Rougier P, et al. Risk factors for chemotherapy-associated liver injuries: a multivariate analysis of a group of 146 patients with colorectal metastases. Surgery 2009;145(4): 362-371.

[20] van Kessel CS, Buckens CF, van den Bosch MA, van Leeuwen MS, van Hillegersberg R, Verkooijen HM. Preoperative Imaging of Colorectal Liver Metastases After Neoadjuvant Chemotherapy: A Meta-Analysis Ann Surg Oncol 2012;19(9): 2805-2813.

[21] Rödel C, Liersch T, Becker H, Fietkau R, Hohenberger W, Hothorn T, et al (German Rectal Cancer Study Group). Preoperative chemoradiotherapy and postoperative chemotherapy with fluorouracil and oxaliplatin versus fluorouracil alone in locally advanced rectal cancer: initial results of the German CAO/ARO/AIO-04 randomised phase 3 trial. Lancet Oncol 2012;13(7): 679-687.

[22] Smalley SR, Benedetti JK, Williamson SK, Robertson JM, Estes NC, Maher T, et al. Phase III trial of fluorouracil-based chemotherapy regimens plus radiotherapy in postoperative adjuvant rectal cancer: GI INT 0144. J Clin Oncol 2006;24(22): 3542-3547.

[23] Folprecht G, Gruenberger T, Bechstein WO, Raab HR, Lordick F, Hartmann JT, et al. Tumour response and secondary resectability of colorectal liver metastases following neoadjuvant chemotherapy with cetuximab: the CELIM randomised phase 2 trial. Lancet Oncol 2010;11(1): 38-47.

[24] Masi G, Vasile E, Loupakis F, Cupini S, Fornaro L, Baldi G, et al. Randomized trial of two induction chemotherapy regimens in metastatic colorectal cancer: an updated analysis. J Natl Cancer I 2011;103(1): 21-30.

[25] Choti MA. Chemotherapy-associated hepatotoxicity: do we need to be concerned? Ann Surg Oncol 2009;16(9): 2391-2394.

[26] Wildi SM, Gubler C, Hany T, Petrowsky H, Clavien PA, Jochum W, et al. Intraoperative sonography in patients with colorectal cancer and resectable liver metastases on preoperative FDG-PET-CT. J Clin Ultrasound 2008;36(1): 20–26.

[27] Sahani DV, Kalva SP, Tanabe KK, Tanabe KK, Hayat SM, O'Neill MJ, et al. Intraoperative US in patients undergoing surgery for liver neoplasms: comparison with MR imaging. Radiology 2004;232(3): 810–814.

[28] Elias D, Goere D, Boige V, Kohneh-Sharhi N, Malka D, Tomasic G, et al. Outcome of post-hepatectomy-missing colorectal liver metastases after complete response to chemotherapy : impact of adjuvant intra-arterial hepatic oxaliplatin. Ann Surg Oncol 2007;14(11): 3188-3194

[29] Tanaka K, Takakura H, Takeda K, Matsuo K, Nagano Y, Endo I. Importance of complete pathologic response to prehepatectomy chemotherapy in treating colorectal cancer metastases. Ann Surg 2009;250(6): 935-942.

[30] Slesser AA, Simillis C, Goldin R, Brown G, Mudan S, Tekkis PP. A meta-analysis comparing simultaneous versus delayed resections in patients with synchronous colorectal liver metastases. Surg Oncol 2013;22(1): 36-47.

[31] Chen J, Li Q, Wang C, Zhu H, Shi Y, Zhao G. Simultaneous versus staged resection for synchronous colorectal liver metastases: a meta-analysis. Int J Colorectal Dis 2011;26(2): 191–199.

[32] Viganó L. Treatment strategy for colorectal cancer with resectable synchronous liver metastases: Is any evidence-based strategy possible? World J Hepatol 2012;4(8): 237–241.

[33] Reddy SK, Pawlik TM, Zorzi D, Gleisner AL, Ribero D, Assumpcao L, et al. Simultaneous resections of colorectal cancer and synchronous liver metastases: a multi-institutional analysis. Ann Surg Oncol 2007;14(12): 3481–3491.

[34] Tsai MS, Su YH, Ho MC, Liang JT, Chen TP, Lai HS, et al. Clinicopathological features and prognosis in resectable synchronous and metachronous colorectal liver metastasis. Ann Surg Oncol 2007;14(2): 786-794.

[35] Mentha G, Majno PE, Andres A, Rubbia-Brandt L, Morel P, Roth AD. Neoadjuvant chemotherapy and resection of advanced synchronous liver metastases before treatment of the colorectal primary. Brit J Surg 2006;93(7): 872-878.

[36] Brouquet A, Mortenson M, Vauthey JN, Rodriguez-Bigas M, Overman MJ, Chang GJ, et al. Surgical strategies for synchronous colorectal liver metastases in 156 consecutive patients:classic, combined or reversed strategy? J Am Coll Surgeons 2010;210(6): 934-941.

[37] Briggs RH, Chowdhury FU, Lodge JP, Scarsbrook AF. Clinical impact of FDG PET-CT in patients with potentially operable metastatic colorectal cancer. Clin Radiol 2011;66(12): 1167-1174.

[38] Andreou A, Brouquet A, Abdalla EK, Aloia TA, Curley SA, Vauthey JN. Repeat hepatectomy for recurrent colorectal liver metastases is associated with a high survival rate. HPB (Oxford) 2011;13(11): 774-782.

[39] Adam R, Wicherts DA, de Haas RJ, Ciacio O, Lévi F, Paule B, et al. Patients with initially unresectable colorectal liver metastases: is there a possibility of cure? J Clin Oncol 2009;27(11): 1829-1835.

[40] Tanaka K, Kumamoto T, Nojiri K, Takeda K, Ichikawa Y, Endo I. Timing of Two-stage Liver Resection during Chemotherapy for Otherwise Unresectable Colorectal Metastases World J Surg 2012;36(8): 1832–1841.

[41] Fiorentini G, Aliberti C, Tilli M, Mulazzani L, Graziano F, Giordani P, et al. Intra-arterial infusion of irinotecan-loaded drug-eluting beads (DEBIRI) versus intravenous therapy (FOLFIRI) for hepatic metastases from colorectal cancer: final results of a phase III study. Anticancer Res 2012;32(4): 1387-1395.

[42] Ansari D, Andersson R. Radiofrequency ablation or percutaneous ethanol injection for the treatment of liver tumors. World J Gastroenterol 2012;18(10): 1003-1008.

[43] Kosmider S, Tan TH, Yip D, Dowling R, Lichtenstein M, Gibbs P. Radioembolization in combination with systemic chemotherapy as first-line therapy for liver metastases from colorectal cancer. J Vasc Interv Radiol 2011;22(6): 780-786.

[44] Kress MS, Collins BT, Collins SP, Dritschilo A, Gagnon G, Unger K. Stereotactic body radiation therapy for liver metastases from colorectal cancer: analysis of safety, feasibility, and early outcomes. Frontiers in Oncology 2012;2: 8. doi: 10.3389/fonc. 2012.00008.

[45] Meinsma R, Fernandez-Salguero P, Van Kuilenburg AB, Van Gennip AH, Gonzalez FJ. Human polymorphism in drug metabolism: mutation in the dihydropyrimidine dehydrogenase gene results in exon skipping and thymineuracilurea. DNA and Cell Biology 1995;14(1): 1-6.

[46] Gustavsson B, Christopher K, Carlsson G, Wettergren Y, Odin E, Lindskog EB, et al. Molecular determinants of efficacy for 5-FU-based treatments in advanced colorectal cancer: mRNA expression for 18 chemotherapy-related genes. Int J Cancer 2009;124(5): 1220-1226.

[47] Yen JL, McLeod HL. Should DPD analysis be required prior to prescribing fluoropyrimidines? Eur J Cancer 2007;43(6): 1011-1016.

[48] Newton KF, Newman W, Hill J. Review of biomarkers in colorectal cancer. Colorectal Dis 2012;14(1): 3-17.

[49] Alagoz M, Gilbert DC, El-Khamisy S, Chalmers AJ. DNA Repair and Resistance to Topoisomerase I Inhibitors: Mechanisms, Biomarkers and Therapeutic Targets. Curr Med Chem 2012;19(23): 3874-3885.

[50] Cecchin E, Innocenti F, D'Andrea M, Corona G, De Mattia E, Biason P, et al. Predictive role of the UGT1A1, UGT1A7, and UGT1A9 genetic variants and their haplotypes on the outcome of metastatic colorectal cancer patients treated with fluorouracil, leucovorin, and irinotecan. J Clin Oncol 2009;27(15): 2457-2465.

[51] Palomaki GE, Bradley LA, Douglas MP, Kolor K, Dotson WD. Can UGT1A1 genotyping reduce morbidity and mortality in patients with metastatic colorectal cancer treated with irinotecan? An evidence-based review. Genetic Medicine 2009;11(1): 21-34.

[52] Dienstmann R, Vilar E, Tabernero J. Molecular Predictors of Response to Chemotherapy in Colorectal Cancer. Cancer J 2011;17(2): 114-12 6.

[53] Braun MS, Richman SD, Quirke P, Daly C, Adlard JW, Elliott F, et al. Predictive biomarkers of chemotherapy efficacy in colorectal cancer: results from the UK MRC FOCUS trial. J Clin Oncol 2008;26(16): 2690-2698.

[54] Ikeguchi M, Arai Y, Maeta Y, Ashida K, Katano K, Wakatsuki T. Topoisomerase I expression in tumors as a biological marker for CPT-11 chemosensitivity in patients with colorectal cancer. Surg Today 2011;41(9): 1196-1199.

[55] Rasheed ZA, Rubin EH. Mechanisms of resistance to topoisomerase I-targeting drugs. Oncogene 2003;22(47): 7296–7304.

[56] Lenz HJ, Zhang W, Shi MM, Jacques C, Barrett JC, Danenberg KD, et al. ERCC-1 gene expression levels and outcome to FOLFOX chemotherapy in patients enrolled in CONFIRM1 and CONFIRM2. J Clin Oncol 2008;26(suppl): abstract 4131.

[57] Yin M, Yan J, Martinez-Balibrea E, Graziano F, Lenz HJ, Kim HJ. ERCC1 and ERCC2 Polymorphisms Predict Clinical Outcomes of Oxaliplatin-based Chemotherapies in Gastric and Colorectal Cancer: A Systemic Review and Meta-analysis. Clin Cancer Res 2011;17(6): 1632-1640.

[58] Lin YL, Liau, JY, Yu SC, Ou DL, Lin LI, Tseng LH, Chang YL, et al. KRAS Mutation Is a Predictor of Oxaliplatin Sensitivity in Colon Cancer Cells. PLOS ONE 2012;7(11) e50701. doi: 10.1371/journal.pone.0050701.

[59] LeGolvan MP, Resnick M. Pathobiology of colorectal cancer hepatic metastases with an emphasis on prognostic factors. Journal of Surg Oncol 2010;102(8): 898-908.

[60] Wanebo HJ, Berz D. The neoadjuvant therapy of colorectal hepatic metastases and the role of biologic sensitizing and resistance factors. J Surg Oncol 2010;102(8): 891-897.

[61] Olayioye MA, Neve RM, Lane HA, Hynes NE. The ErbB signaling network: receptor heterodimerization in development and cancer. EMBO J 2000;19(13): 3159-3167.

[62] Christophi C, Harun N, Fifis T. Liver regeneration and tumor stimulation-A review of Cytokine and angiogenic factors. J Gastrointest Surg 2008;12(5): 966-980.

[63] Chung KY, Shia J, Kemeny NE, Shah M, Schwartz GK, Tse A, et al. Cetuximab shows activity in colorectal cancer patients with tumors that do not express the epidermal growth factor receptor by immunohistochemistry. J Clin Oncol 2005;23(9): 1803-1810.

[64] Tol J, Punt CJA. Monoclonal antibodies in the treatment of metastatic colorectal cancer: a review. Clin Ther 2010;32(3): 437-453.

[65] De Roock W, Piessevaux H, De Schutter J, Janssens M, De Hertogh G, Personeni N, et al. KRAS wild-type state predicts survival and is associated to early radiological response in metastatic colorectal cancer treated with cetuximab. Ann Oncol 2008;19(3): 508-515.

[66] Bokemeyer C, Bondarenko I, Makhson A, Hartmann JT, Aparicio J, de Braud F, et al. Fluorouracil, leucovorin, and oxaliplatin with and without cetuximab in the first-line treatment of metastatic colorectal cancer. J Clin Oncol 2009;27(5): 663-671.

[67] Van Cutsem E, Köhne CH, Láng I, Folprecht G, Nowacki MP, Cascinu S, et al. Cetuximab plus irinotecan, fluorouracil, and leucovorin as first-line treatment for metastatic colorectal cancer: updated analysis of overall survival according to tumor KRAS and BRAF mutation status. J Clin Oncol 2011;29(15): 2011-2019.

[68] De Roock W, Claes B, Bernasconi D, De Schutter J, Biesmans B, Fountzilas G. Effects of KRAS, BRAF, NRAS, and PIK3CA mutations on the efficacy of cetuximab plus chemotherapy in chemotherapy-refractory metastatic colorectal cancer: a retrospective consortium analysis. Lancet Oncol 2010;11(8) 753-762.

[69] Di Nicolantonio F, Martini M, Molinari F, Sartore-Bianchi A, Arena S, Saletti P, et al. Wild-type BRAF is required for response to panitumumab or cetuximab in metastatic colorectal cancer. J Clin Oncol 2008;26(35): 5705-5712.

[70] George B, Scott K. Predictive and Prognostic Markers in Colorectal Cancer. Current Oncol Rep 2011;13(3): 206-215.

[71] Loupakis F, Pollina L, Stasi I, Ruzzo A, Scartozzi M, Santini D, et al. PTEN expression and KRAS mutations on primary tumors and metastases in the prediction of benefit from cetuximab plus irinotecan for patients with metastatic colorectal cancer. J Clin Oncol 2009;27(16): 2622-26299.

[72] Ellis LM, Takahashi Y, Liu W, Shaheen RM. Vascular endothelial growth factor in human colon cancer: biology and therapeutic implications. Oncologist 2000;5(s1): 11-15.

[73] Hirashima Y, Yamada Y, Tateishi U, Kato K, Miyake M, Horita Y, et al. Pharmacokinetic parameters from 3-Tesla DCE-MRI as surrogate biomarkers of antitumor effects of bevacizumab plus FOLFIRI in colorectal cancer with liver metastasis. Int J Cancer 2012;130(10): 2359-2365.

[74] Ince WL, Jubb AM, Holden SN, Holmgren EB, Tobin P, Sridhar M, et al. Association of k-ras, b-raf and p-53 status with the treatment effect of bevacizumab. J Natl Cancer I 2005;97(13): 981-989.

[75] Zoratto F, Rossi L, Zullo A, Papa A, Zaccarelli E, Tomao L, et al. Critical appraisal of bevacizumab in the treatment of metastatic colorectal cancer. OncoTargets Ther 2012;5: 199-211.

[76] Felcht M, Luck R, Schering A, Seidel P, Srivastava K, Hu J. Angiopoietin-2 differentially regulates angiogenesis through TIE2 and integrin signalling. J Clin Invest 2012;122 (6): 1991-2005.

[77] Goede V, Coutelle O, Neuneier J, Reinacher-Schick A, Schnell R, Koslowsky TC, et al. Identification of serum angiopoietin-2 as a biomarker for clinical outcome of colorec-

tal cancer patients treated with bevacizumab-containing therapy. Brit J Cancer 2010;103(9): 1407-1414.

[78] Kopetz S, Hoff PM, Morris JS, Wolff RA, Eng C, Glover KY, et al. Phase II trial of infusional fluorouracil, irinotecan, and bevacizumab for metastatic colorectal cancer: efficacy and circulating angiogenic biomarkers associated with therapeutic resistance. J Clin Oncol 2010;28(3): 453-459.

[79] Tabernero J, Baselga J. Multigene assays to improve assessment of recurrence risk and benefit from chemotherapy in early-stage colon cancer: has the time finally arrived, or are we still stage locked? J Clin Oncol 2010;28(25): 3904-3907.

[80] Sikaroodi M, Galachiantz Y, Baranova A. Tumor markers: the potential of "omics" approach. Curr Mol Med 2010;10(2): 249-257.

[81] García-Bilbao A, Armañanzas R, Ispizua Z, Calvo B, Alonso-Varona A, Inza I, et al. Identification of a biomarker panel for colorectal cancer diagnosis. BioMed Central Cancer 2012;12: 43.

[82] Schwarz RE, Berlin JD, Lenz HJ, Nordlinger B, Rubbia-Brandt L, Choti MA. Systemic cytotoxic and biological therapies of colorectal liver metastases: expert consensus statement. HPB 2013;15(2): 106-115.

[83] Aranda E, Abad A, Carrato A, Cervantes A, García-Foncillas J, García-Alfonso P, et al. Treatment recommendations for metastatic colorectal cancer. Clin Translat Oncol 2011;13(3): 162-178.

[84] Song X, Zhao Z, Barber B, Gregory C, Wang PF, Long SR. Treatment patterns and metastasectomy among mCRC patients receiving chemotherapy and biologics. Curr Med Res Opin 2011;27(1): 123-130.

[85] Fornaro L, Vasile E, Masi G, Loupakis F, Baldi GG, Allegrini G, et al. Outcome of Second-Line Treatment After First-Line Chemotherapy with the GONO FOLFOXIRI Regimen. Clin Colorectal Cancer 2012;11(1): 71-76.

[86] Gravalos C, Salut A,García-Girón C, García-Carbonero R, León AI, Sevilla I, et al. A randomized phase II study to compare oxaliplatin plus 5-fluorouracil and leucovorin (FOLFOX4) versus oxaliplatin plus raltitrexed(TOMOX) as first-line chemotherapy for advanced colorectal cáncer. Clin Translat Oncol 2012;14(8): 606-612.

[87] Nordlinger B, Adam R, Arnold D, Zalcberg JR, Gruenberger T. The role of biological agents in the resection of colorectal liver metastases. Clin Oncol-UK 2012;24(6): 432-442.

[88] Palomares T, Caramés M, García-Alonso I, Alonso-Varona A. Growth Factors and the Redox State as New Therapeutic Targets for Colorectal Cancer. In: Ettarh R. (ed.) Colorectal Cancer Biology. From genes to tumor. Rijeka: InTech;2012. p189-216.

[89] Geva R, Vecchione L, Tejpar S,Piessevaux H, Cutsem EV, Prenen H. Bevacizumab plus chemotherapy as salvage treatment in chemorefractory patients with metastatic colorectal cancer. Oncotargets Ther 2013;6: 53-58.

[90] Grothey A, Sugrue MM, Purdie DM, Dong W, Sargent D, Hedrick E, et al. Bevacizumab beyond first progression is associated with prolonged overall survival in metastatic colorectal cancer: results from a large observational cohort study (BRiTE). J Clin Oncol 2008;26(33): 5326-5334.

[91] Pentheroudakis G, Kotoula V, De Roock W, Kouvatseas G, Papakostas P, Makatsoris T, et al. Biomarkers of benefit from cetuximab-based therapy in metastatic colorectal cancer: interaction of EGFR ligand expression with RAS/RAF, PIK3CA genotypes. BioMed Central Cancer 2013;13(1): 49-63.

[92] García-Foncillas J, Díaz-Rubio E. Progress in metastatic colorectal cancer: growing role of cetuximab to optimize clinical outcome. Clin Translat Oncol 2010;12(8): 533-542.

[93] Fuloria J. Safety profiles of current antiangiogenic therapies for metastatic colorectal cancer. Oncotargets Ther 2012;5: 133-142.

[94] Ballestrero A, Garuti A, Cirmena G, Rocco I, Palermo C, Nencioni A, et al. Patient-tailored treatments with anti-EGFR monoclonal antibodies in advanced colorectal cancer: KRAS and beyond. Curr Cancer Drug Tar 2012;12(4): 316-328.

[95] Zhou SW, Huang YY, Wei Y, Jiang ZM, Zhang YD, Yang Q, Xie DR. No survival benefit from adding cetuximab or panitumumab to oxaliplatin-based chemotherapy in the first-line treatment of metastatic colorectal cancer in KRAS wild type patients: a meta-analysis. PLOS One 2012;7(11). e50925. doi: 10.1371/journal.pone.0050925.

[96] Saridaki Z, Georgoulias V, Souglakos J. Mechanisms of resistance to anti-EGFR mAb treatment in metastatic colorectal cancer. World J Gastroenterol 2010;16(10): 1177-1187.

[97] Grothey A, Allegra C. Antiangiogenesis therapy in the treatment of metastatic colorectal cancer. Ther Adv Med Oncol 2012;4(6): 301-319.

[98] Holash J, Davis S, Papadopoulos N, Croll SD, Ho L, Russell M, et al. VEGF-Trap: a VEGF blocker with potent antitumor effects. PNAS-USA 2002;99(17): 11393-11398.

[99] Van Cutsem E, Tabernero J, Lakomy R, Prenen H, Prausová J, Macarulla T, et al. Addition of aflibercept to fluorouracil, leucovorin, and irinotecan improves survival in a phase III randomized trial in patients with metastatic colorectal cancer previously treated with an oxaliplatin-based regimen. J Clin Oncol 2012;30(28): 3499-3506.

[100] Spratlin J. Ramucirumab (IMC-1121B): MAb inhibition of vascular endothelial growth factor receptor-2. Curr Oncol Rep 2011;13(2): 97-102.

[101] Chu E. An update on the current and emerging targeted agents in metastatic colorectal cancer. Clin Colorectal Canc 2012;11(1): 1-13.

[102] Schwartz JD, Rowinsky EK, Youssoufian H, Pytowski B, Wu Y. Vascular endothelial growth factor receptor-1 in human cancer: concise review and rationale for development of IMC-18F1 (human antibody targeting vascular endothelial growth factor receptor-1). Cancer 2010;116(4s): 1027-1032.

[103] Grothey A, Van Cutsem E, Sobrero A, Siena S, Falcone A, Ychou M, et al. CORRECT Study Group. Regorafenib monotherapy for previously treated metastatic colorectal cancer (CORRECT): an international, multicentre, randomised, placebo-controlled, phase 3 trial. Lancet 2013;381(9863): 303-312.

[104] Schmoll HJ, Cunningham D, Sobrero A, Karapetis CS, Rougier P, Koski SL, et al. Cediranib with mFOLFOX6 versus bevacizumab with mFOLFOX6 as first-line treatment for patients with advanced colorectal cancer: a double-blind, randomized phase III study (HORIZON III). J Clin Oncol 2012;30(29): 3588-3595.

[105] O'Neil BH, Cainap C, Van Cutsem E, Gorbunova VA, Karapetis CS, Berlin J, et al. Randomized phase II open-label study of mFOLFOX6 in combination with linifanib or bevacizumab for metastatic colorectal cancer. J Clin Oncol 2012;30(15s): 3532.

[106] Richardson PG, Eng C, Kolesar J, Hideshima T, Anderson KC. Perifosine, an oral, anti-cancer agent and inhibitor of the Akt pathway: mechanistic actions, pharmacodynamics, pharmacokinetics, and clinical activity. Expert Opin Drug Met 2012;8(5): 623-633.

[107] Kim DD, Eng C.The promise of mTOR inhibitors in the treatment of colorectal cancer. Expert Opin Inv Drugs 2012;21(12): 1775-1788.

[108] Gulhati P, Zaytseva YY, Valentino JD, Stevens PD, Kim JT, Sasazuki T, et al. Sorafenib enhances the therapeutic efficacy of rapamycin in colorectal cancers harboring oncogenic KRAS and PIK3CA. Carcinogenesis 2012;33(9): 1782-1790.

[109] Feng YH, Wu CL, Shiau AL, Lee JC, Chang JG, Lu PJ, et al. MicroRNA-21-mediated regulation of Sprouty2 protein expression enhances the cytotoxic effect of 5-fluorouracil and metformin in colon cancer cells. Int J Mol Med 2012;29(5): 133-142.

[110] Suh DH, Kim MK, Kim HS, Chung HH, Song YS. Unfolded protein response to autophagy as a promising druggable target for anticancer therapy. Ann N.Y. Acad Sci 2012;1271: 20-32.

[111] Carew JS, Kelly KR, Nawrocki ST. Autophagy as a target for cancer therapy: new developments. Cancer Manag Res 2012;4: 357-365.

[112] McAfee Q, Zhang Z, Samanta A, Levi SM, Ma XH, Piao S, et al. Autophagy inhibitor Lys05 has single-agent antitumor activity and reproduces the phenotype of a genetic autophagy deficiency. PNAS-USA 2012;109(21): 8253-8258.

[113] Jegga AG, Schneider L, Ouyang X, Zhang J. Systems biology of the autophagy-lysosomal pathway. Autophagy 2011;7(5): 477-489.

[114] García-Mauriño S, Alcaide A, Domínguez C. Pharmacological control of autophagy: therapeutic perspectives in inflammatory bowel disease and colorectal cancer. Curr Pharm Design 2012;18(26): 3853-3873.

[115] Hong YS, Hong SW, Kim SM, Jin DH, Shin JS, Yoon DH, et al. Bortezomib induces G2-M arrest in human colon cancer cells through ROS-inducible phosphorylation of ATM-CHK1. Int J Oncol 2012;41(1): 76-82.

[116] Kozuch PS, Rocha-Lima CM, Dragovich T, Hochster H, O'Neil BH, Atiq OT, et al. Bortezomib with or without irinotecan in relapsed or refractory colorectal cancer: results from a randomized phase II study. J CLin Oncol 2008;26(14): 2320-2326.

[117] Caponigro F, Lacombe D, Twelves C, Bauer J, Govaerts AS, Marréaud S, et al. An EORTC phase I study of Bortezomib in combination with oxaliplatin, leucovorin and 5-fluorouracil in patients with advanced colorectal cancer. Eur J Cancer 2009;45(1): 48-55.

[118] Benbrook DM, Long A. Integration of autophagy, proteasomal degradation, unfolded protein response and apoptosis. Exp Oncol 2012;34(3): 286-297.

[119] Fábián A, Barok M, Vereb G, Szöllosi J. Die hard: are cancer stem cells the Bruce Willises of tumor biology? Cytometry Part A 2009;75(51): 67-74.

[120] Moitra K, Lou H, Dean M. Multidrug efflux pumps and cancer stem cells: insights into multidrug resistance and therapeutic development. Clin Pharm Ther 2011;89(4): 491–502.

[121] Vaiopoulos AG, Kostakis ID, Koutsilieris M, Papavassiliou AG. Colorectal cancer stem cells. Stem cells 2012;30(3): 363-371.

[122] Prud'homme GJ. Cancer stem cells and novel targets for antitumor strategies. Current Pharmaceutical Design 2012;18(19): 2838-2849.

[123] McDonald SL, Silver AR. On target? Strategies and progress in the development of therapies for colorectal cancer targeted against WNT signalling. Colorectal Dis 2011;13(4): 360-369.

[124] Herszényi L, Hritz I, Lakatos G, Varga MZ, Tulassay Z. The behavior of matrix metalloproteinases and their inhibitors in colorectal cancer. Int J Mol Sci 2012;13(10): 13240-13263.

[125] Dong TT, Zhou HM, Wang LL, Feng B, Lv B, Zheng MH. Salinomycin selectively targets 'CD133+' cell subpopulations and decreases malignant traits in colorectal cancer lines. Ann Surg Oncol 2011;18(6): 1797-1804.

[126] Naujokat C, Steinhart R.Salinomycin as a drug for targeting human cancer stem cells. J Biomed Biotechnol 2012;2012: 1-17.

[127] Ning X, Du Y, Ben Q, Shu J, Li Z. Therapeutic strategies targeting cancer stem cells. Cancer Biol Ther 2013;14(4): 1-9.

[128] Lim YC, Kang HJ, Kim YS, Choi EC. All-trans-retinoic acid inhibits growth of head and neck cancer stem cells by suppression of Wnt/β-catenin pathway. Eur J Cancer 2012;48,(17): 3310-3318.

[129] García-Alonso I, Palomares T, Alonso-Varona A, Díaz-Sanz I, Miró B, Méndez J. All-Trans Retinoic Acid blocks the proliferative effect of growth factors on rat colocarcinoma cells. Brit J Surg 2010;97(S4): 15.

[130] van Gulik TM, van den Esschert JW, de Graaf W, van Lienden KP, Busch OR, Heger M, et al. Controversies in the use of portal vein embolization. Digest Surg 2008;25(6): 436-444.

[131] Bowers KA, O'Reilly D, Bond-Smith GE, Hutchins RR. Feasibility study of two-stage hepatectomy for bilobar liver metastases. Am J Surg 2012;203(6): 691-697.

[132] Abulkhir A, Limongelli P, Healey AJ, Damrah O, Tait P, Jackson J, et al. Preoperative portal vein embolization for major liver resection: a meta-analysis. Ann Surg 2008;247(1): 49-57.

[133] Ribero D, Abdalla EK, Madoff DC, Donadon M, Loyer EM, Vauthey JN. Portal vein embolization before major hepatectomy and its effects on regeneration, resectability and outcome. Brit J Surg 2007;94(11):1386-1394.

[134] Barbaro B, Di Stasi C, Nuzzo G, Vellone M, Giuliante F, Marano P. Preoperative right portal vein embolization in patients with metastatic liver disease. Metastatic liver volumes after RPVE. Acta Radiol 2003;44(1): 98-102.

[135] Wicherts DA, Miller R, de Haas RJ, Bitsakou G, Vibert E, Veilhan LA, et al. Long-term results of two-stage hepatectomy for irresectable colorectal cancer liver metastases. Ann Surg 2008;248(6): 994-1005.

[136] Knoefel WT, Gabor I, Rehders A, Alexander A, Krausch M, Schulte am Esch J, et al. In situ liver transection with portal vein ligation for rapid growth of the future liver remnant in two-stage liver resection. Brit J Surg 2012;100(3): 388-394.

[137] Schnitzbauer AA, Lang SA, Goessmann H, Nadalin S, Baumgart J, Farkas SA, et al. Right portal vein ligation combined with in situ splitting induces rapid left lateral liver lobe hypertrophy enabling 2-staged extended right hepatic resection in small-for-size settings. Ann Surg 2012;255(3): 405-414.

[138] Sindram D, Lau KN, Martinie JB, Lamnitti DA. Hepatic tumor ablation. Surg Clin N Am 2010;90(4): 863-876.

[139] Hoffmann RT, Paprottka P, Jakobs TF, Trumm CG, Reiser MF. Arterial therapies of non-colorectal cancer metastases to the liver (from chemoembolization to radioembolization). Abdom Imagin 2011;36(6): 671-676.

[140] Malik U, Mohiuddin M. External-beam radiotherapy in the management of liver metastases. Sem Oncol 2002;29(2): 196-201.

[141] Van de Wiele C, Maes A, Brugman E, D'Asseler Y, De Spiegeleer B, Mees G, et al. SIRT of liver metastases: physiological and pathophysiological considerations. Eur J Nucl Mol I 2012;39(10): 1646-1655.

[142] Namur J, Citron SJ, Sellers MT, Dupuis MH, Wassef M, Manfait M, et al. Embolization of hepatocellular carcinoma with drug-eluting beads: doxorubicin tissue concentration and distribution in patient liver explants. J Hepatol 2011;55(6): 1332-1338.

[143] Liersch T, Meller J, Kulle B, Behr TM, Markus P, Langer C, et al. Phase II Trial of Carcinoembryonic Antigen Radioimmunotherapy With 131I-Labetuzumab After Salvage Resection of Colorectal Metastases in the Liver: Five-Year Safety and Efficacy Results. J Clin Oncol 2005;23(27): 6763-6770.

[144] Rajkumar VS, Boxer G, Robson M, Muddle J, Papastavrou Y, et al. A comparative study of PDGFR inhibition with imatinib on radiolabeled antibody targeting and clearance in two pathologically distinct models of colon adenocarcinoma. Tumor Biol 2012;33(6): 2019-2029.

[145] Gonçalves AS, Macedo AS, Souto EB. Therapeutic nanosystems for oncology nanomedicine. Clin Translat Oncol 2012;14(12): 883-890.

[146] Garcia-Bennett A, Nees M, Fadeel B. In search of the Holy Grail: folate-targeted nanoparticles for cancer therapy. Biochemical Pharmacology 2011;81(8): 976-984.

[147] Echevarria-Uraga JJ, García-Alonso I, Plazaola F, Insausti M, Etxebarria N, Saiz-López A, et al. Study of the intra-arterial distribution of Fe3O4 nanoparticles in a model of colorectal neoplasm induced in rat liver by MRI and Spectrometry. Int J Nanomed 2012;7: 2399-2410.

[148] Ortiz R, Prados J, Melguizo C, Arias JL, Ruiz MA, Alvarez PJ, et al. 5-Fluorouracil-loaded poly(epsilon-caprolactone) nanoparticles combined with phage E gene therapy as a new strategy against colon cancer. Int J Nanomed 2012;7: 95-107.

[149] Echevarria-Uraga JJ, García-Alonso I, Herrero B, Marin H, Insausti M, Plazaola F, et al. Liver hyperthermia induced by different iron magnetic nanoparticles "ex vivo" and correlation to pathological damage in the tissue. Brit J Surgery 2013;100(S1): 12.

4

Surgical Strategies for Liver Metastases from Colorectal Cancer

Nikola Kolev, Valentin Ignatov, Anton Tonev,
Tanya Kirilova, Georgi Ivanov,
Alexander Zlatarov and Krassimir Ivanov

1. Introduction

Colorectal carcinoma is one of the more common types of cancer around the world. For patients in UICC stage I (i.e., those who have pT1/2 tumors and do not have any lymph node metastases), the probability of surviving 5 years is 90% [2]. The prognosis of patients in stages II (pT3/4 tumors without lymph node metastases) and III (tumors with lymph node metastases) has improved steadily in recent years. At present, the 5-year survival in these two groups is 80% and 60% [1].

Approximately, 1.2 million cases of CRC occur yearly worldwide, with 412, 900 new cases diagnosed in Western Europe alone and 150, 000 in the United States. [1, 2] Resection of colorectal liver metastases (CRLM) is the only treatment offering the possibility of cure and has been shown to provide clear survival benefits. [3] Unfortunately, only 10% to 20% of patients with CRLM are eligible for this procedure upfront. On the other hand, during the last 10 years, major advances in the management of CRLM have taken place involving principally three different fields: oncology (new and more effective chemotherapeutic agents), interventional radiology (portal embolization and radiofrequency), and surgery (better instruments and newer techniques). These advances as part of a multidisciplinary team approach have gradually but effectively increased the resectability rate to 20%-30% of cases with a 5-year survival of 35%-50%. [3]

Nonetheless, distant metastases eventually arise in about 20% of patients who are stage II or III at the time of diagnosis [3]. About 35% of all patients already have distant metastases when the diagnosis is made. Patients with untreated hepatic metastases have a very poor prognosis.

In a prospective, observational study carried out on 484 patients from 1980 to 1990, the median time to death was 6.9 months [4]. Adson and colleagues, in the 1970's, were the first to show that patients could be cured by the resection of hepatic metastases [5]. Since then, resection has become established as a standard treatment. For this review, we selectively searched the literature for articles containing the words "colorectal liver metastases, " "chemotherapy, " and "surgery, " paying special attention to studies carried out on larger groups of patients and to randomized clinical trials. [6]

Most favorable outcomes were observed in patients with pedicle lymph node involvement (5-year survival rate 25% vs 0% for patients with celiac and/ or para-aortic lymph node metastases), and in patients younger than 40 years (5-year survival rate 45% vs 10% for older patients). [7, 8] In relation to our results and those reported by others, we recommend combining hepatectomy with lymphadenectomy only for young CLM patients presenting with pedicle lymph node involvement, in the absence of disease progression after preoperative chemotherapy. On the other hand, patients presenting with celiac or para-aortic lymph node involvement should not be subjected to this oncosurgical treatment strategy. Even concomitant pulmonary metastases should not be considered a contraindication to surgery. Patients with only pulmonary metastases as a site of extrahepatic disease have a particularly good outcome after complete metastasectomy of both liver and lung disease. Five-year survival rates ranged from 22% to 50% in patients with metastases limited to the lungs. [8] Also, selected patients with complex multiorgan metastases have been associated with prolonged survival after a multimodality treatment. Patients with simultaneous hepatic and extrahepatic disease (EHD) do, however, need to be selected for surgery. Elias et al stated that EHD, when resectable, is no longer a contraindication to hepatectomy. [18] More importantly, the total number of metastases, whatever their location, has a strong prognostic effect than the site of the metastases. In addition, a study conducted at our centre demonstrated that patients with concomitant EHD who were resected experienced a lower 5-year survival than those without EHD (28% vs 55%, *P*<.001). Five poor prognostic factors were identified with multivariate analysis: EHD location other than lung metastases, EHD concomitant to colorectal liver metastases recurrence, CEA-level>10 ng/ml, >6 colorectal liver metastases and right colon cancer. The five-year survival ranged from 64% (0 factors) to 0% (>3factors). [19]

We aim to report the new trends in strategies about surgical treatment of colorectal liver metastases and our experience according to surgical and oncological outcome in patients, operated for IV stage colorectal cancer.

2. Criteria for resectability

Currently available data have led to a change in the indications for resecting hepatic metastases of colorectal carcinoma. Previously, the indication was based on tumor-biological and clinical characteristics. The new criterion is the feasibility of complete resection of both intra- and extrahepatic disease. R0-resectable hepatic metastases, in patients without any extrahepatic metastases, should be resected. [12] As the determination of resectability is becoming ever more complex, all patients with hepatic metastases of colorectal carcinoma should be presented to an experienced hepatobiliary surgeon before the beginning of treatment. Postoperative hepatic function can be predicted more precisely with the aid of CT volumetry. This technique enables prediction of the remaining volume of hepatic tissue after surgery to within 10% of the actual value. [9, 11]

Metastases are considered resectable when the following criteria are met:

- exclusion of a non-resectable extrahepatic tumor manifestation,
- parenchymal involvement <75%,
- <3 hepatic veins and <7 hepatic segments involved,
- no hepatic insufficiency, no Child B or C cirrhosis,
- no severe accompanying diseases.

Metastases are considered non-resectable or marginally resectable when an R0 resection is not possible. Metastases are also considered marginally resectable in the setting of, for example, extra-hepatic tumor manifestations, technical impediments to surgery, or inadequate expected residual liver mass. For these patients, intensified preoperative chemotherapy can be considered. The feasibility of secondary resection should be evaluated at each re-staging under chemotherapy. [15]

3. New treatment strategies

Today, patients with metastatic CRC should be treated by multidisciplinary teams including surgeons, oncologists and radiologists. Evidence of the benefit of perioperative chemotherapy over surgery alone [22] and the potential benefit of adjuvant chemotherapy (after liver resection) [23] caused a rethink among the experts particularly in terms of the timing of the administration of chemotherapy for CRC patients with initially resectable liver and lung metastases. Poor prognostic factors for patients with liver metastases are multiple metastases, >5 cm in diameter, synchronous presentation, lymph node-positive primary and high tumor marker levels. [17] Thus, even when the metastases are technically resectable (in terms of number, location and size), when facing a patient with more than one of the poor prognostic factors listed above, the current trend is to refer patients for neoadjuvant chemotherapy before surgery. The data from the EORTC study showed quite clearly that nearly all patients were able to tolerate neo-adjuvant chemotherapy. Also, analysis of the PFS curves from the EORTC–EPOC trial shows that the main difference comes after the first 2 months when the curves drop down and then move out in parallel, suggesting that the benefit conferred by perioperative chemotherapy might be a consequence of a reduction in the occurrence of early cancer relapse as a consequence of preoperative chemotherapy. [16] An exception to preoperative chemotherapy is, however, those patients with a single resectable metachronous metastasis who could be directly referred to surgery, [14] with the recognition that this accounts for <10% of patients seen in routine clinical practice. All other patients with resectable metastases should be treated up front with chemotherapy, with the caveats that the patient is able to receive chemotherapy and the position of the lesion is not going to be lost. On the other hand, it has also become a standard strategy to give postoperative adjuvant chemotherapy to all resected patients (if possible) based on the data for the resected patients in the EORTC–EPOC trial. [22] For patients who are non-responders, there are two treatment strategies available: 1) change to a new chemotherapy protocol or 2) liver resection before the metastatic disease becomes unresectable. At this point it is important to mention that, the decision to perform either treatment strategy should always be decided by a multidisciplinary. Currently, it has become mandatory to select the systemic therapy regimen based on biological predictive factors, such as KRAS mutation status. This strategy has had a double impact: first of all, it has helped to optimize the choice of first-line treatment, in turn decreasing the risk of immediate disease progression; secondly, it has also helped to better select the second-line 'rescue' treatment strategies with the possibility of resection. [27] However, considering that surgery is still the only treatment that has curative potential per se, in some situations this can be the treatment of choice, even if resistance to medical treatment generally means that the patient has a unfavorable tumor biology. The situation is much simpler for patients whose metastases are initially unresectable, where systemic therapy is administered until an adequate response has been achieved. [24]

4. Primarily resectable hepatic metastases

For operable hepatic metastases, hepatic resection is the treatment of choice. The reported 5-year-survival rates that have been achieved after the resection of isolated hepatic metastases with curative intent range from 25% to 50% [1–4, 6–8]. Hepatic metastases, however, are primarily resectable in only about 20% of patients [4]. For the remaining 80%, resection is contraindicated by the presence of diffuse hepatic metastases, non-resectable extra-hepatic disease, or impaired liver function. It is now generally accepted that the contraindications for hepatic resection that were defined in the 1980's are no longer applicable. At that time, the presence of 4 or more tumor nodules, metastases exceeding 5 cm in size, extra-hepatic disease, or a tumor-free resection margin of less than 1 cm [9] was held to contraindicate hepatic resection. Many subsequent studies have confirmed that these are, indeed, relevant prognostic factors for survival after the resection of hepatic metastases of colorectal carcinoma, yet long-term survival is still possible when hepatic resection is performed despite the presence of these supposed contraindications. There have also been technical improvements in the treatment of hepatic metastases of colorectal carcinoma. Diagnostic assessment has become markedly more sensitive through the use of modern types of CT and MRI scanners and the introduction of PET-CT (5, 10–14]. Furthermore, surgical dissecting techniques and the development of potent systemic chemotherapy protocols have been optimized [15–18]. As a result, 5-year survival rates after the resection of hepatic metastases of colorectal carcinoma have improved markedly. [6] Today, even patients with more than three metastases or with metastases larger than 5 cm in diameter can be cured with appropriate surgical treatment, as found in a recent analysis [7]. One hundred and two patients were tumor-free 10 years after the resection of hepatic metastases of colorectal carcinoma, and only one patient among them developed a recurrent tumor thereafter.

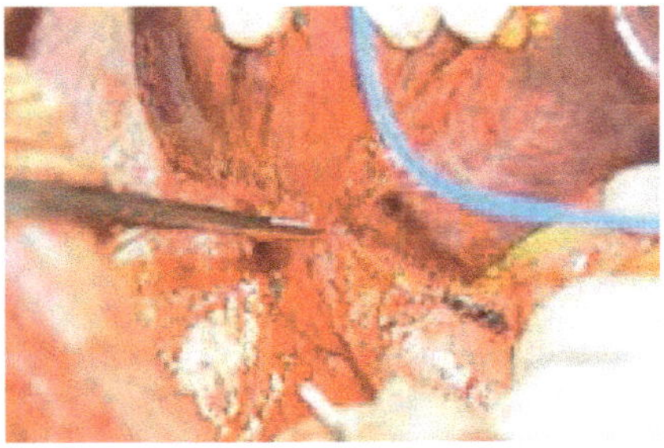

Right and retro-hepatic mobilization

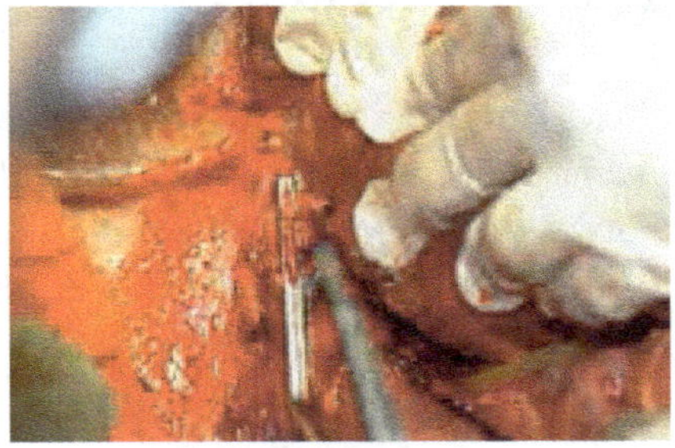

Hepatic vein division

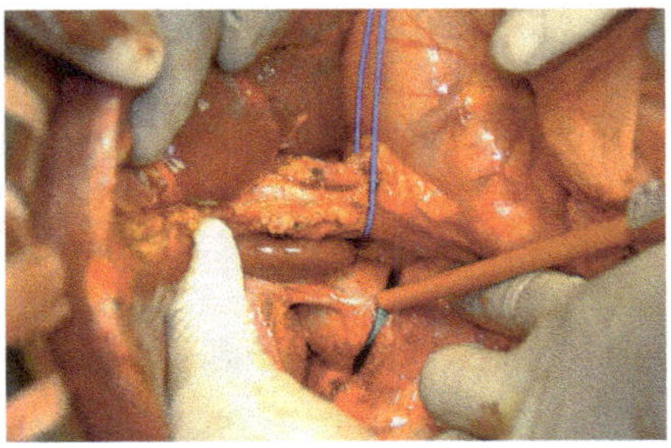

Total vascular exclusion of the liver – infra-hepatic

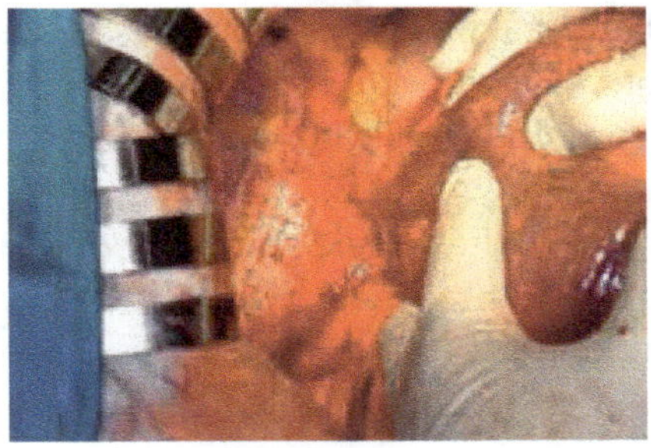

Total vascular exclusion of the liver – supra-hepatic

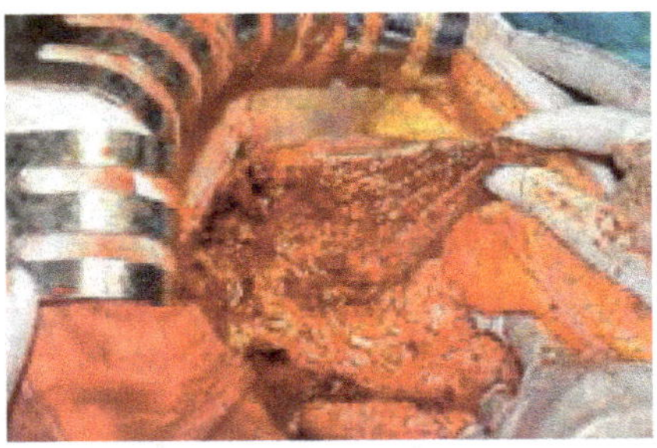

Right hepatectomy

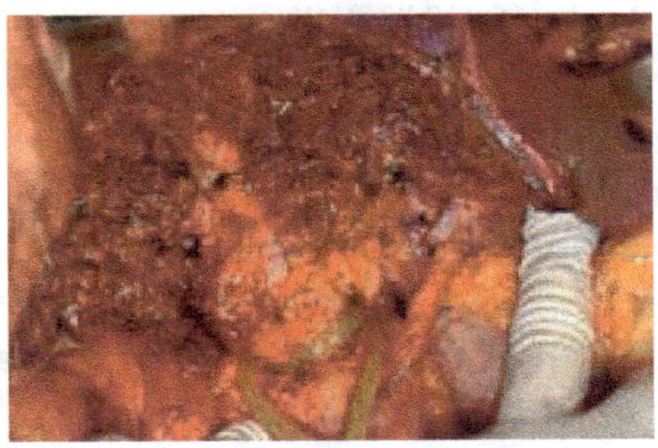

Mesohepatectomy

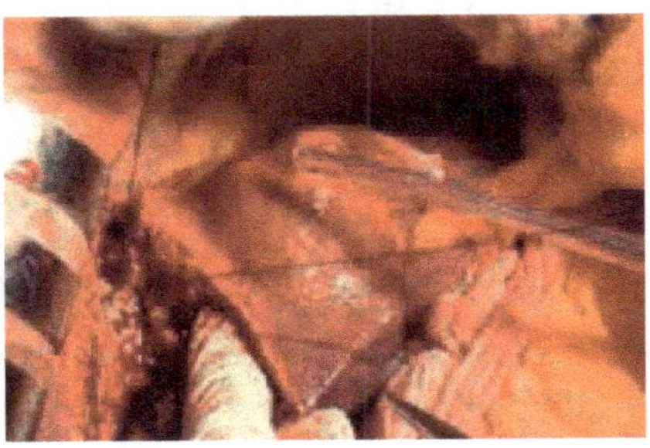

Left hepatectomy

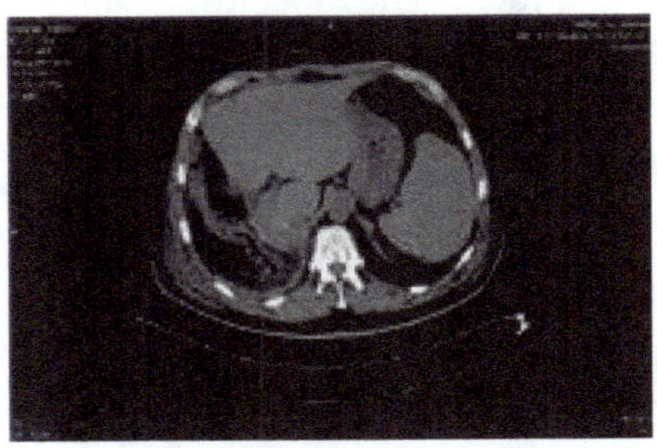

Postoperative CT scan – left lobe hypertrophy

Figure 1. Different types of liver resections

5. Perioperative complications

Hepatic resections can now be performed safely and effectively. The mortality of hepatic resection was about 5% as late as 1990, while recent articles on the subject generally document figures between 1% and 2%. This reduction of mortality has been achieved even though the resections themselves have become ever more extensive. [3]

6. Long-term results after hepatic resection

More than 40% of appropriately selected patients with colorectal carcinoma who undergo the resection of hepatic metastases survive for at least 5 years thereafter [5, 6, 8, 9]. This is particularly true of patients whose surgery was performed more recently. As many as two-thirds of patients later develop a recurrent tumor, and half of them have a recurrent tumor in the liver [23]. In one of the largest studies performed to date, which included 1001 patients, showed that the benefit of surgery extends not just to patients who have undergone an R0 resection (5-year survival: 37%), but also to those who have undergone an R1 resection, i.e., a resection with positive margins, up to 20% of whom are still alive 5 years after surgery. [31]

7. Prognostic parameters

Many different prognostic scores are used to predict the patient's risk of recurrence and chances of long-term survival on the basis of preoperatively measured parameters. The three most commonly used scoring systems in hepatic surgery are those of Nordlinger, Fong, and Iwatsuki [2, 9, 24]. Although these scoring systems differ with respect to certain individual parameters, they share the common feature that a low score (i.e., the presence of no more than a few risk factors) is correlated with a low risk of recurrence, while the chance of long-term survival is less than 10% when all risk factors are present. No preoperatively measurable prognostic parameter can identify with any certainty the patients who will not benefit from surgical treatment. The most important prognostic factor, according to all studies, is a tumor-free resection margin [10, 11, 25, 26].

8. Expanded application of resection for CRLM

Liver resection is the current preferred treatment for CRLM patients and should be undertaken whenever feasible and potentially curative (R0), regardless of prognostic factors and presence of extra hepatic metastases. The main limiting factors to perform curative resection of CRLM are: presence of bilobar or bulky disease and presence of extra hepatic disease. Resection in patients with multiple or bulky lesions may result in insufficient residual hepatic tissue (i.e., less than 30% functional parenchyma). [19]

9. Neoadjuvant chemotherapy in patients with resectable CRLM

Despite major survival improvements achieved with successful primary hepatectomy for CRLM, [7-13, 20] many of these patients experience disease recurrence. Data indicate that pre or post-operative chemotherapy may provide a meaningful benefit, although controlled trials are needed. Tanaka et al [21] reported a retrospective analysis of patients with multiple CRLMs, wherein use of neoadjuvant chemotherapy was an independent predictor of survival by multivariate analysis. In 71 patients undergoing hepatectomy for more than five bilobar liver tumors, 3- and 5-year survival rates were superior ($P<.05$, log-rank) in the neoadjuvant chemotherapy group (n=48; 67.0% and 38.9%) than in the hepatectomy-alone group (n=23; 51.8% and 20.7%). Furthermore, neoadjuvant treatment reduced the need for extended (>4 segments) hepatectomies (39 of 48 neoadjuvant vs 23 of 23 control patients). Data from the LiverMetSurvey [5] also indicate a survival improvement with neoadjuvant treatment. In 207 patients with more than five metastases resected, 5-year survival was better with neoadjuvant treatment, although not significantly (20% vs 15%) and among 1, 045 patients who had only one liver metastasis resected, 5-year survival rates were 49% and 57% with and without neoadjuvant chemotherapy, respectively. Similar results were reported in a metanalysis by Mitry et al, [22] which showed a strong trend toward better diseasefree survival with adjuvant 5-FU treatment (HR 0.76, P=5.8), and a trend toward favorable overall survival (HR 0.76, P=9.8). In addition, a phase III randomized study (The EORTC Intergroup) examined perioperative FOLFOX4 (5-fluorouracil (5-FU), leucovorin, oxaliplatin) chemotherapy for patients with potentially resectable CRLM.23 A total of 364 patients with up to four CRLM were randomized between perioperative FOLFOX4 (oxaliplatin 85 mg/mI and LV5FU2), six cycles before and six cycles after surgery (CT), vs surgery alone (S). Eleven of 182 patients were ineligible in each arm, mostly due to more advanced disease; 31 and 30 patients in the CT and S arms, respectively, could not undergo resection. At a median follow-up of 3.9 years, progression-free survival (PFS) was significantly better with CT in the group of resected patients, although the trial was formally not positive in the intentionto- treat (ITT) analysis (HR 0.79, P=.058). In terms of postoperative chemotherapy in resectable patients with CRLM data from United States and Europe show better survival in patients receiving adjuvant chemotherapy after resection of CRC liver metastases. [24] Use of adjuvant or neoadjuvant systemic treatment is widely recognized as standard of care in cases of liver resection, and was the focus of single-center studies with XELOX/FOLFOX25 and XELOX plus bevacizumab.26 So far, only one study has as yet shown a clear benefit. [27] In this randomized trial, 109 patients (75 assessable) with one to three hepatic lesions received hepatic arterial floxuridine plus intravenous 5-FU (n=30) or no further therapy (n=45) after hepatectomy. The 4-year recurrence-free rates (46% vs 25%) and 4-year liver recurrence-free rates (67% vs 43%) were significantly better in the adjuvant therapy group. Median survival differences were not statistically significant (64% vs 49%), however, the trial was insufficiently powered to evaluate overall survival. [33]

10. Strategies for improving resectability

At present, only 10% to 20% of patients with hepatic metastases of colorectal carcinoma can be considered candidates for resective surgery. Opportunities for resection are often limited by an unfavorable anatomical site of the metastasis (-es), poor function of the remaining hepatic parenchyma, and/or the patient's poor general condition. Multiple strategies have been developed in order to increase the percentage of patients whose metastases are resectable.

Liver surgery has progressed in parallel to the improvements in chemotherapy and interventional radiology. Bad-located tumors (situated deeply or close to critical vascular or biliary structures) can now be safely resected thanks to the availability of sophisticated instruments such as the ultrasonic dissector, argon gas diathermy and new techniques such as the one of low-central venous pressure anaesthesia that allows an almost bloodless field. With the routine use of intraoperative ultrasound examination precise localization of liver lesions and planning of the resection is done aiming at removing all possible lesions with a clear margin and at the same time preserve the maximum of liver parenchyma. This improvement in surgical planning and techniques has been directly responsible for the low hospital mortality. The risk of liver resection for CRLM has decreased in specialized hepatobiliary centres probably below the figures observed after colorectal surgery. The mortality of elective liver resection on non-cirrhotic livers is estimated to be around 1% [35, 36] at a time when patients' age and disease complexity are increasing, in addition to the associated changes of SOS and CASH often present in chemotherapy patients undergoing surgery. The experience of the centre has a major impact on outcome: the mortality and morbidity of liver resections decreased inversely to the number of cases performed in the institution. [37] It has been shown in US that patients resected at high volume centres (>25 cases/year) for liver cancer have not only a better perioperative outcome, but also a better long-term survival, [38] and similar results concerning the correlation between high volume surgery and specialization and outcome were observed in Europe. [39]

11. Preoperative chemotherapy ("down-staging")

When hepatic metastases of colorectal carcinoma are unresectable, systemic chemotherapy is indicated. About 20% of metastases respond to treatment with 5-fluorouracil (5-FU) and folic acid [4]. When these are used in combination with newer drugs, such as oxaliplatin or irinotecan (CPT-11), the response rate rises as high as 60% [29]. Folprecht et al. reviewed the available studies on the "down-staging" of hepatic metastases of colorectal carcinoma and found that resectionrates are correlated with response rates [4]. The first major clinical series of this type was published in 1996 by Bismuth et al. [13] and updated in the years thereafter [14, 30]. The 5-year-survival was 40% (95% confidence interval: 33% to 68%) and was thus comparable to that of patients with primarily resectable hepatic metastases. A major bias in the studies of neoadjuvant chemotherapy published to date arises from patient selection. In the available prospective studies of patients with "isolated" hepatic metastases (i.e., no extrahepatic metastases), the criteria for nonresectability differ from one study to another and are often poorly defined. The hepatotoxicity of all currently used chemotherapeutic drugs argues against their use as neoadjuvant treatment for patients with primarily resectable hepatic metastases. Oxaliplatin can cause sinusoidal obstruction ("blue liver"), while irinotecan can induce fatty liver or steatohepatitis [31–34]. These changes are associated with significantly more frequent perioperative complications. Vauthey et al. found that steatohepatitis after irinotecan use is associated with a significantly higher 90-day mortality [15].

12. Systemic chemotherapy in patients with non-resectable CRLM

Systemic chemotherapy is currently the main treatment approach for non-resectable CRLM. Incorporation of drugs such as oxaliplatin and irinotecan have led to an improvement of median survival as well as response rates compared with those achieved previously with 5-fluoracil (5-FU)/leucovorin-based regimens. Development of oral fluoropyrimidines has also improved treatment options in these patients. Median survival duration after systemic chemotherapy alone is approximately 20 months, [28, 29] however, only 1% to 2% of such patients remain alive at 5 years. [3, 30] On the other hand, the improved efficacy of newer regimens in down staging tumors is rendering more patients resectable. [14]

13. Accompanying chemotherapy

There is no longer any doubt that patients benefit from hepatic resections that are performed with curative intent. The current discussion concerns the question whether they also benefit from accompanying adjuvant or neo-adjuvant chemotherapy. The first encouraging data on adjuvant chemotherapy after hepatic resection were published by Kemeny et al., who compared local intra-arterial therapy combined with systemic 5-FU chemotherapy to adjuvant treatment with 5-FU alone. A trend was found toward improved progression-free survival in the group that additionally received regional therapy (37.4 versus 17.2 months, $p = 0.06$) [20, 44]. Nonetheless, the overall survival was no better in this group. This finding could not be replicated in a German study of intraarterial chemotherapy administered in the hepatic artery [21]. There are currently two further options for systemic chemotherapy: neo-adjuvant and adjuvant postoperative chemotherapy. For adjuvant chemotherapy, data are only available on 5-FU based treatment. Portier et al., in the AURC 9002 trial, describe an improved 5-year tumor-free survival of 33.5% among patients receiving adjuvant 5-FU bolus therapy, compared to 26.7% treated with resection alone [22]. These 5-FU patients' overall survival was no better than that of their counterparts without 5-FU, but the study size was, in any case, inadequate to detect a moderate benefit. An unplanned subgroup analysis revealed that patients with a greater tumor burden (diameter >5cm, or 3 or more tumor nodules) survived longer if they received adjuvant chemotherapy. Likewise, a pooled analysis of a number of studies, including the FFCD study, found a trend toward a benefit from adjuvant 5-FU treatment, in terms of both progression-free survival and overall survival [23]. These data appear promising, especially because there have been further improvements in chemotherapeutic regimens since they were published. Further evidence that adjuvant 5-FU treatment confers a survival benefit after the resection of hepatic metastases of colorectal carcinoma comes from a cohort study of 792 patients by Parks et al. [24]: The median survival time was 47 months, compared with 36 months without 5-FU. This year (2010), Nordlinger et al. have published the results of the

EORTC 40 983 trial, in which neoadjuvant therapy with FOLFOX (folic acid, 5-FU, and oxaliplatin) before and after hepatic resection was compared with resection alone. There were 182 patients in each of the study's two groups (with and without neoadjuvant therapy). The declared study endpoint of a significantly improved progression-free 3-year survival was not met in the intent-to-treat analysis. Tumor-free survival was 28.1% after surgery alone and 35.4% in the FOLFOX group [25]. The study did, however, show a significantly improved tumor-free 3-year survival when all patients whose data could be completely evaluated were taken into account (as opposed to the intent-to-treat analysis). Data on overall survival are currently unavailable. It should also be mentioned that the chemotherapy group had a higher rate of postoperative complications, but their postoperative mortality was no higher. Thus, in our view, preoperative chemotherapy should remain reserved, at least for now, to patients whose hepatic metastases are marginally resectable. This group includes patients whose tumor burden is high because of multiple hepatic metastases and extrahepatic tumor manifestations. Our view is founded on the documented survival benefit that can be achieved in patients who have a large burden of initially unresectable hepatic metastases by down-staging their tumors with chemotherapy, in order to render them resectable. [29]

14. Portal-vein embolization

In some cases, the resection of one or more hepatic metastases is technically feasible, yet cannot be performed because the amount of liver tissue remaining after resection would be too small. To minimize the risk of postoperative hepatic insufficiency, ipsilateral hepatic atrophy and contralateral hepatic hypertrophy can be induced preoperatively by selective embolization of the hepatic portal vein, or else by ligation of the branch of the portal vein that leads to the hepatic lobe containing the metastasis.

14.1. Definitions

Future liver remnant (FLR) is the liver that will be left in place after surgery and that was not targeted by embolization. The FLR must hypertrophy after portal vein embolization (PVE). Most teams wait 4 weeks before surgery. FLR hypertrophy must be measured by way of computed axial tomography (CAT) examination after injection of iodine with volumetric measurements of the FLR segments, with the results compared with the measurements performed before PVE using the same technique. Hypertrophy can be quantified as FLR hypertrophy, which is defined as the difference between FLR after a waiting period from 3 to 6 weeks after PVE minus FLR before PVE divided by FLR before PVE. The waiting period must be long enough to allow hypertrophy and as short as possible to avoid tumor growth, which precludes surgery. Hypertrophy can also be quantified by increased FLR ratio. The FLR ratio is defined as (FLR volume—tumor in the FLR)/ (total liver volume—total tumor volume) [8]. Technical success of PVE is defined by a complete occlusion of portal branches feeding the future resected liver segments. Branches of the FLR must be patent with hepatopetal flow. In the late phase of control portography, parenchymography must be visible only in the FLR. Clinical success is considered to occur when the patient reaches the volumetric criteria for liver resection. Patients with Tumors that Developed in Normal Underlying Liver Parenchyma PVE is recommended when the FRL-to-total liver ratio is 25 to 30 [7, 10, 11]. The indication of PVE can be extended to a 40% FLR ratio in patients having received chemotherapy or showing abnormal indocyanine green test results (or other abnormal liver function tests) [10, 12, 13]. Portal-vein embolization should always be considered when the residual hepatic volume without it would be less than 30% of the normal size of the liver, and when at least two contiguous hepatic segments are free of metastases. For technical surgical reasons, the left lateral segments 2 and 3 are particularly suitable for this approach. As long as the liver is not cirrhotic, portal-vein embolization results in a 40% to 60% hypertrophy of the contralateral hepatic lobe. It remains unclear at present whether the stimulus to hypertrophy that portal-vein embolization provides might also accelerate the growth of tumor nodules [16, 35]. In any case, the data regarding morbidity, mortality, and long-term survival are comparable to those of standard hepatic resections [16, 36–39].

Patients with Tumors that Develop in Chronic Liver Disease and Cirrhosis States

In such cases, the decision is based either on liver volume or on liver volume plus estimation of overall liver function by indocyanin green retention rate at 15 min. An FRLR of 40% is recommended when the ICCG 15 is between 10% and 20%. When the ICCG 15 is[20%, an FRLR of 50% is recommended [12–14].

Patients with Tumors Invading the Biliary Tree Associated with Cholestasis

Because biliary obstruction has impaired liver regeneration and hypertrophy, the biliary tree of the FRL must be drained first, and PVE can be performed secondarily. The indication is an FRLR\40% [15].

Contraindication for PVE [11]

PVE is contraindicated in the following types of patients:

1. Tumors invading the portal vein
2. Portal hypertension (blocked to free hepatic veinpressure gradient[12 mmHg)
3. Coagulation disorders (PT\60%, platelet count\50 G/l)
4. Even if previous transarterial chemoembolization (TACE) may improve PVE results [16], a minimum of 3-week delay between TACE and PVE is recommended.

Patients should be informed that this procedure is not an antitumoral treatment but a treatment made to increase safety or to enable a surgical procedure. Minor complications are encountered in 20% to 25% of cases and are mainly associated with slight fever and abdominal discomfort and pain. Major complications are infrequent and mainly include infection and subcapsular hematoma, hemobilia, and portal vein thrombosis 9\2% of cases). Mortality due to PVE has not been reported. When tumors (usually small nodules) are present in the nonembolized lobe, it must be explained to the patient that those lesions might increase in size more quickly due to PVE [17]. Patients must also be told that the efficacy of the procedure can be estimated approximately 4 weeks after

PVE by way of CAT with injection of contrast media and liver volumetry.

14.2. Embolization method

Access to the portal system should be done under ultrasound guidance to puncture a peripheral branch [8]. Access can be obtained by way of controlateral approach (i.e., puncture of the left portal branch and embolization of theright portal branches) or ispsilateral approach (puncture of the right portal branch to embolize right portal branches. The advantage of the controlateral approach is easier catheterization, but there is a risk of damage to the FLR. Five-French materials (catheter or introductory sheath) are usually recommended. The catheter should be placed at the splenomesenteric confluence to perform a portography to visualize portal anatomy, including its variations, and to localize segment IV branches. Measurement of portal pressure is not routinely performed in patients with normal liver. In cirrhotic patients, measuring the portal and central venous pressures is useful to determine whether the patient has a portostemic gradient[12 mmHg in, which case the patient is at major risk of perisurgical complications [18, 19]. These patients are not eligible for PVE. The aim of embolization is complete obstruction of the targeted branches and redistribution of flow to the FLR branches only. Final portography is mandatory to verify this objective. A final pressure measurement should be obtained at the end of the procedure in patients with chronic liver disease to document portal pressure increase, which is usually approximately 3 mmHg. Embolization of segment IV branches is recommended in patients with tumors who are undergoing extended right hepatectomy. However, if embolization of that segment causes risk of reflux into the portal branch of the FRL, such embolization must not be performed because any major reflux into FRL portal branches might preclude surgery.

15. Two-stage hepatic resection

A further way of enabling curative resection of patients with extensive bilobar hepatic metastases of colorectal carcinoma is so-called two-stage hepatic resection [17]. This technique is suitable for patients with bilateral hepatic metastases who can undergo neither complete tumor resection, nor tumor resection combined with a local ablative procedure, because of the risk of postoperative hepatic insufficiency. Most, but not all, of the tumor burden is resected in a first operation, and then the remaining tumor nodules are resected in a second one, after liver tissue has regenerated. The decision whether to operate in one or two stages depends on the quantity and quality of the extratumoral hepatic tissue. The second operation is usually performed three to four weeks after the first, to allow time for the residual liver tissue to become adequately hypertrophic. [40]

16. Extreme liver surgery

Involvement of major vascular structures (vena cava or hepatic veins) by liver metastases has been considered as a contraindication to surgery for colorectal liver metastases. However, at

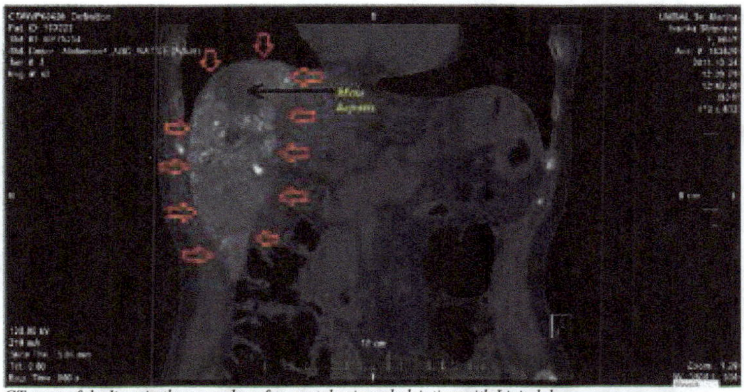

CT-scan of the liver in the same day after portal vein embolsiation with Lipiodol.

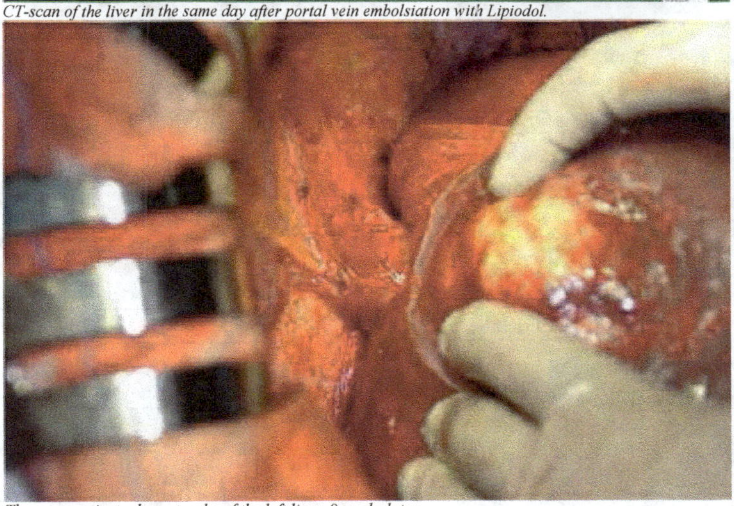

The same patient – hypertrophy of the left liver, 8 weeks later

Figure 2. Portal vein embolization and liver hypertrophy.

the present time this clinical situation is no longer considered as contraindication due to the experience gained with total vascular exclusion (TVE) of the liver combined with vascular reconstruction. These techniques have made the surgery possible even for this group of patients, without exposing them to the risk of massive intraoperative blood loss and gas embolism. TVE consists on hepatic inflow and outflow occlusion. [46-48] This can be achieved by clamping the portal vein/ hepatic artery as well as the supra and infra hepatic vena cava. Alternatively, the hepatic veins are isolated and clamped in addition to the vascular portal structures. The latter technique is more advantageous as it can preserve the caval flow, however, in cases of caval infiltration by metastatic lesion/s this technique is not feasible. On the other hand, if hemodynamic instability is encountered while the vena cava is clamped, a veno-venous bypass should be installed to overcome this complication. Although, it is believed that the hepatic blood flow can be interrupted safely up to 60 minutes, when vascular resection/ reconstruction is necessary, a 60 minute duration of ischemia may be not sufficient. [47] Hence, hypothermic perfusion of the liver should be instituted. The combination of TVE with in situ hypothermic perfusion was evaluated in our center. [68] It is found that this combination was

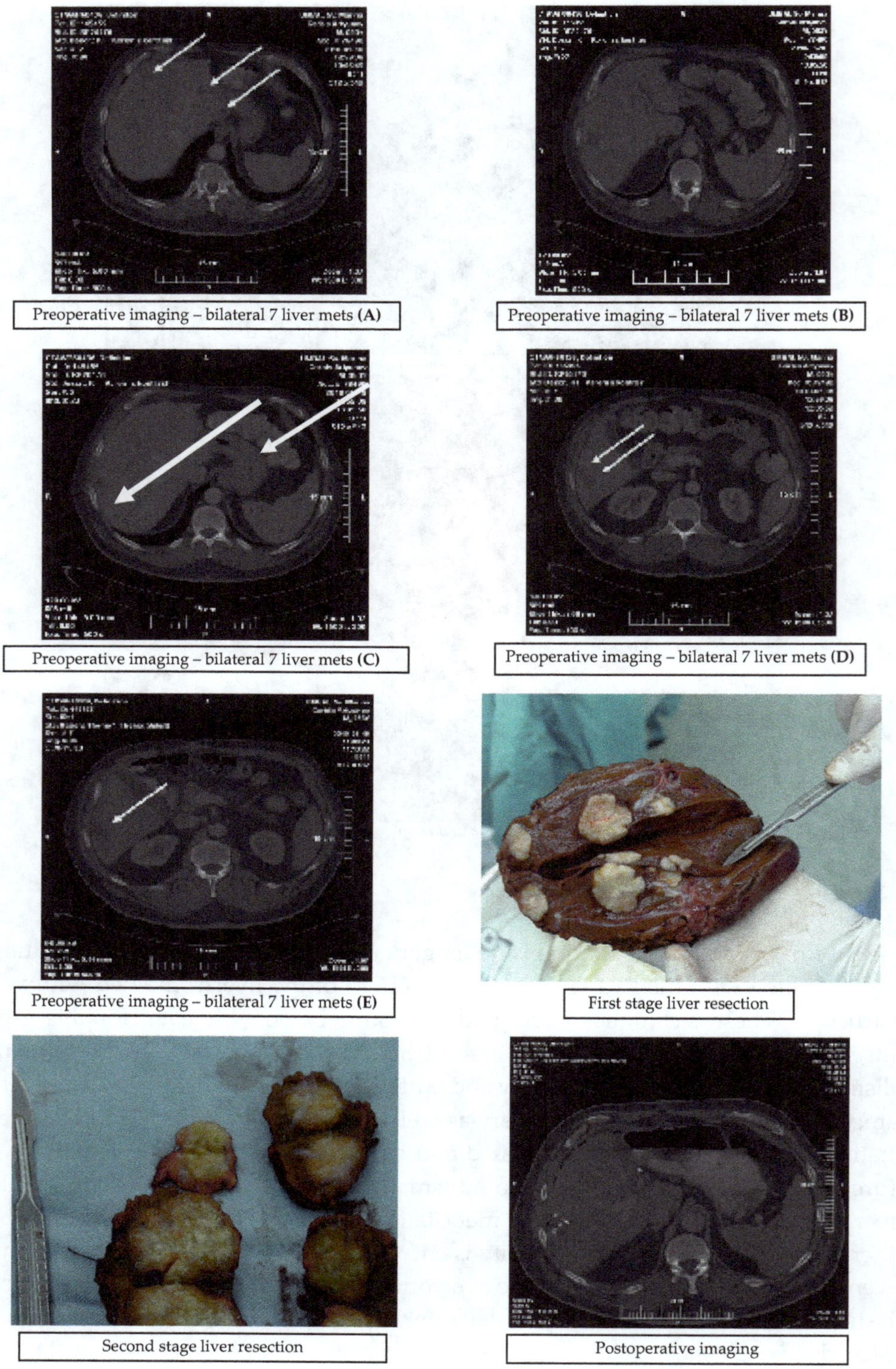

Figure 3. Two stage hepatectomy.

associated with a better liver tolerance to ischemia, a better liver function, and a significantly lower rate of complications compared to standard TVE >60 min. In some cases, a combined liver and vascular resection may be required. An experience with such cases (combined liver and vena cava resection) has shown that a 5-year survival of 38.3% can be obtained even for this group of patients. [49] In conclusion, using TVE and vascular reconstruction techniques, surgery in cases with involvement of the vena cava or hepatic veins is not necessarily contraindicated. However, a very careful evaluation and selection of the cases should be done, making sure that the risks involved do not counterbalance the desired benefits. [42]

17. Timing of surgery

Optimal duration chemotherapy and timing of liver surgery in responding patients have not been definitively established. For patients not considered resectable, in the clinical setting, most surgeons perform liver resection as soon as metastases become operable. Similarly, there is still debate, whether chemotherapy should precede resection when metastases are synchronous, particularly when the primary tumor is in place and the surgery involves the resection of the primary tumor as well as a simultaneous major liver resection. At the present, many surgeons believe that the chemotherapy is a better choice for patients with synchronous liver metastases, although these conclusions come from retrospective or surgical series from a single center. Capussotti and colleagues have published several papers on this topic. [40-43] There is only one randomized study [23] which has evaluated the results of preoperative chemotherapy and demonstrating an absolute difference in favor of chemotherapy. However, this study has a drawback as it was not possible to separate the benefits of preoperative chemotherapy from those of adjuvant postoperative chemotherapy. Another issue is the impact which the disease progression while on chemotherapy has on the timing of surgery. Disease progression during neoadjuvant chemotherapy indicates a poor prognosis. In a cohort of 131 patients undergoing rescue hepatectomy, 5-year survival rates were 8% if disease progressed during preoperative chemotherapy, 30% if disease was stable, and 37% in responders. [14] These findings suggest that hepatectomy for CRC metastases should be undertaken as soon as technically feasible and underscore the importance of collaboration between medical oncologists and surgeons in achieving that goal. Medical oncologists should be referring patients for surgery before tumor progression, and surgeons need to consider tumor evolution in addition to resectability. Thus, patients with biologically aggressive tumors unlikely to benefit from resection may be spared surgery upfront and can instead consult with the medical oncologist for a better regimen likely to induce tumor response or stabilization. [44]

18. Local tumor destruction and hybrid techniques

In recent years, local ablative methods such as cryotherapy and radiofrequency ablation (RFA) have come into more common use for the *in situ* destruction of hepatic metastases. Among these methods, RFA has been studied the best. It can be performed percutaneously, laparoscopically, or at open surgery and is currently used for tumors up to 5 cm in diameter. Lencioni et al. recently reported a multicenter study of 423 patients with a total of 615 metachronous metas - tases of colorectal carcinoma who were treated with RFA. The average tumor size was 2.7 cm [18]. In this patient group, 25% had local tumor progression, and the 1-, 3-, and 5-year survival rates were 86%, 47%, and 24%. These figures correspond to those of Abdalla et al., who found that tumor progression is more probable after RFA than after surgical resection [19, 43]. In general, RFA is associated with low morbidity and mortality. As no prospective data are yet available for a comparison of local ablative techniques to hepatic resection with curative intent, the procedure cannot be recommended as an alternative to hepatic resection, though it does play a role as an additional, complementary method of achieving complete tumor destruction in patients whose lesions are not otherwise R0-resectable.

19. Radiofrequency thermal ablation (RFA)

RFA is the most widely used technique for local destruction of CRLM and has gained popularity because of its relative easy usage, and its effectiveness as an adjuvant treatment.48 For the treatment of CRLM, RFA can be used as: 1) a definitive treatment per se; 2) a complementary procedure to surgery, or 3) in the treatment of recurrent metastatic disease after surgery. Results so far show that RFA must be restricted to cases in which the size of the dominant lesion is less than 3 cm or when a maximum of three tumours are present.49 In a study on percutaneous RFA for CRLM, local control was achieved in 78% of tumours <2.6 cm, but only in 47% of tumours 2.6-4.0 cm and 32% of tumours >4.0 cm.42 The anatomic location of a metastasis is an additional limitation of RFA. In the vicinity of a large hepatic vessel, the heat sink effect significantly increases the risk of incomplete ablation. Also, the risk of thermal injury is increased when nodules are close to main biliary structures or to extrahepatic organs. In these cases, new RFA techniques or additional procedures, such as hepatic inflow occlusion or intraductal cooling, have to be considered. [50, 51] Because of the high local recurrence rates, and of the anatomical limitations described above, there is still no place for RFA in patients with resectable colorectal metastases. Surgical RFA for small resectable CRLM could only be acceptable in a randomized trial comparing resection with surgical RFA, [52] and it was shown that hepatic resection is still the treatment of choice for CRLM and that RFA alone provides survival only slightly superior to non-surgical treatment. [53] This is the case also for patients with solitary liver metastases who are treated with RFA (higher LR rate and shorter recurrence free and overall survival). [54] Radiofrequency ablation has been proposed to treat a limited number of small metastases, simultaneously with right PVE. [46, 47] Although this strategy is theoretically appealing because it limits the number of surgical operations, its effectiveness compared to two-step hepatectomies is doubtful. The place of RFA in the treatment of CRM is limited: it is most useful for early recurrences detected as small lesions after resection, because it is not mandatory to stop the chemotherapy, except for the use of bevacizumab, and because RFA allows a ''test of time'' that helps to select out patients with very aggressive/ disseminated disease that would not benefit from repeated surgery.

19.1. Frequency of complications

19.1.1. Mortality

A total of 21 deaths were reported in 11 series, [41] with overall mortality varying from 0% to 5.2%. Four deaths were related to cirrhosis. Eleven occurred in patients undergoing resections, eight of which were major hepatectomies. Eight deaths were related to liver failure, four of which were subsequent to major hepatectomy with IRFA on the remnant liver for bilobar disease. Five deaths were caused by myocardial infarct; one of these related to a carcinoid crisis and another to a haemorrhage. Four deaths resulted from portal thrombosis, three of which occurred in cirrhotic patients. One of these patients had been treated by IRFA alone. Four deaths were related to septic complications; two of these referred to pulmonary infections, one to infection of the ascites and one to multiple deep abscesses. Lastly, three deaths were reported after postoperative haemorrhaging; one was caused by liver failure after an intrahepatic haematoma in a cirrhotic setting, one resulted from myocardial infarction following a haemorrhage in a large metastasis treated by IRFA, and one patient was treated by major hepatectomy and two IRFA sessions and died of cardiac arrest after postoperative bleeding.31

19.1.2. Infections

Abdominal infections were reported in 49 patients in 21 series. [41] Diagnosis of infection was delayed by up to 5 months. Seventeen liver abscesses were reported, of which one was fatal and were related to IRFA. Only one case of biliary digestive anastomosis was observed. Ten cases of perihepatic abscesses at resection sites were reported. Twelve were following digestive system-associated procedures. These abscesses were treated by percutaneous drainage and antibiotics. One patient needed re-operation and died from septic shock. Seven cases of wound infection were reported; two were re-operated. Lastly, one case of peritonitis after infection of the ascites was reported and was fatal.

19.1.3. Biliary complications

Twenty-five early (30 postoperative days) and 14 delayed (sometimes for >4 months18) biliary complications [42] were reported in 10 series. Twelve biliary leakages occurred, 10 of which were early. Six occurred in resection combined with IRFA. One early leakage was caused by a prophylactic cholecystectomy, but two delayed leakages were associated with a biliary stenosis. Fifteen intrahepatic bile collections were described, one of which induced duodenal compression. One article gave details of the treatment of eight biliomas: all eight were drained percutaneously and two recurred after drain clamping. Two were related to biliary stenoses and were treated by intrahepatic stenting; the other six patients underwent endoscopic sphincterotomy. Eleven biliary stenoses associated with jaundice and biliary dilatation were reported, of which five were early. These were complicated by biliomas, biliary leakage and cholangitis. In their prospective study, some authors [43] did not observe a correlation between central or peripheric localization of the tumour and the frequency of biliary complications.

19.1.4. Liver failure

Liver failure was reported in 24 patients in 11 articles [41] and was fatal in eight patients. Fourteen liver failures occurred after IRFA combined with major resection. Six liver failures occurred in cirrhotic patients; three of these failures occurred after IRFA alone. Two liver failures were subsequent to portal thrombosis.

19.1.5. Vascular complications

Different types of vascular complication were described in in a total of 22 patients. Associated procedures such as cholecystectomy or colectomy induced six haemorrhages, two of which were fatal and one required re-operation after prophylactic cholecystectomy. Three haemorrhages from the needle track were treated during surgery by compression. In three cirrhotic patients, haemorrhage occurred in the necrosis induced by the IRFA; one patient died as a result. [25]

Treatment of two juxta-portal lesions induced haemorrhages from arterial injuries. 25, 26 In one patient, an arterio-portal fistula appeared in an area of necrosis 6 weeks later and was treated by a transfemoral embolization. [18] Similarly, a false aneurysm occurred in one patient 6 months after IRFA and led to a haemorrhage. Five portal thromboses were reported, [19, 25, 34] four of which were complete and fatal. Three of these occurred in cirrhotic patients treated with Pringle vascular occlusion.

19.1.6. Skin burns

Eight dispersive pad skin burns were reported in four articles. Skin burns occurred when RFA ran for >30 min on high power and within large and multiple skin pads. One skin burn occurred in a patient with bilateral hip prostheses.30 One third-degree skin burn required surgical treatment. [38]

19.1.7. Visceral damage

Two instances of thermal gastric damage [41] and one of acute cholecystitis near the gallbladder were observed after IRFA during surgery and were treated immediately.

19.1.8. Comparison with hepatectomy

The morbidity of hepatectomy depends on the extent and complexity of the hepatic resection. Intraoperative RFA as a standalone treatment is indicated for unresectable tumours in patients in whom major hepatectomy would leave a low level of functional hepatic reserve. Mortality and morbidity rates in major hepatic resection are 0–5% and 20–50%, respectively. [45] Rates of liver failure after major hepatectomy preceded by portal embolization are 4–10% vs.2.6% after IRFA [46, 47] combined with hepatic resection. There is reported mortality of 2.3% and morbidity of 19.8% in patients treated by resection and combined IRFA, and estimates their results to be comparable with those of resection alone. [31] Morbidity rates after major hepatic resection and IRFA combined with hepatic resection are comparable, even if IRFA is indicated in tumours unresectable by hepatectomy alone. [48]

The past 10 years have represented a period of learning for surgeons who deal with liverme-tastases with the aim of treating more patients by combining IRFA with resection. The benefit: risk ratio is now well known and surgeons have access to the knowledge they need to make more informed choices about whether to resect, ablate or renounce treatment on a lesion-by-lesion basis. Surgeons who are skilled in intraoperative ultrasound diagnosis and guidance are now not only able to choose whether or not to perform surgery, but are also able to perform IRFA and do not need to involve a radiologist. Specific complications related to IRFA are rare, especially if the lesion is <35 mm in diameter and is located far from a main biliary duct and no additional septic procedures are used. The surgeon can decide to ablate a lesion in a more difficult situation, but this carries greater risk. Combining resection with IRFA leads to higher morbidity, especially in difficult patients with numerous bilateral lesions, but this may be necessary to achieve R0 (microscopically negative) resection margins.

20. Hepatic re-resection in case of recurrent tumor

The resection of hepatic metastases of colorectal carcinoma is followed by tumor recurrence in up to two thirds of cases, and about half of these recurrences are found in the liver [12, 23, 27, 28]. In general, whenever there is a chance of a curative resection, resection should be considered for recurrent tumors as well. The operative morbidity and mortality of hepatic reresection in experienced centers are no greater than those of primary resection. In a study on second operations in 94 patients with recurrent hepatic metastases of colorectal carcinoma, 38% of the patients were alive 5 years after surgery [12]. Thus, whenever complete resection of the tumor is possible, surgery is indicated even for patients with recurrent hepatic metastases.

21. Conclusion

The results of surgical treatment of metastatic colorectal carcinoma have improved markedly in recent years. The reasons for this include developments in medical imaging, in perioperative and surgical treatment, and in chemotherapy, with the introduction of potent new protocols. Clinicopathological factors such as tumor size, number of tumor nodules, and extrahepatic tumor manifestations no longer contraindicate hepatic resection. The main consideration at present is the need to achieve a complete R0 resection. Accompanying chemotherapy should be considered, especially for patients with an unfavorable risk profile. Neoadjuvant chemotherapy is reserved for patients with marginally resectable metastases. The resectability or nonresectability of hepatic metastases is a matter that must be evaluated by a surgeon who is experienced in the treatment of hepatic metastases. Hepatic resection of colorectal liver metastases after downsizing by chemotherapy provides the only chance of long term survival for patients with initially unresectable colorectal liver metastases. Additional surgical techniques can be combined to chemotherapy to further improve resectability. The only absolute contraindication for resection is the inability to completely resect all metastases, avoiding postoperative liver failure by leaving enough functional liver parenchyma. The presence of poor prognostic factors no longer limits the indications for resection. Neoadjuvant treatment with chemotherapeutic agents such as irinotecan and oxaliplatin, hepatic artery infusion combined with systemic therapy and biologic agents (bevacizumab, cetuximab) play an important role in increasing the number of patients eligible to secondary resection. However, with the progressive use of neoadjuvant chemotherapy further studies are necessary to answer questions such as the risk: benefit ratio in maximizing response rates versus vascular changes in the liver (current opinion still divided concerning their importance). These questions remain challenging and should not be underestimated. The perfecting of surgical techniques together with safer procedures, as well as the improvement in chemotherapy regimens have allowed doctors to offer patients with liver metastasis the possibility of curative treatment or longterm survival. Factors that were previously considered contraindications for the surgery, such as number of metastases, synchronous metastases and even the presence of extrahepatic disease, must be considered only as prognostic factors and must not prevent the patient from having the opportunity of being treated.

Author details

Nikola Kolev[1], Valentin Ignatov[1], Anton Tonev[1], Tanya Kirilova[2], Georgi Ivanov[1], Alexander Zlatarov[1] and Krassimir Ivanov[1]

1 Department of General and Operative Surgery, University Hospital "St. Marina", Varna, Bulgaria

2 Department of Gastroenterology, University Hospital "St. Marina", Varna, Bulgaria

References

[1] Jemal A, Murray T, Ward E, Hao Y, Xu J, Murray T, et al. Cancer statistics, 2005. CA Cancer J Clin. 2005;55:10-30.

[2] International Agency for research on cancer: GLOBOCAN 2002 data. [Accessed 2006 Nov 16]. Available from: http:// www-dep.iarc.fr

[3] Stangl R, Altendorf-Hofmann A, Charnley RM, Scheele J. Factors influencing thenatural history of colorectal liver metastases. Lancet. 1994;343:1405-10.

[4] Mentha G, Majno P, Terraz S, Rubbia-Brandt L, Gervaz P, Andres A, et al. Treatment strategies for the management of advanced colorectal liver metastases detected synchronously with the primary tumour. EJSO. 2007;33:76-83.

[5] Livermetsurvey. International registry of liver metastases of colorectal cancer. [Accessed 2010 Mar].

[6] Choti M, Sitzmann J, Tiburi M, Sumetchotimetha W, Rangsin R, Schulick RD, et al. Trends in long term survival following liver resection for hepatic colorectal metastases. Ann Surg. 2002;235:759-66.

[7] Abdalla EK, Vauthey JN, Ellis LM, Ellis V, Pollock R, Broglio KR, et al. Recurrence and outcomesfollowing hepatic resection, radiofrequency ablation, and combined resection/ablation for colorectal liver metastases. Ann Surg. 2004;239:818-27.

[8] Fong Y, Fortner J, Sun RL, Brennan MF, Blumgart LH. Clinical score for predicting recurrence after hepatic resection for metastatic colorectal cancer: analysis of 1001 consecutive cases. Ann Surg. 1999;230:309-18.

[9] Nordlinger B, Jaeck D, editors. Traitment de metastases hépatiques as cancers colorectaus. Paris: Springer-Verlag; 1992.

[10] Gayowski TJ, Iwatsuki S, Madariaga JR, Selby R, Todo S, Irish W, et al. Experience in hepatic resection of colorectal cancer – analysis of clinical and pathological risk factors. Surgery. 1994;116:703-71.

[11] Minagawa M, Maltuuchi M, Torzilli G, Takayama T, Kawasaki S, Kosuge T, et al. Extension of the frontiers metastases from colorectal cancer: Long-term results. Ann Surg. 2000;231: 487-99.

[12] Ercolani G, Grazi GL, Ravaioli M, Cescon M, Gardini A, Varotti G, et al. Liver resection for multiple colorectal metastases: influence of parenchymal involvement and total tumor volume versus number or location on long term survival. Arch Surg. 2002;137:1187-92.

[13] Scheele J, Stangl R, Altendorf-Hofmann A. Hepatic metastases from colorectal carcinoma: impact of surgical resection on the natural history. Br J Surg. 1990;77:1241-6.

[14] Adam R, Delvart V, Pascal G, Valeanu A, Castaing D, Azoulay D, et al. Rescue surgery for unresectable colorectal liver metastases downstaged by chemotherapy: a model to predict longterm survival. Ann Surg. 2004;240:644-58.

[15] Rodgers M, Mccall J. Surgery for colorectal liver metastases with hepatic lymph node involvement: A Systematic review. Br J Surg. 2000;87:1142-55.

[16] Adam R, De Haas RJ, Wicherts DA, Aloia TA, Delvart V, Azoulay D, et al. Is hepatic resection justified after chemothera- py in patients with colorectal liver metastases and lymph node involvement? J Clin Oncol. 2008;26:3672-80.

[17] Pfannschmidt J, Dienemann H, Hoffmann H. Surgical resection of pulmonary metastases from colorectal cancer: a systematic review of published series. Ann Thorac Surg. 2007;84:324-38.

[18] Elias D, Liberale G, Vernerey D, Pocard M, Ducreux M, Boige V, et al. Hepatic and extrahepatic colorectalmetastases: when resectable, their localization does not matter, but their total number has a prognostic effect. Ann Surg Oncol. 2005;12: 900-9.

[19] Adam R, Haas RJ, Wicherts D, et al. Concomitant extrahepatic in patients with colorectal liver metastases: when is there a place for surgery? Ann Surg. 2011. In press.

[20] Adam R, Pascal G, Azoulay D, Tanaka K, Castaing D, Bismuth H. Liver resection for colorectal metastases: the third hepatectomy. Ann Surg. 2003;238:871-83.

[21] Tanaka K, Adam R, Shimada H, Azoulay D, Lévi F, Bismuth H. Role of neoadjuvant chemotherapy in the treatment of multiple colorectal metastases to the liver. Br J Surg. 2003;90:963-9.

[22] Mitry E, Fields AL, Bleiberg H, Labianca R, Portier G, Tu D, et al. Adjuvant chemotherapy after potentially curative resection of metastases from colorectal cancer: A pooled analysis of two randomized trials. J Clin Oncol. 2008;26:4906-11.

[23] Nordlinger B, Sorbye H, Glimelius B, Poston GJ, Schlag PM, Rougier P, et al. Perioperative chemotherapy with FOLFOX4 and surgery versus surgery alone for resectable liver metastases from colorectal cancer (EORTC Intergroup trial 40983): a randomised controlled trial. Lancet. 2008;371: 1007-16.

[24] Parks R, Gonen M, Kemeny N, Jarnagin W, D'Angelica M, DeMatteo R, et al. Adjuvant chemotherapy improves survival after resection of hepatic colorectal metastases: analysis of data from two continents. J Am Coll Surg. 2007;204:753-61.

[25] Gruenberger B, Scheithauer W, Punzengruber R, Zielinski C, Tamandl D, Gruenberger T. Importance of response to neoadjuvant chemotherapy in potentially curable colorectal cancer metastases. BMC Cancer. 2008;8:120.

[26] Kemeny MM, Adak S, Gray B, Macdonald JS, Smith T, Lipsitz S, et al. Combined-modality treatment for resectable metastatic colorectal carcinoma to the liver: Surgical resection of hepatic metastases in combination with continuous infusion of chemotherapeutic-An Intergroup Study. J Clin Oncol. 2002;20:1499-505.

[27] Thirion P, Wolmark N, Haddad E, Buyse M, Piedbois P. Survival impact of chemotherapy in patients with colorectal metastases confined to the liver: A reanalysis of 1458 non-operable patients randomized in 22 trials and 4 meta-analysis. Meta-Analysis Group in cancer. Ann Oncol. 1999;10:1317-20.

[28] Hobday TJ, Kugler JW, Mahoney MR, Sargent DJ, Sloan JA, Fitch TR, et al. Long-term survivors of metastatic colorectal cancer treated with chemotherapy only: A North central Cancer Treatment group review. J Clin Oncol. 2002;20: 4574-80.

[29] Giacchetti S, Itzhaki M, Gruia G, Adam R, Zidani R, Kunstlinger F, et al. Long-term survival of patient with unresectable colorectal cancer liver metastases following infusional chemotherapy with 5-fluorouacil, leucovorin, oxaliplatin and surgery. Ann Oncol. 1999;10:663-9.

[30] Folprecht G, Grothey A, Alberts S, Raab HR, Kuhne CH. Neoadjuvant treatment of unresectable colorectal liver metastases: Correlation between tumor response and resection rates. Ann Oncol. 2005;16:1311-9.

[31] Ychou M, Viret F, Kramar A, Desseigne F, Mitry E, Guimbaud R, et al. Tritherapy with fluorouracil/leucovorin, irinotecan and oxaliplatin (FOLFIRINOX): a phase II study in colorectalcancer patients with non-resectable liver metбstases. Cancer Chemother Pharmacol. 2008;62:195-201.

[32] Van Cutsem E, Kцhne CH, Hitre E, Zaluski J, Chang Chien CR, Makhson A, et al. Cetuximab and chemotherapy as initial treatment for metastatic colorectal cancer. N Engl J Med. 2009;360:1408-17.

[33] Bokemeyer C, Bondarenko I, Makhson A, Hartmann JT, Aparicio J, De Braud F, et al. Fluorouracil, leucovorin, and oxaliplatin with and without cetuximab in the first-line treatment of metastatic colorectal cancer. J Clin Oncol. 2009;27:663-71.

[34] Ocvirk J, Brodowicz T, Wrba F, Ciuleanu TE, Kurteva G, et al. Cetuximab plus FOLFOX6 or FOLFIRI in metastatic colorectal cancer: CECOG trial. World J Gastroenterol. 2010;16:3133-43.

[35] Folprecht G, Gruenberger T, Bechstein WO, Raab HR, Lordick F, Hartmann JT, et al. Tumour response and secondary respectability of colorectal liver metastases following neoadjuvant chemotherapy with cetuximab: the CELIM randomized phase 2 trial. The Lancet Oncol. 2010;11:38-47.

[36] Adam R, Aloia T, Levi F, Wicherts DA, De Haas RJ, Paule B, et al. Hepatic resection after rescue cetuximab treatment for colorectal liver metastases previously refractory to conventional systemic therapy. J Clin Oncol. 2007;25: 4593-602.

[37] De Baere T, Roche A, Elias D, Lasser P, Lagrange C, Bousson V. Preoperative portal vein embolization for extension of hepatectomy indications. Hepatology. 1996;200:559-63.

[38] Madoff DC, Abdalla EK, Gupta S, Wu TT, Morris JS, Denys A, et al. Transhepatic ipsilateral rightportal vein embolization extended to segment IV: improving hypertrophy and resection outcomes with spherical particles and coils. J Vasc Interv Radiol. 2005;16:215-25.

[39] Abdalla EK, Barnett CC, Doherty D, Curley SA, Vauthey JN. Extended hepatectomy in patients with hepatobiliary malignancies with and without preoperative portal vein embolization. Arch Surg. 2002;137:675-80.

[40] Razafindratsira T, Isambert M, Evrard S Complications of intraoperative radiofrequency ablation of liver metastases. HPB (Oxford). 2011 Jan;13 (1):15-23.

[41] Vauthey JN, Chaoui A, Do KA, Bilimoria MM, Fenstermacher MJ, Charnsangavej C, et al. Standardized measurement of the future liver remnant prior to extended liver resection: methodology and clinical associations. Surgery. 2000;127: 512-9.

[42] Azoulay D, Castaing D, Smail A, Adam R, Cailliez V, Laurent A, et al. Resection of nonresectable liver metastases from colorectal cancer after percutaneous portal vein embolization. Ann Surg. 2000;231:480-6.

[43] Madoff DC, Abdalla EK, Vauthey JN. Portal vein embolization in preparation for major hepatic resection: evolution of a new standard of care. J Vasc Interv Radiol. 2005;16:779-90.

[44] Elias D, De Baere T, Roche A, Ducreux M, Leclere J, Lasser P. During liver regeneration following right portal embolization the growth rate of liver metastases is more rapid than that of the liver parenchyma. Br J Surg. 1999;86:784-8.

[45] Kokudo N, Tada K, Seki M, Ohta H, Azekura K, Ueno M, et al. Proliferative activity of intrahepatic colorectal metastases after preoperative hemihepatic portal vein embolization. Hepatology. 2001;34:267-72.

[46] Elias D, Santoro R, Ouellet JF, Osmak L, De Baere T, Roche A. Simultaneous percutaneous right portal vein embolization and left liver tumour radiofrequency ablation prior to a major right hepatic resection for bilateral colorectal metastases. Hepatogastroenterology. 2004;51:1788-91.

[47] Terraz S, Constantin C, Majno P, Spahr L, Mentha G, Becker CD. Image-guided multipolar radiofrequency ablation of liver tumours: initial clinical results. Eur Radiol. 2007;17:2253-61.

[48] Lencioni R, Cioni D, Crocetti L, Franchini C, Pina CD, Lera J, et al. Early-stage hepatocellular carcinoma in patients with cirrhosis: long-term results of percutaneous image-guided radiofrequency ablation. Radiology. 2005;234:961-7.

[49] Berber E, Pelley R, Siperstein AE. Predictors of survival after radiofrequency thermal ablation of colorectal cancer metastases to the liver: a prospective study. J Clin Oncol. 2005;23:1358-64.

[50] Solbiati L, Livraghi T, Goldberg SN, Ierace T, Meloni F, Dellanoce M, et al. Percutaneous radiofrequency ablation of hepatic metastases form colorectal cancer: long-term results in 117 patients. Radiology. 2001;221:159-66.

[51] De Baere T, Bessoud B, Dromain C, Ducreux M, Boige V, Lassau N, et al. Percutaneous radiofrequency ablation of hepatic tumors during temporary venous occlusion. Am J Roentgenol. 2002;178:53-9.

[52] Elias D, Sideris L, Pocard M, Dromain C, De Baere T. Intraductal cooling of the main bile ducts during radiofrequency ablation prevents biliary stenosis. J Am Coll Surg. 2004;198:717-21.

[53] Mulier S, Ni Y, Jamart J, Ruers T, Marchal G, Michel L. Local recurrence after hepatic radiofrequency coagulation. Multivariate meta-analysis and review of contributing factors. Ann Surg. 2005;242:158-71.

[54] Aloia TA, Vauthey JN, Loyer EM, Ribero D, Pawlik TM, Wei SH, et al. Solitary colorectal liver metastases: resection determines outcome. Arch Surg. 2006;141:460-7.

[55] Wicherts DA, Miller R, de Haas RJ, Bitsakou G, Vibert E, Veihan LA et al. Long-term results of two-stage hepatectomy for irresectable colorectal cancer liver metastases. Ann Surg. 2008;248:994-1005.

[56] Martin R, Paty P, Fong Y, Grace A, Cohen A, De Matteo R et al. Simultaneous liver and colorectal resections are safe for synchronous colorectal liver metastasis. J Am Coll Surg. 2003;197:233-41; discussion 41-2.

[57] Reddy SK, Pawlik TM, Zorzi D, Gleisner AL, Ribeiro D, Assumpção L et al. Simultaneous resections of colorectal cancer and synchronous liver metastases: a multi-institutional analysis. Ann Surg Oncol. 2007;14:3481-91.

[58] Brouquet A, Mortenson MM, Vauthey JN, Abdalla EK. Surgical strategies for synchronous colorectal liver metastases in 156 consecutive patients: classic, combined or reverse strategy? J Am Coll Surg. 2010;210:934-41.

[59] Mentha G, Majno PE, Andres A, Rubbia-Brandt L, Morel P, Roth AD. Neoadjuvant chemotherapy and resection of advanced synchronous liver metastases before treatment of the colorectal primary. Br J Surg. 2006;93:872-8.

[60] Poultsides GA, Servais EL, Saltz LB, Patil S, Kameny NE, Guillem JG et al. Outcome of primary tumor in patients with synchronous stage IV colorectal cancer receiving combination chemotherapy without surgery as initial treatment. J Clin Oncol. 2009;27:3379-84.

[61] Tebbutt NC, Norman AR, Cunningham D, Andreyev J. Intestinal complications after chemotherapy for patients with unresected primary colorectal cancer and synchronous metastases. Gut. 2003;52:568-73.

[62] Adam R, Pascal G, Castaing D, Azoulay D, Delvart V, Paule B et al. Tumor progression while on chemotherapy: a contraindication to liver resection for multiple colorectal metastases? Ann Surg. 2004;240:1052-61; discussion 61-4.

[63] Herman P, Machado MAC, Diniz AL, Coimbra FJF, Sallum RA, Montagnini AL. Surgical treatment of colorectal cancer hepatic metastases; experience of A. C. Camargo Cancer Hospital - São Paulo. Appl Cancer Res. 2006;26:88-93.

5

Role of Magnetic Resonance Imaging in Locally Advanced Rectal Cancer

Roberta Fusco, Mario Sansone, Mario Petrillo,
Antonio Avallone, Paolo Delrio,
Fabiana Tatangelo and Antonella Petrillo

1. Introduction

This chapter will give an overview of the magnetic resonance imaging (MRI) modalities used in locally advanced rectal cancer (LARC) staging with an emphasis on the role of MRI and its significance for planning an effective therapeutic strategy for the individual patient.

Specifically, the aim of this chapter is to present a brief review about:

1. Methodologies of Magnetic Resonance Imaging in LARC staging
   - a. Morphologic MRI
   - b. Functional MRI
     - i. Dynamic Contrast Enhanced MRI (DCE-MRI)
     - ii. Diffusion Weighted MRI (DW-MRI)
2. The role of MRI in diagnosis, staging, evaluation of response of neoadjuvant treatment, follow-up post surgery.

This chapter will be organised in the following sections. First, in order to better define the role of MRI in LARC management, we will briefly describe the epidemiological scenario and therapeutic options, with an emphasis on issues in which MRI is relevant. Second, we will describe morphologic and functional MRI including DCE-MRI and DW-MRI. Finally, a systematic review of the literature concerning MRI, CT and PET for LARC management will be presented.

2. Epidemiology

Colorectal cancer is the third most common cancer worldwide [1], which includes cancers of the colon, rectum, rectosigmoid junction and anus. Specifically, in men it represents the third commonest neoplasm after prostate and lung cancers while in women it is the second major cause of morbidity and mortality, following breast cancer.

In recent years, mortality rates have decreased due to several factors, including less exposure risk factors, more possibility of prevention and "early diagnosis" followed by an effective management of the disease. In particular, major changes in therapeutic management are given by the standardization of operative procedures and the introduction of adjuvant and neoadjuvant therapy [2-7], able to reduce recurrence risk and tumor size.

Cancers are characterized by profound spatial and temporal heterogeneity in their biologic characteristics. Most invasive cancers typically have alterations in cell physiology that promote malignant growth [2-7]. Rectal cancer is the result of a complex interaction between genetic and environmental factors and it is defined as a tumor whose aboral margin measured with the rigid rectoscope is 16 cm or less from the anocutaneous line. This distance serves to classify rectal cancer into tumours of the upper third (12–16 cm), the middle third (6–12 cm), and the lower third (<6 cm) [26] according to the Union for International Cancer Control (UICC).

The mesorectal fascia is an important anatomic landmark for the diagnostic evaluation of local tumor extent [26]. It is a connective tissue sheath that surrounds the rectum and the perirectal fatty tissue and acts as a natural barrier for tumor spread.

A locally advanced tumor often describes a tumor extending beyond the rectal wall with infiltration to surrounding organs or structures, and/or perforation of the visceral peritoneum. It includes bulky T3 tumors with threatened circumferential margins or T4 tumors, tumors with growth onto the peritoneal surface. A radiological T4 tumor is considered when detected growing outside the mesorectal fascia, while a T3 tumor refers to a tumor invading through muscularis propria [26].

These tumors have traditionally been looked upon as "unresectable", although previous staging, due to the wide tumor extension. However, when it is possible, these tumors cannot be resected without leaving microscopic or gross residual disease at the local site because of tumor adherence or fixation to that site.

3. Therapeutic options

In LARC accurate and detailed anatomic information in tumor extent is essential not only for the selection of the patients for neoadjuvant chemotherapy and radiation therapy to achieve tumor shrinkage but also for the optimal surgical procedure planning. Moreover, the treatment for patients with locally advanced and recurrent rectal cancer differs significantly from patients with rectal cancer restricted to the mesorectum.

Adequate preoperative imaging of the pelvis is therefore important to identify those patients who are candidates for multimodality treatment, including preoperative chemoradiation protocols, intraoperative radiotherapy, and extended surgical resections. Much effort should be made to select patients with these advanced tumors for treatment in specialized referral centers. This has been shown to reduce morbidity and mortality and improve long-term survival rates.

Two main therapeutic options can be considered according to different pathological stages presented [13-35]:

1. Total mesorectal excision (TME): using this surgical technique, the rectum is resected together with all surrounding lymphatic pathways, lymph nodes, mesorectal fatty tissue, and the mesorectal fascia while the parietal pelvis fascia and the pelvic splanchnic nerves are spared. This surgical technique minimizes the chance of tumor being left inside;
2. Adjuvant/neoadjuvant therapy: the aims of adjuvant or neoadjuvant therapy are to enable or facilitate total tumor resection even in advanced disease, to prevent local tumor recurrence, and to minimize the risk of distant metastases.

The majority of patients with primary rectal cancer have a tumor located within the mesorectal fascia, which is generally treated with total mesorectal excision (TME). Results of TME surgery are excellent with a significant reduction in local recurrences when preoperative short-term radiotherapy (5 x 5 Gy) is delivered one week prior to surgery [27]. In ≈10% of all rectal cancer patients the tumor extends into or beyond the enveloping fascia of the mesorectal compartment.

Often these tumors infiltrate adjacent structures and therefore have a higher risk to develop a local recurrence [28].

Patients with these primary locally advanced or recurrent rectal cancer are difficult to treat with surgery alone, but outcome has significantly improved using multimodality treatment. Although preoperative and adjuvant therapy is important in these patients, the mainstay of treatment in rectal cancer is complete surgical removal of the tumor. In both locally advanced and recurrent rectal cancers, this involves not only the removal of the total mesorectum, but en bloc resection of involved structures is often needed.

Although postoperative chemoradiotherapy (CRT) has long been recommended for locally advanced and node positive rectal cancer patients, preoperative treatment is now widely used worldwide. In many European centers, radiotherapy only was used as neoadjuvant treatment for locally advanced rectal cancer, but the addition of chemotherapy has recently demonstrated to improve local control in two large randomized trials [30,31]. Addition of 5-FU and leucovorin to preoperative radiation slightly increased the amount of acute toxicity in T3 to T4 resectable rectal cancer patients [32]. However, it increased the number of complete responses and decreased the local recurrence rate after 5 years.

Not only new chemotherapeutic drugs, but also a vascular endothelial cell growth factor-(VEGF-) specific monoclonal antibody in combination with chemoradiation was recently reported by Willet et al [32] to lead to considerable downstaging of the tumor. Other modalities such as the use of intensity-modulated radiotherapy (IMRT), which has the potential of more accurate delivery of higher radiotherapy dosages, thus avoiding the damage of critical structures surrounding the tumor, are being tested in rectal cancer.

Total pelvic exenteration (TPE) is a widely used technique for resection of locally advanced or recurrent rectal tumors invading the bladder and/or prostate. Longterm survival with excellent local control is possible after TPE for primary locally advanced rectal cancer [33-35]. The majority of resections in primary cancer are without microscopic or macroscopic residual tumor mass, which clearly justifies the use of TPE in selected patients with primary disease. Although current guidelines for colorectal cancer surgery advocate TPE, only one third of the patients in a recent study based on SEER (survival, epidemiology and end results) data underwent the appropriate surgical resection.

These patients had a clinically significant overall survival benefit with no increase in short-term mortality compared with similar patients who did not receive a multi-visceral resection. Local control in rectal cancer patients is related to the dose of irradiation, but because of toxicity to radiosensitive organs (such as small bowels), the external radiation dose should not exceed 60 Gy. A combination of external radiation and intraoperative radiation therapy (IORT) allows the safe delivery of higher effective doses of irradiation than can be delivered with external-beam only techniques. IORT is used when resection margins are narrow or involved with tumor cells and can be applied very specifically to an area at risk, under direct visual control, and with the ability to shield the surrounding structures from radiation. The biological effectiveness of single-dose IORT is considered to be as effective as 2 to 3 times the equivalent dose of fractionated radiotherapy.

3. Role of MRI vs other modalities

3.1. Generalities

Imaging techniques play a pivotal role in the strategies for management of locally advanced rectal cancer patients. The role of diagnostic imaging is to perform a loco-regional staging as accurate as possible in both evaluation of infiltration and extension degrees of disease. Image features also enable preoperative assessment of important prognostic outlines, which may guide patient selection for neoadjuvant therapies. Moreover, imaging plays an important role in therapeutic assessment, surveillance after surgery, and evaluation of suspected disease fall-out. To date, imaging innovations have led to improvements in spatial and contrast resolution, increased data acquisition speeds, and enabled complex image to achieve excellence in anatomic resolution.

There are many different imaging modalities suitable for rectal cancer staging, tumour location and restaging but not all of them have the same accuracy for each indication. An optimal visualization of tumor volume and of its surrounding anatomical structures is necessary for any local cancer treatment. This issue is particularly important for radiotherapy treatment planning in order that a geographical miss can be avoided and the tumor adequately treated.

Among the imaging methods available Magnetic Resonance Imaging (MRI) is currently the modality of choice because of its capacity to perform local staging, since it enables evaluation of anatomic aspects and prognostic factors that are key to choosing the appropriate surgical approach and determining the need for neoadjuvant treatment.

3.2. MRI physical basics

MRI is an imaging technique based on the different magnetic properties of tissues in the body. The exposure to a high intensity magnetic field determines the alignment of the hydrogen nuclei (protons) along the magnetic field axis itself. The emission of radio frequency pulses causes a shift from this alignment, which tends to reconstitute as soon as the impulse is interrupted. This phenomenon leads to a variation in energy level of the charges, which can be translated into a signal whose decoding is the basis of the generation of magnetic resonance images. All this is based on specific parameters that describe these steps of energy levels (including the so-called "relaxation times T1 and T2"), as well as on the concentration of protons within a given tissue.

Pulses sequences are used to obtain the different MR images, sequences consisting of radio frequency pulses with different characteristics in terms of duration, frequency and type of sampling of the resulting signal.

In the various biological tissues, the characteristics of the magnetic resonance signal are influenced mainly by the content of hydrogen atoms (whose nuclei are composed of only one proton). Since water is the most abundant molecule in the body and contains hydrogen atoms, it can be reasonably stated that the increase or the decrease of water in a given tissue is almost always at the basis of changes in signal intensity when using sequences of magnetic resonance imaging.

Where tissue contrast depends primarily on electron density, the tissue contrast obtained by MRI can be extensively varied by imaging the intrinsic tissue properties, as spin-lattice and spin-spin relaxation times, protons density, magnetization transfer, separately or in combination, using a number of pulse sequences, which in turn can be altered by an essentially infinite number of different experimental conditions. These MR parameters can be exploited and tailored to facilitate optimal tumor visualization and evaluation. Another feature of MRI is that cortical bone does not give rise to an MR signal and therefore appears hypointense. This is because cortical bone contains calcium and there are few hydrogen protons to provide an MR signal. Furthermore, MRI can obtain detailed anatomical images in any desired plane, also acquiring 3D or volumetric image sets. Therefore, the superior soft tissue definition provided by MRI, together with its unrestricted multiplanar, volumetric, vascular and functional information has benefits for 3D treatment planning.

3.3. Comparison of MRI and CT

Computed Tomography (CT) scanning is an imaging technique able to reproduce a 3D image of internal organs by irradiating X-ray. In LARC treatment CT shows the effective tumor size and its possible dissemination to internal organs. Although CT imaging provides excellent definition between structures with different electron density or X-ray attenuation characteristics, it distinguishes poorly between structures with similar electron density such as different soft tissue structures, including tumors, unless there is an obvious fat or air interface [60]. The major advantage of MRI compared with CT is in its superior ability to demonstrate and characterize soft tissues that have similar electron densities. In this manner, MRI may provide better delineation not only of the tumor extent, but also of the adjacent critical soft tissue organs. This will allow conformal planning to enhance its therapeutic ratio by more accurately targeting the tumor, avoiding the organs at risk and subsequently improving local control.

3.4. Comparison of MRI and PET/CT

In LARC patient management detection of tumor sites throughout the body is needed with high sensitivity and specificity in order to have accurate information about the local extent. As discussed in the previous section, an accurate tumour visualization can be performing using MRI techniques. An additional value should be given to consider the combination of Positron Emission Tomography (PET) and CT [61]. PET/CT is a diagnostic procedure that allows to obtain morphological images of the human body provided by CT and images of the tissue metabolic processes provided by PET by means of a co-registration system.

Tissues appear differently on PET and on CT images. CT displays anatomy with high spatial resolution, but with low contrast resolution for soft tissues, while PET visualizes pathological sites with high contrast resolution but a limited spatial resolution and surrounding normal anatomical structures are hardly visualized. The combination of metabolic activity with anatomic localization achievable with PET/CT improve accuracy over that of PET or CT alone [62].

4. Role of MRI in LARC

In the recent years MRI has undergone significant transformations resulting from technological innovation that have taken place as the introduction of high-field magnets, powerful gradients, multi-channel phased array coils and endorectal coils improvement. These technological developments have certainly allowed the executing of high quality diagnostic studies due to the high spatial resolution and contrast obtained, to the possibility of identification and distinction of rectal wall layers, and to the possibility of assessing perirectal and sphinteric structures. Mainly, superficial endorectal coils are currently able to identify various layers of lower rectum wall. MRI is thus the ideal technique for rectal cancer staging, combining the capabilities of an accurate loco-regional staging to the outlook and multi-planar properties.

In conclusion, MRI can currently stage with high accuracy the T parameter (related to the degree of tumor infiltration) due to the possibility offered by the endorectal coil to recognize the wall layers, resulting also extremely useful in planning surgery and in prognostic stratification, owing to the ability to accurately identify mesorectum and the distance between mesorectal fascia and neoplasia. Furthermore the high temporal resolution of last generation devices allows to perform perfusion and dynamic studies after gadolinium administration that allow to detection of the residual tumor after neoadjuvant therapy and to diagnose recurrences, distinguishing them from fibrosis.

4.1. Morphological MRI

As regards the topographic relationship of the tumor with the mesorectal fascia can be adequately established with morphologic MRI [26]. The advent of powerful gradient systems and, above all, the development of high-resolution phased array surface coil systems in recent years brought the breakthrough in the staging of rectal cancer by MRI. The use of these phased-array surface coils combines a very high spatial resolution with a large FOV that allows not only detailed evaluation of the intestinal wall but also depicts surrounding anatomy including the mesorectal fascia.

A standard phased-array morphologic MRI protocol for LARC staging (including T-N stage and CRM evaluation) consists of T2-weighted coronal, transversal and sagittal turbospin-echo MR sequences with high spatial resolution (Fig. 1) [26].

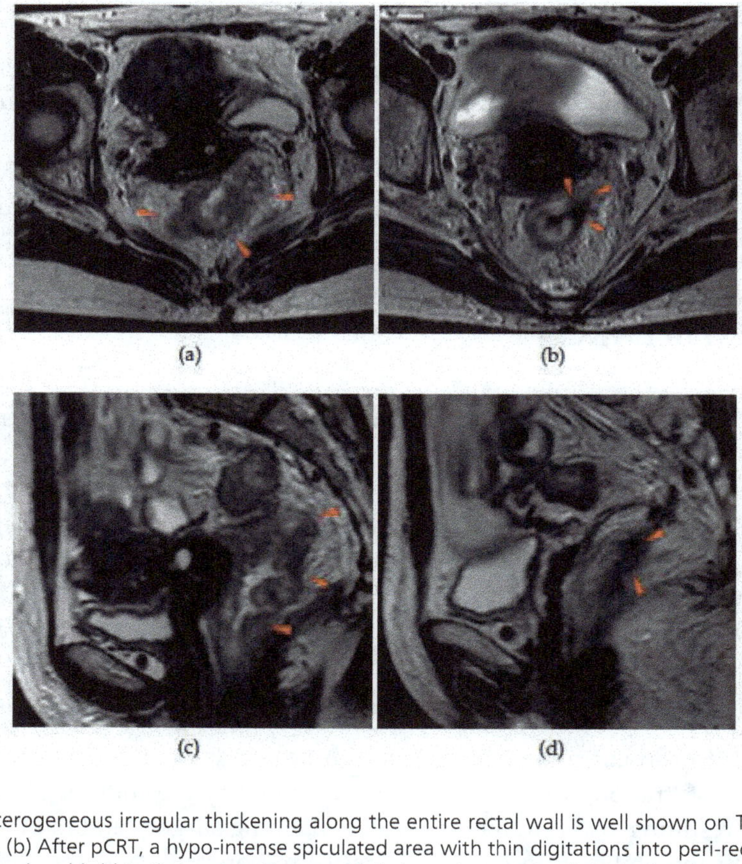

(a) (b) (c) (d)

Figure 1. (a) A heterogeneous irregular thickening along the entire rectal wall is well shown on T2w axial pre-pCRT scan (arrowheads). (b) After pCRT, a hypo-intense spiculated area with thin digitations into peri-rectal fat is visible on T2w axial scan (arrowheads). (c) In the same patient, multiple irregular rectal wall thickening are shown on T2w sagittal pre-pCRT scan (arrowheads). (d) A single hypo-intense area, showed also in (b) is pointed by arrowheads, suspecting for a residual post-pCRT tumor focus (arrowheads).

An adequate, state-of-the-art MRI staging classification is capable to predict whether a tumor-free CRM is likely to be achieved or not [26]. In this way one would be able to differentiate patients with minimal mesorectal infiltration in whom neoadjuvant therapy is not mandatory from patients who would definitely benefit from neoadjuvant therapy because the mesorectal fascia is infiltrated or at risk.

The common use of total mesorectal excision (TME) and the shift from a postoperative to a preoperative chemo-radiotherapy (pre-CRT) approach have substantially reduced the risk of local recurrences, increasing curative resection and the rate of anal sphincter preservation and improving local control and overall survival rates [13-18].

4.2. Functional MRI

Although morphological tumour assessment performed by MRI has been repeatedly shown to be the most accurate modality in evaluating the presence of a positive circumferential resection margin (CRM), MRI is considered not to be conclusive in pre-CRT tumor response evaluation since histopathological downstage is not always associated with tumour effective reduction [17]. The main difficulty regarding post-chemoradiation MRI includes discrimination of active tumour and post-treatment fibrosis, particularly when differentiating stage T2 and stage T3 carcinomas, according to different recurrence and overall survival rates between Low Risk (T1/T2N0) and Intermediate Risk (T3/N0) as reported by Gunderson et al. [23-24].

Several studies have shown the potential of functional [diffusion- or perfusion] weighted imaging to predict the response to adjuvant or neoadjuvant therapy [5–7,19].

In fact, it has long been known that the pathophysiology and aggressiveness of a tumor are determined not only by the macroscopic tumor extent but also by other factors such as tumor microcirculation and angiogenesis.

4.2.1. DCE-MRI

Previous considerations support a Dynamic Contrast Enhanced-Magnetic Resonance Imaging (DCE-MRI) approach that could gain a renewed role to MRI adding functional data to the morphological examination. DCE-MRI has been reported by many authors as a tool potentially able to permit an evaluation of pre-CRT effectiveness basing on the strict relationship between tumor growth and angiogenesis [6-7,24-25].

DCE-MRI is gaining a large consensus as a technique for diagnosis, staging and assessment of therapy response for different types of tumours, due to its capability to detect highly active angiogenesis. It is well known that angiogenesis is a key factor in the growth and dissemination of cancer; characterization of the angiogenic status of the tumour on an individual patient basis could allow for a more targeted approach to treatment of rectal cancer [24].

More specifically, in the case of rectal cancer, previous trials have provided the proof of principle that inhibition of angiogenesis has the potential to enhance the effectiveness of the treatment for this disease. In vivo imaging techniques capable to assess tumour perfusion have the potential to improve the management of treatment for patients with rectal cancer [6-7,24-25].

Angiogenesis is a key factor for the growth and dissemination of solid tumors and is a prognostic marker in CRC. Neovascularization arises early in the adenoma–carcinoma sequence via upregulation of vascular endothelial growth factor. Tumor angiogenesis is characterized by structurally abnormal blood vessels that are thin, fragile, tortuous, and hyperpermeable. They have a chaotic, heterogeneous intratumoral distribution. Abnormal vascularity often extends beyond the tumor boundaries into surrounding tissues.

DCE-MRI techniques inform on tissue perfusion and vascular leakage (Fig. 2). T1- or relaxivity-based MR sequences are sensitive to the presence of dilute contrast medium in the extravascular– extracellular space. In most tumors, low-molecular-weight contrast media readily diffuse from the blood into the extravascular– extracellular space at a rate determined by perfusion and the capillary permeability and surface area.

The most commonly used model for analyzing DCE-MRI data uses two compartments where the contrast agent resides (blood plasma and extravascular– extracellular space). K^{trans} (volume transfer constant between the blood plasma and the extravascular–extracellular space, the washin rate, measured in minutes−1) and k_{ep} (rate constant between the extravascular–extracellular space back to the blood plasma, the washout rate, measured in minutes−1) determine the transport between these two compartments.

Physiologically, K^{trans} indicates a variable combination of the flow and permeability properties. For blood vessels where leakage is rapid (that is, when the extraction fraction during the first pass of the contrast agent is high, as typically is found in tumors), perfusion will determine contrast agent distribution and K^{trans} approximates to tissue blood flow per unit volume. There are circumstances in which transport out of the vasculature does not significantly deplete intravascular contrast medium concentration (that is, tissues with lower first-pass extraction fraction). This is typically found after treatment with chemotherapy or late after radiotherapy and in fibrotic lesions, and in these situations, K^{trans} approximates to the product of permeability and the surface area (permeability surface area product).

4.2.2. Diffusion-weighted imaging DWI-MRI

At present, the use of diffusion-weighted imaging (DWI) incorporated into a standard MR protocol is gradually increasing because of its proven benefit not only for tumor detection/ characterization but also for monitoring treatment response (8–12). Diffusion-weighted imaging measures water diffusion characteristics, which are dependent on multiple factors such as cell density, vascularity, viscosity of extracellular fluid, and cell membrane integrity (12). By quantifying these properties and expressing them as an apparent diffusion coefficient (ADC), DWI could potentially be used as an imaging biomarker to better select patients with poor prognosis who will truly benefit from a more aggressive neoadjuvant treatment (8-12). In literature it was demonstrated that ADC values of rectal cancers significantly correlate with prognostic factors including the MRF status, the nodal stage and the histological differentiation grade.

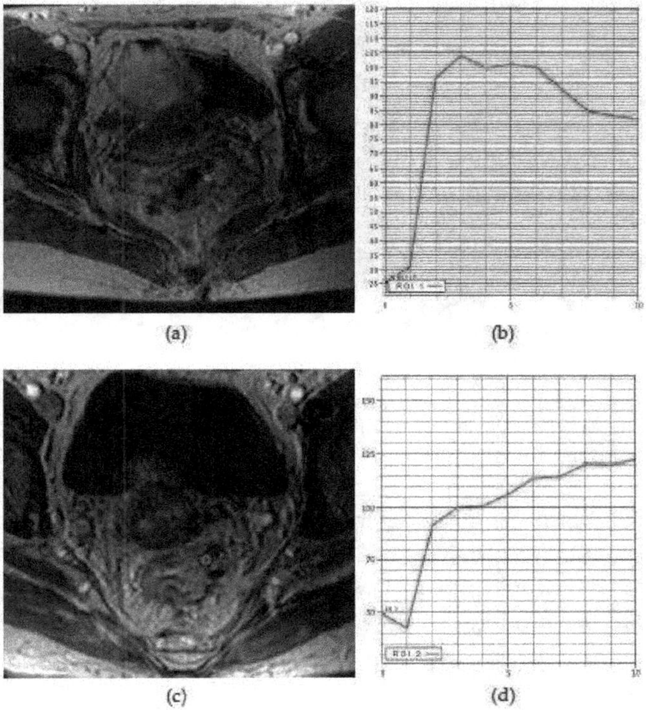

Figure 2. T1w post-contrast scan obtained on the same patient in fig. 8, before (a)-(b) and after (c)-(d) pre-CRT. The analysis of TIC calculated on a ROI, drawn outside the rectal wall where on T2w scans (fig. 8) tumor clearly spreads into peri-rectal fat pad, confirm this suspect showing a rapid CA intake and a fast discharge (b). After pre-CRT, on the same areas showed on T2w scans (fig. 8) no pathological CA uptake is present confirming that hypo-intense tissue visible on T2w scans are tumor nests but only residual inflammation due to pre-CRT. This patient was considered as a Responder. Histopathology showed a TRG 1.

The movement of water molecules in biologic tissues is restricted because their motion is modified and limited by interactions with cell membranes and macromolecules. Water-molecule motion in tissues can be assessed by applying diffusion- weighting gradients to T2-weighted sequences. This process entails the application of two balanced gradients placed symmetrically about a focusing 180° pulse. Water molecules that have not moved during the time taken to apply the first gradient will have acquired phase shifts that are exactly cancelled out by the proceeding second gradient; thus, there is no net additional signal loss induced by the application of the paired diffusion gradients. For water molecules that have moved during the application of the first gradient, however, the acquired phase shifts will not be cancelled out by the second gradient; residual phase incoherence will result in net losses of signal. Hence, the motion of water molecules is detected as attenuation of the measured signal intensity on DWI (Fig. 3).

The sensitivity of the DWI sequence to water motion can be varied by changing the parameter known as the b value (measured in s/mm2), which is proportional to the gradient amplitude, duration of the applied gradient, and time interval between the paired gradients. DWI can be

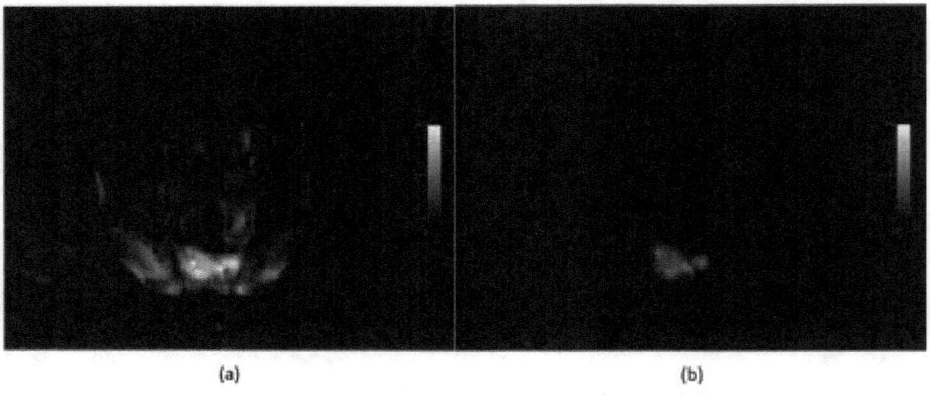

Figure 3. (a) Axial diffusion weigthed imaging b=0, (b) Axial diffusion weigthed imaging b=800. Hyperintensity diffusion weigthed imaging is consistent with the diagnosis of tumor.

exploited in clinical practice to provide indirect assessments of tissue properties such as cellularity, gland formation, perfusion, and cell death. In general, the greater the cell density per high power field, the more impeded will be tissue water diffusion. Diffusion-weighted signal is derived from the motion of water molecules within the extravascular–extracellular space and intravascular space with some component from intracellular space water. The relative contribution of each space to the derived signal varies from tissue to tissue. In highly vascular tumors, intravascular water diffusion will account for a significant proportion of the diffusion-weighted signal. In highly glandular tissues, such as the pancreas and salivary glands, significant signal contributions arise from glandular water.

By performing DWI using different b values, quantitative analysis is possible with the calculation of the apparent diffusion coefficient (ADC, measured in μm/s). Areas of restricted diffusion show low ADC values. ADC values are inversely correlated with tumor cellularity and reductions in ADC correlate with response to cytotoxic therapy.

Areas retaining high signal intensity on high-b-value images usually (but not always) indicate highly cellular tissues such as tumors. Normal tissues including lymph nodes, spleen, nervous tissues, adrenal glands, bowel mucosa, and endometrium may show the same findings. Lower-signal-intensity regions are seen in most organized normal tissues, cystic spaces, and vessels. However, high signal intensities on high-b-value images are not always reliable indicators of increased cellularity on their own. Occasionally, fluid, edema, or mucinous materials remain of high signal intensity because of high proton density. This observation is called T2-shine through, but this effect can be detected easily by noting corresponding high signal on ADC maps.

There is growing interest in the application of DWI for the evaluation of CRC. DWI aids in detection of lesions, particularly when lesions are small. High-b-value DWI may be a useful tool for detecting and defining tumor extent.

DWI has been shown to be feasible as an early marker of treatment response because cell death and vascular alterations typically occur before size changes. Increases in ADC values with treatment reflect decreases in cellularity and thus provide indirect assessment of chemotherapy induced cell death. It has been reported that transient decreases in ADC may occur early in treatment related to cellular swelling, reduction in blood flow, or reduction in the extravascular– extracellular space due to dehydration. However, early decreases in ADC values are not consistently seen, and it has recently been reported that increases in ADC value with therapy response occur within 3–7 days in responding CRC patients treated with chemotherapy.

Responders had a lower ADC at presentation than non responders. Higher pretreatment ADC values in nonresponders may reflect necrotic tumors that are more resistant to therapy because of concomitant hypoxia. Similarly, for CRC liver metastases, a higher pretreatment ADC is also predictive of poor response.

5. A systematic review

5.1. Methodologies

A systematic literature search was performed to identify English-language studies and articles concerning different diagnostic imaging methodologies available in locally advanced rectal cancer disease after radiation therapy. Data were identified using PubMed database with the following keywords: "locally advanced rectal cancer, magnetic resonance imaging, CT planning, PET imaging". This yielded 309 titles. Articles, reviews and studies that did not present data about specificity and sensibility of tests treated were excluded. Due to the small number of studies for each imaging modality, there was not set a minimum number of patients as an inclusion criteria. For this reason, a total number of 12 titles were considered as studies included in the research.

Details regarding the number of patients, imaging modality investigated, the accuracy values and parameters examined of the studies were recorded. Cascini et al. [41] evaluated ^{18}F-FDG PET to assess the effect of chemoradiation therapy in thirty-three patients with LARC proved disease. They correlate the change in tumor ^{18}F-FDG standardized uptake value (SUV) during and after preoperative radiotherapy with the pathologic response achieved.

The accuracy of CT and MRI in restaging rectal cancer after preoperative chemoradiation in order to plan optimal therapy was performed in Martellucci et al. [42] study, in which thirty-seven consecutive patients undergoing neoadjuvant therapy were evaluated. Considering the depth of invasion after treatment only in neoplasia with stage T3 they found CT agree with histopathology in 19 cases and MRI in 10/12 cases.

Denecke et al. [46] compare CT, MRI and FDG-PET examining a total of twenty-three patients with T3/4 rectal cancer. Response criteria were a change in T category and tumour volume for CT and MRI and a change in glucose uptake for FDG-PET. Their results in sensitivity and specificity suggest that PET is superior to CT and MRI in predicting response to preoperative multimodal treatment of LARC.

A prospective analysis to evaluate tumor response with ^{18}F-FDG PET in twenty-seven patients with biopsy-proven rectal adenocarcinoma was conducted by Leibold et al. [47]. They found of the total 27 patients, 11 (41%) had pathologic complete response; 16 (59%) had suboptimal response. They evaluate the ability of change in 4 specific PET parameters to predict pathologic response: the maximum SUV in the region of interest, SUV_{max}; the average SUV throughout the entire region of interest, SUV_{avg}; the summed metabolic rate of the tumor, TLG; the virtual graded global assessment of response, VRS.

Chien-Chih Chen et al. [37] evaluated the correlation between pathological verified tumor stage and clinical stage predicted by MRI. The overall predictive accuracy in T stage was 52%, whereas overstaging and understaging occurred in 38% and 10% of patients, respectively. Another study regard the MRI accuracy was conducted by Dresen et al. [45] using T2- weighted MR images obtained before and after radiation therapy and correlating findings with histopathology results.

Kristiansen et al. [39] investigated the possibility of using PET/CT to predict the histopathologic response in 30 patients with LARC treated with a combination of radiotherapy and concurrent Uftoral® and leucovorine. PET/CT correctly identified six of eight patients, specificity 75%, with complete pathologic response.

To evaluate the correlation between the change of SUV_{max} and of apparent diffusion coefficient (ADC) before and after neoadjuvant therapy, thirty patients with locally advanced rectal cancer were recruited in Ippolito et al. [40] analysis, in which all the patients underwent a whole body ^{18}F-FDG PET/CT scan and a pelvic MR examination including DW imaging for staging therapy.

Table 1 summarizes the main characteristics of the examined methodologies in locally advanced rectal cancer studies.

Study	Modality	No.Patients	Parameters
C. C. Chen et al. [37]	MRI	50	TNM
T. Denecke et al. [46]	MRI	23	TNM
	CT	23	TNM
	PET	23	SUV
G. L. Cascini et al. [41]	PET	33	SUV
C. Capirci et al. [38]	PET/CT	45	SUV
C. Kristiansen et al. [39]	PET/CT	30	TRG,SUV
R. Rosenberg et al. [44]	PET/CT	30	SUV
A. Suppiah et al. [36]	MRI	49	TNM
R. C. Dresen et al. [45]	MRI	67	TNM
T. Leibold et al. [47]	PET	27	SUV,TLG,VRS
D. Ippolito et al. [40]	MRI	30	ADC
	PET/CT	30	SUV
J. Martellucci et al. [42]	MRI	20	TNM
	CT	37	TNM
M. J. M. Duréndez et al. [43]	PET/CT	41	SUV

Table 1. Summary of the main characteristics of includes studies about different methodologies used in LARC diseases. Per each study the table reports: imaging modality used; number of patients examined; parameters examined; sensitivity and specificity methodology values.

5.2. Summary ROC curves and Forest Plots

In order to assess individual methodology in LARC treatment, Summary Receiver Operating Characteristic (SROC) curves have been realized, Fig. 4. ROC curves is a statistic technique for displaying, organizing and selecting classifiers based on their performance.

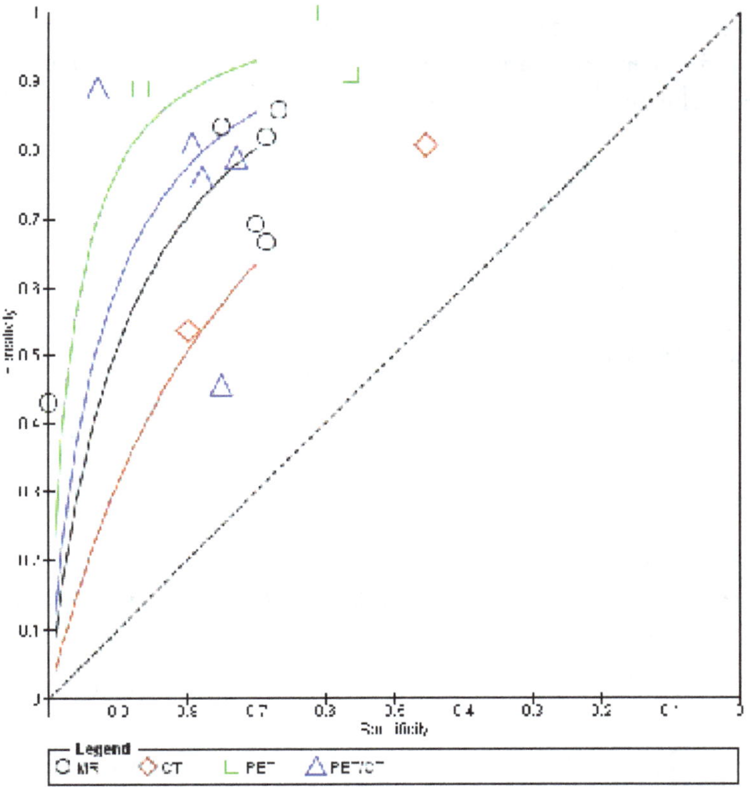

Figure 4. Estimated Summary ROC curves and original data points for four imaging techniques. MRI= magnetic resonance imaging, CT= computed tomography, PET= Positron emission tomography, PET/CT= positron emission tomography and computed tomography.

ROC analysis was performed through the study of the function that links the probability to obtain a true-positive result in the disease like class, i.e. the sensitivity, to the probability to obtain a false-positive result in the non-diseased class, linked to the specificity. In this way a graphical 2D representation that shows the false-positive proportion in x-axis and true-positive proportion in y-axis, relatively to values obtained from each test applied.

For each modality, a model was obtained that was adjusted for significant variables that were set to 1, indicating the ideal design versus 0, as appropriate, Fig. 4. The position of the summary ROC curve indicates the difference in diagnostic performance among the imaging modalities. A summary ROC curve located near the upper left corner indicate rte better diagnostic modality, while a summary ROC curve for a worthless modality is represented by the bisector, also named change line.

Another additional graphical representation realized is the Forest Plot, Fig. 5, which shows the sensitivity and specificity estimates of the results for each study. It is composed of a plot of the measure of effect for each of these studies incorporating confidence intervals represented by horizontal bars. The confidence interval expresses the precision level associated with the parameter estimation: the more is small, the more indicates that the prediction is accurate. In this analysis confidence intervals are computed with a probability of containing the true effect size equal to 95%. The blue square represents the point estimate, i.e. the sensitivity or specificity.

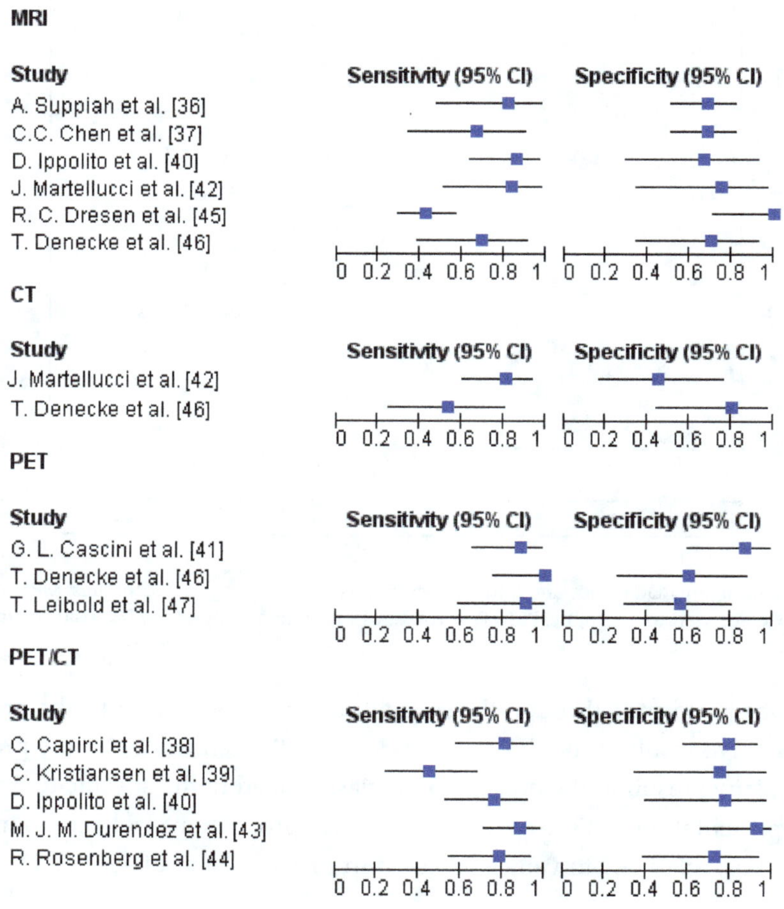

Figure 5. Forest Plot of MRI, CT, PET and PET/CT sensitivity and specificity estimates and their confidence intervals (95%).

5.3. Discussion

The objective of this statistical analysis was to evaluate the diverse methodologies (MRI, PET, PET/CT, CT) in LARC management. In particular, in our analysis we considered the accuracy in assessing the therapy response.

Although, the ROC curves analysis showed that PET has the best accuracy in term of sensitivity and specificity it should be noticed that only three studies have been retrieved from the literature.

However, in agreement with the intuitive considerations MRI and PET/ CT showed a high diagnostic accuracy and their results are also more reliable than PET because the statistical analysis has been carried out on a larger number of studies (6 studies for MRI with a total of 239 patients and 5 studies for PET/CT with a total of 176 patients).

The number of studies for CT is very small to draw detailed conclusions.

In conclusion we could state that a greater number of studies should be performed in the future for each modalities to improve the reliability of any conclusion.

Author details

Roberta Fusco[1,3], Mario Sansone[2], Mario Petrillo[3], Antonio Avallone[4], Paolo Delrio[3], Fabiana Tatangelo[3] and Antonella Petrillo[1]

1 Department of Diagnostic Imaging, Radiant and Metabolic Therapy, "Istituto Nazionale dei Tumori Fondazione G. Pascale " – IRCCS, Naples, Italy

2 Department of Electrical Engineering and Information Technologies University 'Federico II' of Naples, Italy

3 Department of Radiology, Second University of Naples, Italy

4 Gastrointestinal Medical Oncology, "Istituto Nazionale dei Tumori Fondazione G. Pascale " – IRCCS, Naples, Italy

References

[1] Jemal A, Siegel R, Xu J, Ward E. Cancer statistics, 2010. CA Cancer J Clin 2010;60(5): 277–300.

[2] Folkman J Tumor angiogenesis: therapeutic implications. N Engl J Med 1971;285:1182–1186.

[3] Choi HJ, Hyun MS, Jung GJ, Kim SS, Hong SH. Tumor angiogenesis as a prognostic predictor in colorectal carcinoma with special reference to mode of metastasis and recurrence. Oncology 1998; 55:575–581.

[4] Dvorak HF, Brown LF, Detmar M, Dvorak AM. Vascular permeability factor/vascular endothelial growth factor, microvascular hyperpermeability, and angiogenesis. Am J Pathol 1995;146:1029–1039.

[5] Dzik-Jurasz A, Domenig C, George M et al (2002) Diffusion MRI for prediction of response of rectal cancer to chemoradiation. Lancet 360 (9329):307–308

[6] Devries AF, Griebel J, Kremser C et al (2001) Tumor microcirculation evaluated by dynamic magnetic resonance imaging predicts therapy outcome for primary rectal carcinoma. Cancer Res 61(6):2513–2516

[7] DeVries AF, Kremser C, Hein PA et al (2003) Tumor microcirculation and diffusion predict therapy outcome for primary rectal carcinoma. Int J Radiat Oncol Biol Phys 56(4):958–96

[8] Koh DM, Padhani AR. Diffusion-weighted MRI: a new functional clinical technique for tumor imaging. Br J Radiol 2006;79: 633–635.

[9] Koh DM, Collins DJ. Diffusion-weighted MRI in the body: applications and challenges in oncology. AJR Am J Roentgenol 2007; 188:1622–1635.

[10] Patterson DM, Padhani AR, Collins DJ. Technology insight: water diffusion MRI-a potential new biomarker of response to cancer therapy. Nat Clin Pract Oncol 2008;5:220–233.

[11] Padhani AR, Liu G, Koh DM, et al. Diffusion-weighted magnetic resonance imaging as a cancer biomarker: consensus and recommendations. Neoplasia 2009;11:102–125.

[12] deSouza NM, Riches SF, Vanas NJ, et al. Diffusion-weighted magnetic resonance imaging: a potential non-invasive marker of tumour aggressiveness in localized prostate cancer. Clin Radiol 2008;63:774–782.

[13] Avallone A, Delrio P, Guida C, Tatangelo F, Petrillo A, Marone P, Cascini LG, Morrica B, Lastoria S, Parisi V, Budillon A, Comella P. (2006). Biweekly oxaliplatin, raltitrexed, 5-fluorouracil and folinic acid combination chemotherapy during preoperative radiation therapy for locally advanced rectal cancer: a phase I-II study, Brit J Cancer 94(12): 1809–1815.

[14] Avallone A, Delrio P, Pecori B, Tatangelo F, Petrillo A, Scott N, Marone P, Aloi L, Sandomenico C, Lastoria S, Iaffaioli VR, Scala D, Iodice G, Budillon A., Comella P. (2011). Oxaliplatin plus dual inhibition of thymidilate synthase during preoperative pelvic radiotherapy for locally advanced rectal carcinoma: long-term outcome, Int J Radiat Oncol 79(3): 670–676.

[15] Delrio P, Avallone A, Guida C, Lastoria S, Tatangelo F, Cascini GM, Marone P, Petrillo, A, Budillon A, Marzo MD, Palaia R, Albino V, Rosa VD, Parisi V. (2005). Multidis-

ciplinary approach to locally advanced rectal cancer: results of a single institution trial, Suppl Tumori 4(3): S8.

[16] Delrio P, Lastoria S, Avallone A, Ravo V, Guida C, Cremona F, Izzo F, Palaia R, Ruffolo F, Puppio B, Guidetti GM, Cascini GL, Casaretti R, Tatangelo F, Marone P, Rossi GB, Budillon A, Petrillo A, Rosa VD, Comella G, Morrica B, Tempesta A, Botti G, Parisi V. (2003). Early evaluation using PET-FDG of the efficiency of neoadjuvant radiochemotherapy treatment in locally advanced neoplasia of the lower rectum, Tumori 89(4 Suppl): 50–53.

[17] Petrillo A, Catalano O, Delrio P, Avallone A, Guida C, Filice S, Siani A. (2007). Post-treatment fistulas in patients with rectal cancer: MRI with rectal superparamagnetic contrast agent, Abdom Imaging 32(3): 328–331.

[18] Petrillo A, Filice S, Avallone A, Delrio P, Guida C, Tatangelo F, Marone P, Nunziata A, Siani A. (2006). Staging of locally advanced rectal cancer (LARC): proposal of 96 Rectal Cancer – A Multidisciplinary Approach to Management Dynamic Contrast Enhanced Magnetic Resonance Imaging in Rectal Cancer 23 a one-stop magnetic resonance (MR) imaging-based protocol, Eur Radiol Supplements 16: 321–494.

[19] Sansone M, Fusco R, Petrillo A, Petrillo M, Bracale M. (2011). An expectation-maximisation approach for simultaneous pixel classification and tracer kinetic modelling in dynamic contrast enhanced-magnetic resonance imaging, Med Biol Eng Comput 49(4): 485–495.

[20] Fusco R, Sansone M, Petrillo M, Antonella Petrillo. Influence of parameterization on tracer kinetic modeling in DCE-MRI. Journal of Medical and Biological Engineering, Uncorrected Proof Available online 7 Sep 2012, doi: 10.5405/jmbe.1097

[21] Fusco R, Sansone M, Maffei S, Petrillo.A. Dynamic Contrast-Enhanced MRI in Breast Cancer: A Comparison between Distributed and Compartmental Tracer Kinetic Models. Journal of Biomedical Graphics and Computing, Journal of Biomedical Graphics and Computing, vol. 2, no. 2, p. p23, Aug. 2012.

[22] Gunderson LL, Sargent DJ, Tepper JE, O'Connell MJ, Allmer C, Smalley SR, Martenson JA, Haller D. G.,Mayer, R. J., Rich, T. A., Ajani, J. A., Macdonald, J. S. & Goldberg, R.M. (2002). Impact of T and Nsubstage on survival and disease relapse in adjuvant rectal cancer: a pooled analysis, Int J Radiat Oncol 54(2): 386–396.

[23] Gunderson LL, Sargent DJ, Tepper JE, Wolmark N, O'Connell MJ, Begovic M, Allmer C, Colangelo L, Smalley SR, Haller DG, Martenson JA, Mayer RJ, Rich TA, Ajani JA, MacDonald JS, Willett CG, Goldberg RM. Impact of T and N stage and treatment on survival and relapse in adjuvant rectal cancer: a pooled analysis, J Clin Oncol 2004; 22(10): 1785–1796.

[24] Goh V, Padhani AR, Rasheed S. Functional imaging of colorectal cancer angiogenesis, Lancet Oncol 2007; 8(3): 245–255.

[25] Kremser C, Trieb T, Rudisch A, Judmaier W, de Vries A. Dynamic t(1) mapping predicts outcome of chemoradiation therapy in primary rectal carcinoma: sequence implementation and data analysis, JMagn Reson Imaging 2007; 26(3): 662–671.

[26] Beets-Tan RG, Beets GL. Rectal cancer: review with emphasis on MR imaging. Radiology. 2004 Aug;232(2):335-46.

[27] Kapiteijn E, Marijnen CA, Nagtegaal ID, et al. Preoperative radiotherapy combined with total mesorectal excision for resectable rectal cancer. N Engl J Med 2001;345:638–646

[28] Vermaas M, Ferenschild FT, Nuyttens JJ, et al. Preoperative radiotherapy improves outcome in recurrent rectal cancer. Dis Colon Rectum 2005;48:918–928

[29] Gerard JP, Conroy T, Bonnetain F, et al. Preoperative radiotherapy with or without concurrent fluorouracil and leucovorin in T3–4 rectal cancers: results of FFCD 9203. J Clin Oncol 2006;24:4620–4625

[30] Bosset JF, Collette L, Calais G, et al. Chemotherapy with preoperative radiotherapy in rectal cancer. N Engl J Med 2006;355:1114–1123

[31] Bosset JF, Calais G, Daban A, et al. Preoperative chemoradiotherapy versus preoperative radiotherapy in rectal cancer patients: assessment of acute toxicity and treatment compliance. Report of the 22921 randomised trial conducted by the EORTC Radiotherapy Group. Eur J Cancer 2004;40:219–224

[32] Willett CG, Boucher Y, di Tomaso E, et al. Direct evidence that the VEGF-specific antibody bevacizumab has antivascular effects in human rectal cancer. Nat Med 2004;10:145–147

[33] Vermaas M, Ferenschild FT, Verhoef C, et al. Total pelvic exenteration for primary locally advanced and locally recurrent rectal cancer. Eur J Surg Oncol 2007;33(4):452–458

[34] Wiig JN, Poulsen JP, Larsen S, Braendengen M, Waehre H, Giercksky KE. Total pelvic exenteration with preoperative irradiation for advanced primary and recurrent rectal cancer. Eur J Surg 2002;168:42–48

[35] Luna-Perez P, Delgado S, Labastida S, Ortiz N, Rodriguez D, Herrera L. Patterns of recurrence following pelvic exenteration and external radiotherapy for locally advanced primary rectal adenocarcinoma. Ann Surg Oncol 1996;3:526–533

[36] Suppiah A, Hunter IA, Cowley J, Garimella V, Cast J, Hartley JE, Monson JRT. Magnetic resonance imaging accuracy in assessing tumour down-staging following chemoradiation in rectal cancer. Colorectal Disease 22 April 2008;11:249-253.

[37] Chen CC, Lee RC, Lin JK, Wang LW, Yang SH. How Accurate is Magnetic Resonance Imaging in Restaging Rectal Cancer in Patients Receiving Preoperative Combined Chemoradiotherapy? Disease of the Colon & Rectum 17 February 2005;48:722-728.

[38] Capirci C, Rampin L, Erba PA, Galeotti, Crepaldi G, Banti E, Gava M, Fanti S, Mariani G, Muzzio PC, Rubello D. Sequential FDG-PET/CT reliably predicts response of locally advanced rectal cancer to neo-adjuvant chemo-radiation therapy. Nucl Med Mol Imaging 2007;34:1583-1593.

[39] Kristiansen C, Loft A, Berthelsen AK, Graff J, Lindebjerg J, Bisgaard C, Jakobsen A. PET/CT and Histopathologic Response to Preoperative Chemoradiation Therapy in Locally Advanced Rectal Cancer. Disease of the Colon & Rectum 2008;51:21-25.

[40] Ippolito D, Monguzzi L, Guerra L, Deponti E, Gardani G, Messa C, Sironi S. Response to neoadjuvant therapy in locally advanced rectal cancer: assessment with diffusion-weighted MR imaging and 18FDG PET/CT. Abdominal Imaging 20 January 2012.

[41] Cascini GL, Avallone A, Delrio P, Guida C, Tatangelo F, Marone P, Aloj L, De Martinis F, Comella P, Parisi V, Lastoria S. 18F-FDG PET Is an Early Predictor of Pathologic Tumor Response to Preoperative Radiochemotherapy in Locally Advanced Rectal Cancer. The journal of nuclear medicine August 2006;47(8):1241-1248.

[42] Martellucci J, Scheiterle M, Lorenzi B, Roviello F, Cetta F, Pinto E, Tanzini G. Accuracy of transrectal ultrasound after preoperative radiochemotherapy compared to computed tomography and magnetic resonance in locally advanced rectal cancer. Journal of Colorectal Deseases 3 February 2012;27:967-973.

[43] Murcia MJ, Duréndez L, Frutos Esteban J, Luján MD, Frutos G, Valero JL, Navarro Fernández L, Mohamed Salem G, Ruiz Merino MA, Claver Valderas. The value of 18F-FDG PET/CT for assessing the response to neoadjuvant therapy in locally advanced rectal cancer. Nucl Med Mol Imaging 19 October 2012;40:91-97.

[44] Rosenberg R, Herrmann K, Gertler R, Künzli B, Essler M, Lordick F, Becker K, Schuster T, Geinitz H, Maak M, Schwaiger M, Siewert JR, Krause B. The predictive value of metabolic response to preoperative radiochemotherapy in locally advanced rectal cancer measured by PET/CT. Colorectal Disease 3 December 2008;24:191-200.

[45] Dresen RC, Beets GL, Rutten HJT, Engelen SME, Lahaye MJ, Vliegen RFA, de Bruïne AP, Kessels AGH, Lammering G, Beets-Tan RGH. Locally Advanced Rectal Cancer: MR Imaging for Restaging after Neoadjuvant Radiation Therapy with Concomitant Chemotherapy Part I. Are We Able to Predict Tumor Confined to the Rectal Wall? Radiology July 2009;252(1):71-80.

[46] T. Denecke, B. Rau, K.-T. Hoffmann, B. Hildebrandt, J. Ruf, M. Gutberlet, M. Hünerbein, R. Felix, P. Wust, H. Amthauer. Comparison of CT, MRI and FDG-PETin response prediction of patients with locally advanced rectal cancer after multimodal preoperative therapy: Is there a benefit in using functional imaging? European Journal of Radiology 2 April 2005;15:1658-1666.

[47] Leibold T, Akhurst TJ, Chessin DB, Yeung HW, Macapinlac H, Shia J, Minsky BD, Saltz LB, Riedel E, Mazumdar M, Paty PB, Weiser MR, Douglas WW, Larson SM,

Guillem JG. Evaluation of 18F-FDG-PET for Early Detection of Suboptimal Response of Rectal Cancer to Preoperative Chemoradiotherapy: A Prospective Analysis. Official Journal of the society of surgical oncology 2011;18:2783-2789.

[48] Chau I, Allen M, Cunningham D, Tait D, Brown G, Hill M, Sumpter K, Rhodes A, Wotherspoon A, Norman AR, Hill A, Massey A, Prior Y. Neoadjuvant systemic fluorouracil and mitomycin C prior to synchronous chemoradiation is an effective strategy in locally advanced rectal cancer. British Journal of Cancer 2003;88:1017-1024.

[49] Corner C, Khimji F, Tsang Y, Harrison M, Glynne-Jones R, Hughes R. Comparison of conventional and three-dimensional conformal CT planning techniques for preoperative chemoradiotherapy for locally advanced rectal cancer. The British Journal of Radiology !4 December 2009;84:173-178.

[50] Ruby JA, Leibold T, Akhurst TJ, Shia J, Saltz LB, Mazumdar M, Riedel ER, Larson SM, Guillem JG. FDG-PET Assessment of Rectal Cancer Response to Neoadjuvant Chemoradiotherapy Is Not Associated With Long-Term Prognosis: A Prospective Evaluation. Diseases of the colon and rectum 2012;55(4):378-386.

[51] Kuo LJ, Chern MC, Tsou MH, Liu MC, Jian JJM, Chen CM, Chung YL, Fang WT. Interpretation of Magnetic Resonance Imaging for Locally Advanced Rectal Carcinoma After Preoperative Chemoradiation Therapy. Disease of the Colon & Rectum 7 December 2004;48(23-28).

[52] Yeung JMC, Kalff V, Hicks RJ, Drummond E, Link E, Phil D, Taouk Y, Michael M, Ngan S, Lynch AC, Heriot AG. Metabolic Response of Rectal Cancer Assessed by 18-FDG PET Following Chemoradiotherapy is Prognostic for Patient Outcome. Diseases of the colon & rectum 2011;54:518-525.

[53] Mezzi G, Arcidiacono PG, Carrara S, Perri F, Petrone MC, De Cobelli F, Gusmini S, Staudacher C, Del Maschio A, Testoni PA. Endoscopic ultrasound and magnetic resonance imaging for re-staging rectal cancer after radiotherapy. World Journal of Gastroenterology 28 November 2009;44:5563-5567.

[54] Patel UB, Taylor F, Blomqvist L, George C, Evans H, Tekkis P, Quirke P, Sebag-Montefiore D, Moran B, Heald R, Guthrie A, Bees N, Swift I, Pennert K, Brown G. Magnetic Resonance Imaging–Detected Tumor Response for Locally Advanced Rectal Cancer Predicts Survival Outcomes: MERCURY Experience. Journal of Clinical Oncology 2011;1-11.

[55] Johnston DF, Lawrence KM, Sizer BF, Arulampalam THA, Motson RW, Dove E, Lacey N. Locally advanced rectal cancer: histopathological correlation and predictive accuracy of serial MRI after neoadjuvant chemotherapy. The british journal of radiology 2009;82:332-336.

[56] Shanmugan S, Arrangoiz R, Nitzkorski JR, Yu JQ, Li T, Cooper H, Konski A, Farma JM, Sigurdson ER. Predicting Pathological Response to Neoadjuvant Chemoradio-

therapy in Locally Advanced Rectal Cancer Using18FDG-PET/CT. Society of Surgical Oncology 7 March 2012;19:2178-2185.

[57] Itatani Y, Akiyoshi T, Kuroyanagi H, Yamakawa K, Noaki R, Konishi T, Fujimoto Y, Ueno M, Oya M, Suenaga M, Yamaguchi T. Total mesorectal excision of initially unresectable locally advanced rectal cancer infiltrating the pelvic wall after treatment with FOLFOX4 plus bevacizumab and preoperative chemoradiation: report of a case. Surg Today 12 November 2011;42(75-79).

[58] O'Neill BDP, Brown G, Heald RJ, Cunningham D, Tait DM. Non-operative treatment after neoadjuvant chemoradiotherapy for rectal cancer. The lancet oncology July 2007;8:625-633.

[59] Fusco R, Sansone M, Petrillo M, Avallone A, Delrio P, Antonella Petrillo (2011). Dynamic Contrast Enhanced Magnetic Resonance Imaging in Rectal Cancer, Rectal Cancer - A Multidisciplinary Approach to Management, Giulio Aniello Santoro (Ed.), ISBN: 978-953-307-758-1, InTech, Available from: http://www.intechopen.com/books/rectal-cancer-a-multidisciplinary-approach-to-management/dynamic-contrast-enhanced-magnetic-resonance-imaging-in-rectal-cancer.

[60] Beets-Tan RG, Beets GL, Borstlap SC, Oei Tk, Teune TM, von Meyenfeldt MF, et al. Preoperative assessment of local tumour extent in advanced rectal cancer: CT or high- resolution MRI? Abdominal Imaging 2000;25(5):533-41.

[61] Wiering B, Ruers TJ, Oyen WJ. Role of FDG_PET in the diagnosis and treatment of colorectal liver metastases. Expert Rev Anticancer Ther 2004; 4: 607-13.

[62] Park IJ, Kim HC, Yu CS, et al. Efficacy of PET/CT in the accurate evaluation of primary colorectal carcinoma. Eur J Surg Oncol 2006; 32:941-947.

6

Single-Incision Laparoscopic Colectomy: A New Era in the Treatment of Colorectal Cancer?

Fabio Cianchi, Fabio Staderini and Benedetta Badii

1. Introduction

The laparoscopic technique has been enthusiastically applied to the resection of colorectal cancer for more than 15 years [1]. There is evidence that laparoscopy for colorectal cancer offers the opportunity for a meticulous dissection of the mesocolon and mesorectum under direct vision while facilitating a true no-touch technique [2]. Additional benefits, such as less postoperative pain, reduced need for postoperative analgesia, less ileus, shorter hospital stay, less blood loss, and better cosmesis are also well documented [3,4].

During recent years, great effort has been made to minimize parietal trauma for cosmetic reasons and to further reduce surgery-related pain and morbidity. New techniques, such as natural orifice transluminal endoscopic surgery (NOTES) [5] have been developed in order to reach the goal of "scarless" surgery. Although NOTES actually allows for no scarring of the body surface, it has several disadvantages and limitations with the currently available instruments, including limited access, less familiar working angles and operative approaches. Furthermore, it is associated with possible complications caused by opening of the stomach, colon or vagina, and may not be fully suitable or safe for advanced procedures, such as colectomies [6].

Single incision laparoscopic surgery (SILS) is currently regarded as the next major advance in minimally invasive surgical approaches to colorectal disease that is more feasible for generalized use [7-10]. SILS reduces the invasiveness of laparoscopic conventional surgery (LCS) by decreasing the number of incisions and ports through the abdominal wall. This theoretically could provide important clinical advantages, including less postoperative pain, reduction of port-site associated morbidity (such as wound infection, bleeding, visceral injury and port site herniation), quicker recovery and shorter hospital stay. The small incision through the abdominal wall allows for "scarless" surgery as the wound is usually hidden within the umbilicus, thus providing potentially better cosmesis. Moreover, SILS permits surgeons to use familiar standard laparoscopic instruments but also perform complex procedures, such as colorectal operations, which require extraction of large surgical specimens or intestinal anastomosis.

2. Technical aspects of SILS

SILS was first reported in 1992 by gynecologists who performed single-incision hysterectomy [11]. The performance of the first transumbilical cholecystectomy was published in 1999 [12] and the first single-incision appendectomy was reported in 1998 [13]. The use of SILS in colorectal surgery was first reported in 2008 by Remzi and co-workers [8] and Bucher and colleagues [14].

Since these first reports, it has been evident that SILS raises a number of specific new challenges compared with LCS. The skills required for SILS are different from those needed in conventional multiport laparoscopy, even for experienced laparoscopic surgeons [15]. The handling of straight instruments in parallel with the laparoscope through a small single incision decreases the freedom of movement for the surgeon, and complicates the holding of the laparoscope for the assistant and instruments for the surgeon. The most outstanding technical challenges involved in SILS are the following:

1. Loss of triangulation with straight instruments: the loss of this dogmatic principle of laparoscopic surgery often imposes the need to operate with crossed hands and does not allow an ergonomically favorable position for the surgeon and assistants. The inherent technical challenge is that the visual axis becomes more axial or in-line, so a movement of the camera often results in a inadvertent movement of an adjacent instrument, thus increasing the difficulty of performing even relatively simple tasks.

2. Restricted number of working instruments and thus difficulty of achieving correct exposure and the necessary traction to tissues.

3. Restricted external working space: the multiple instruments and laparoscopes required for a procedure are competing for the same space at the fulcrum of the entry port, causing external hand collisions and difficulty with instrument tip manipulation internally.

4. Difficulty in maintaining pneumoperitoneum.

5. Requirement of training and adjustment.

New operative hardware is being developed to facilitate the technique [16]. Many of the big healthcare manufacturers have developed multilumen access devices to allow for the insertion of several instruments through a single large fascial incision (Figure 1).

Initially, these devices offered three openings with limited gas inflow and outflow, but we are now seeing revision of the devices, incorporating more access ports so standard laparoscopic dissection techniques can be utilized. Newly designed equipment, such as

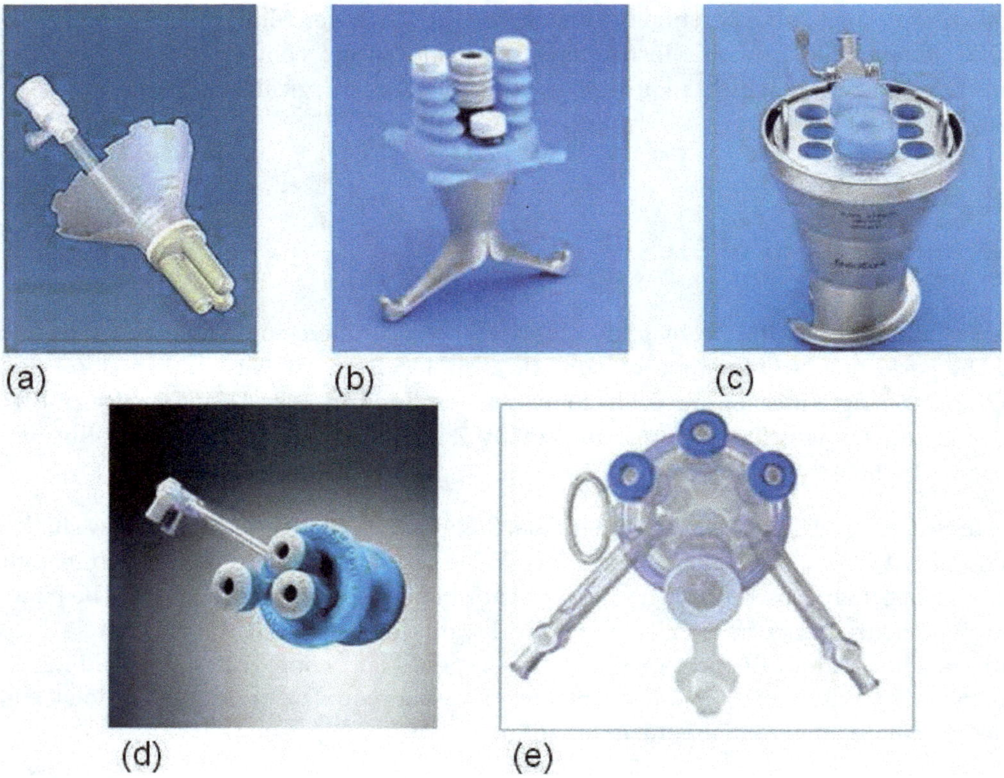

Figure 1. Single port systems: (a) Uni-x (Pnavel Systems, Morganville, New Jersey, USA); (b) X-Cone (Karl Storz, Tuttlingen, Germany); (c) Endo-Cone (Karl Storz, Tuttlingen, Germany); (d) SILS Port (Covidien, Norwalk, Connecticut, USA); (e) Olympus TriPort + (Advanced Surgical Concepts, Bray, Ireland.

articulating or curved instruments and flexible scopes, have been introduced to recreate triangulation (Figure 2).

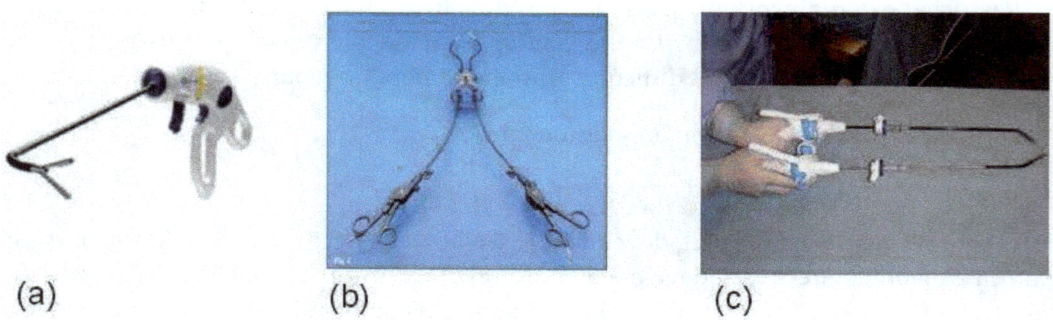

Figure 2. Articulating and curved instruments for SILS: (a) SILS Hand Instrument (Covidien, Norwalk, Connecticut, USA); (b) The Cuschieri Coaxial Deviating Instruments (Karl Storz, Tuttlingen, Germany); (c) Cambridge Endo Instruments (Cambridge Endoscopic Devices, Framingham, Massachusetts, USA).

Moreover, the introduction of an extra-long, 5 mm laparoscope allows placement of the camera on a different plane from the other instruments and help in moving the operator's hand further apart to avoid handle collision (Figure 3) [17]. All these devices have made single site surgery easier and more efficient.

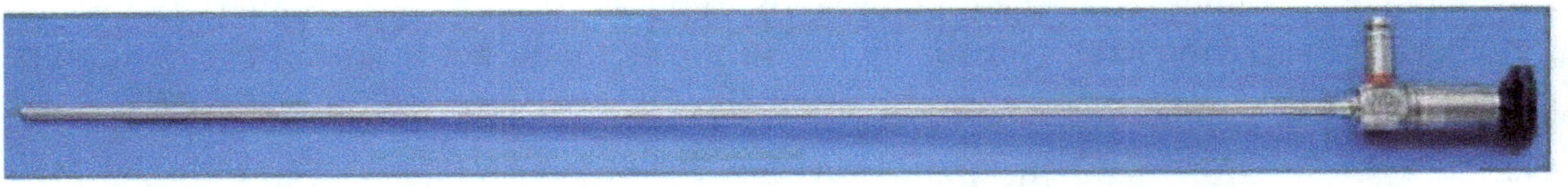

Figure 3. Extra-long, 5 mm, 30° laparoscope (Karl Storz, Tuttlingen, Germany).

3. Feasibility and safety of single-incision colectomy

All the challenges encountered with single-port surgery are magnified with colorectal procedures. Unlike laparoscopic cholecystectomy or appendicectomy, which involve surgery in only one abdominal quadrant, single-incision laparoscopic colectomy often requires operating in different abdominal quadrants. In addition, the need for adequate oncological margins and the creation of a tension-free anastomosis are essential. Although the use of this new approach for complex colorectal procedures might understandingly be viewed as difficult to implement, over the past few years there has been significant interest in SILS for colonic resections in both benign and malignant conditions. In fact, between 2008 and 2012, a nearly 7-fold increase occurred in the number of articles related to single-port colorectal surgery [18-20]. Unfortunately, the currently available literature relating to the technique includes mostly case reports or small case series describing the feasibility, safety and technical difficulties of different operations [21-42]. There are very few studies comparing SILS to LCS and there is a need for randomized controlled trials to definitively establish that SILS is no different from standard laparoscopic surgery in terms of completion rates, complications and oncological adequacy but with the advantage of being more cosmetic with subsequently reduced morbidities including pain [43]. The studies published to date have a number of other flaws limiting their impact. These include low sample size, selection bias and difficulty in blinding the patients enrolled. The vast majority of studies involve a very carefully selected SILS cohort of uncomplicated cases, which significantly limits their generalization.

The most significant datum emerging from the literature is that colonic SILS has been offered to date to a highly selected group of patients [18,19]. This selection is based on two main parameters: body mass index (BMI) that is an indirect measure of visceral fat, and tumor site, that is directly linked to the type of surgical procedure.

It is well known that visceral fat is one the most critical factors in the identification of the correct surgical plane in laparoscopic surgery [44]. This concept is obviously amplified in SILS and visceral obesity is reported as the primary cause of conversion to multiport laparoscopy in most studies [45]. Therefore it is understandable that most patients who are candidates for this type of surgery had a low BMI. Makino et al. [18] have reviewed 23 studies with a total of 378 patients undergoing single-port colectomy. The mean value of BMI was 25.5 kg/m^2 in these patients. Similar results have been found by Fung et al. [19] in their recent review. These authors have analyzed 38 colonic SILS articles containing 565 patients and the median BMI was 25.8 kg/m^2. On the basis of these findings, some studies have suggested the use of preoperative abdominal computed tomography to predict accurately the pattern of visceral fat, allowing better selection of patients for SILS colectomy and reducing the number of conversions [44].

The other factor that has markedly influenced the currently available data on SILS for colorectal cancer is the type of surgical procedure. Makino et al. [18] have reported that 279 (73.8%) of the 378 procedures analyzed in their review were right hemicolectomy, followed by sigmoidectomy (n = 27), performed essentially for diverticular disease, and anterior resection of the rectum (n = 20). Moreover, a high number of published studies have specifically limited the analysis of safety, feasibility and short-term results to only single-port right hemicolectomy [14,25,32-38,42,45-48], thus demonstrating that this type of procedure is the least complex to perform with the single-port technique at the beginning of the experience. Actually, right hemicolectomy involves surgery only in one/two quadrants while left procedures require operating in a multitude of different and opposite abdominal quadrants, from the hypochondrium for splenic flexure mobilization to the pelvis for a total mesorectal excision (TME). Moreover, in right hemicolectomy the surgeon has the possibility of creating an extracorporeal intestinal anastomosis through umbilical access while in left colectomies and anterior resection of the rectum the anastomosis is intracorporeal, thus augmenting the complexity of the procedure.

These considerations clearly show that there is an inevitable case-selection bias in assessing the outcomes of colo-rectal SILS from published studies. Although randomized controlled trials comparing single-port and multi-port right hemicolectomy have not been reported yet, the most significant data available to date relate to this type of procedure. In 2012, the two largest experiences with single-port right hemicolectomies in a single institution have been reported. Waters et al. [49] analyzed the short-term outcomes with single-incision right hemicolectomy in 100 patients. Operative indications were oncological in 92 patients, 57 for adenocarcinoma and 35 for polyps not suitable for endoscopic removal. Morbidity (13%) and mortality (1%) rates were acceptable as well as operative time (median value, 105 minutes) and conversion rate to multiport or open procedures (2% and 4%, respectively). Most importantly, there was no compromise of oncological adequacy with no positive tumor margins and a mean number of 18 lymph nodes retrieved and examined in the surgical specimens. Interestingly, patients with a wide range of BMI measurements were offered single-incision right hemicolectomy, with the largest approaching superobesity at a BMI of 46 kg/m^2 and a mean patient BMI of 28. Unfortunately, no results regarding postoperative pain, cosmetic results or direct comparison with the multi-port laparoscopic approach were reported.

Chew et al. [50] have reported the short outcomes of single-incision laparoscopic hemicolectomy in 40 consecutive patients. These results were compared with those of 104 conventional laparoscopic hemicolectomies. Indications for surgery were oncological in the majority of patients in the two groups. The authors found that single-incision right hemicolectomy is a feasible and safe procedure with equivalent outcomes in terms of operative time, oncological adequacy, postoperative morbidity, and conversions when compared with conventional laparoscopic right hemicolectomy. In particular, there were no differences in lymph node retrieval (median value of 18 and 19 lymph nodes for multi-port and single-port surgery, respectively) and resection margin clearance.

The data regarding left sided procedures, in particular anterior resection of the rectum for cancer, are much more limited. This is mainly due to the complexity of these procedures, in particular some surgical steps such as mobilizing the splenic flexure and dissection of the mesorectum. The fairly great distance of the spleen and the deep pelvis from the umbilicus amplify the difficulty of creating instrument triangulation, especially when standard, straight laparoscopic instruments are used. Even adequate traction of the rectum and stapling procedures have been associated with technical difficulties and adjunctive methods of traction and suspension such as transparietal suture, are frequently needed to achieve adequate surgical exposure [51-56]. Bulut et al. [57] have recently reported their early experience in single-incision surgery for rectal cancer treatment. This study was conducted on 10, highly selected patients: the mean tumor diameter was very small (3.2 cm), BMI was ≤25 in all patients and 8 of them were females, thus providing the advantages of a wide pelvis and relative lack of visceral fat. Although the authors stated that single-incision surgery for rectal cancer can be performed safely in this kind of patient, the overall mean operation time was quite long (240 min) and 6 patients received stomas (4 had diverting ileostomy after anterior resection of the rectum and 2 had colostomy after Hartmann procedure and abdominoperineal resection). Moreover, mesorectum excision was classified as nearly complete in 4 patients and the median number of examined lymph nodes was quite low, namely 14.

One of the most challenging maneuvers in single-incision rectal surgery is maintaining an adequate operative field during TME. Uematsu et al. [54] have proposed a new rectum-suspending system composed of a suspending bar and a bowel clamp with an extracorporeal magnetic tool. This apparatus, along with single access through the right iliac fossa instead of the umbilicus, allowed the authors to perform TME and transect the rectum by ensuring a proper tension. Nevertheless, the proposed new technique is actually complex and, as the authors stated, is not recommended for males with narrow pelvis or obese individuals or when mobilization of the splenic flexure is required because of the distance between the spleen and the single access through the right iliac fossa. Altogether, these data clearly show that some unresolved issues still remain in performing SILS for the treatment of rectal cancer.

There are more data, which are somewhat more reliable regarding other less complex left-sided procedures, such as left hemicolectomy or sigmoidectomy [52,58-60]. In fact, sigmoidectomy is the most frequent procedure performed for benign left-side pathology, predominantly diverticular disease or large colonic polyps not suitable for endoscopic removal. Recently, Vestweber et al. [61] have reported the largest series of patients undergoing single-incision colorectal surgery in a single institution. One hundred and fifty out of 244 procedures were sigmoidectmy (n = 145) with left hemicolectomies (n = 4) and high anterior resection of the rectum (n = 1). Most of these patients were operated on for diverticular disease (n = 142) followed by colonic polyps (n = 4) and colonic cancer (n = 4). The mean operative time for left-sided procedures was 146 ± 48 min and in all cases standard straight, non-articulating laparoscopic instruments along with ultrasonic or radiofrequency dissector/sealer were used. It seems that the authors did not experience any particular technical problems in performing these types of procedures that do not actually need wide splenic flexure mobilization or mesorectal dissection. The fairly higher incidence of early postoperative complications (12.6%) than rates stated in the literature, was imputed to the high rate of severe, complicated diverticular disease rather than to the complexity of single-incision procedure.

The literature concerning subtotal colectomy or proctocolectomy (with or without ileoanal anastomosis), at this time consists only of case reports and a few small case series [62-68]. The predominant indication for this type of operation has been ulcerative colitis followed by polyposis coli [64,65,67]. Overall, 36 single-incision total colectomies have been reported in the literature: these studies have demonstrated the feasibility and safety of single-incision technique even in these more complex colonic procedures but cannot provide any comparative results with traditional laparoscopy. It is likely that cosmetic results will be magnified by single-incision total colectomy since patients suffering from ulcerative colitis or polyposis coli are usually young and may prefer a small incision hidden in the umbilicus. If an ileostomy is scheduled, the single incision is usually performed in the right lower quadrant of the abdomen and the terminal ileum is brought out through this port-site, thus minimizing the traumatic and cosmetic impact of the procedure.

4. Comparison between single-incision and conventional laparoscopic colectomy

As all these data indicate, there are still several limitations to an analysis of the adequacy of single-incision technique in the treatment of colorectal cancer. The most important limiting factor in the interpretation of reported outcomes is the careful selection of patients, with an almost 3-fold predominance of right-sided pathology, a low to average BMI and non-bulky colonic disease. If this case-selection bias is taken into account and the oncological adequacy of a single-incision procedure is hypothetically accepted, this innovation would be justified only in the presence of clear short-term benefits over conventional laparoscopic colonic surgery. These benefits should comprise a lower complication rate, reduced postoperative pain, faster recovery and better cosmesis.

To date, only two randomized trials have compared short-term outcomes after single-incision and conventional laparoscopic colectomies for colon cancer. In 2011, Huscher et al. [69] reported the results of a study conducted on 32 patients, with 16 in the single-incision and 16 in the conventional laparoscopic group. Although the authors confirmed the safety and technical feasibility of single-incision colectomy, they did not show any superiority of the procedure over conventional laparoscopy in terms of postoperative morbidity, resumption of oral liquid/solid food intake and length of hospital stay.

More recently, Poon et al. [70] reported findings from a randomized controlled trial, which enrolled 50 patients, 25 in each study group. As expected, the patients were carefully selected in regard to BMI (median value, 23.2 kg/m^2) and tumor size (< 4 cm). On the contrary, there was a predominance of left-sided procedures, with 14 anterior resections, 1 sigmoidectomy, 2 left hemicolectomies and only 8 right hemicolectomies in the single-incision group. The authors did not find any statistically significant difference in operative outcome and oncological adequacy between the single-incision and the conventional laparoscopic group. Interestingly, they found a lower postoperative pain score and shorter median hospital stay in the single-incision group. Although these findings emerge from a randomized controlled trial, they cannot be considered definitive due the low number of patients involved in the study.

Two recent meta-analyses have addressed the issue of comparison between SILS and LCS for both benign and malignant colorectal diseases [71,72]. Both studies have been published in 2012 and thus have included all the comparative studies published to date with the exception of the above mentioned randomized trial by Poon et al. Notwithstanding the heterogeneity of the analyzed studies (14 by Zhou et al. and 15 by Yang et al) in terms of type of procedures performed, indication for surgery, different patient inclusion and exclusion criteria, neither meta-analysis found any significant difference in the incidence of postoperative complications or operative time between single-incision and conventional laparoscopic colectomy. Importantly, they show that patients undergoing single-incision colectomy had a significantly shorter length of hospital stay, significantly shorter incision length, significantly less estimated blood loss, and significantly more lymph nodes harvested during oncological resections. Unfortunately, the two pooled analyses were not able to compare the pain score due to lack of data, the differences in scoring methods and in postoperative care and pain management in the available reported data. However, at least three studies [48,73,74] show a significant decrease in pain scores for patients undergoing single-incision colectomy compared to conventional laparoscopy. The decreased pain score is likely due to less surgical trauma as a consequence of eliminating the additional ports at separate sites on the abdominal wall. There is no meta-analysis regarding cosmetic results due to absence of adequate information on this interesting outcome in the individual studies. Only one study reported cosmetic score results with an advantage for SILS over LCS [23]. However, it is logical to assume that a shorter final incision length in single-incision surgery results in improved cosmetic satisfaction for the majority of the patients.

Another important issue emerging from the literature data is that experienced laparoscopic surgeons have performed almost all single-incision colectomies. This implies that SILS is offered not only to a select group of patients but is also performed by a select group of surgeons. It might appear premature to propose a complex and technically challenging evolution of conventional laparoscopy colectomy when this has yet to be fully accepted as a gold standard in the treatment of colorectal cancer [75]. It must be considered that in 2010, only about 20% of colorectal resections in England and in other countries were performed laparoscopically [76]. Therefore, although the principles of SILS are highly attractive, they might not, at this moment, be transferable and proposed to the general community of surgeons.

The last but not least important concern about single-incision colectomy regards the costs. It is logical to expect an initial increase in costs associated with SILC over conventional laparoscopic surgery since the additional equipment such as single-incision access ports or flexible/articulating instruments are still relatively new. In their analysis of single-incision right-hemicolectomy, Waters et al. [46] found a marginal increase in direct operative cost of US $310 to $410 per case. If patients have a shorter length of hospital stay, and consequently, a quicker return to work and normal activity after single-incision surgery, it is likely there will be an improvement in the cost-effectiveness of SILS in the future.

5. Conclusion

Most of the current studies on single-incision colectomy for cancer are observational and lack statistical power due to the relatively low number of patients studied. Although meta-analyses can increase the statistical power by pooling results of all available trials, only randomized, controlled studies can provide high levels of evidence. To date, only two randomized controlled studies have compared short-term results between single-incision and conventional laparoscopic surgery and, unfortunately, even these studies have enrolled a very low number of patients. Bearing in mind these limitations, we can still glean several important factors from these published series:

1. Colonic SILS is technically demanding but the introduction of new specialized equipment including multilumen ports, angled scopes, articulated instruments and instruments of variable length, will eventually reduce this difficulty.

2. Principles of colonic SILS are attractive and applicable in carefully selected groups of patients, namely with right-sided pathology, low BMI and non-bulky tumors.

3. In the hands of experienced laparoscopic surgeons, colonic SILS in the above mentioned patients has been demonstrated to be safe and feasible with rates of surgery-related complications and mortality, operative time and oncological adequacy comparable with those of conventional laparoscopy.

4. Two meta-analyses and one randomized controlled study provide evidence in support of some advantages of SILS over conventional laparoscopy, namely, shorter length of hospital stay, significantly shorter incision length and significantly less estimated blood loss; other hypothesized benefits, such as reduction in postoperative pain and improvement of cosmesis remain unproven.

Further high-powered randomized studies comparing SILS and LCS by using standardized outcome assessment tools are needed to confirm or not the above-mentioned results. But one thing is certain: we will not see the same dramatic clinical advantages with the passage from LCS to SILS as we saw with the advent of laparoscopic technique over open surgery.

Furthermore, the more complex the procedure performed by single-incision surgery, the more likely are there to be advantages in comparison with conventional laparoscopic procedures.

In this prospective, a possible field of investigation might be the assessment of systemic stress response of single-incision versus conventional laparoscopy in colorectal surgery. The reduced parietal trauma and manipulation of the peritoneum could decrease the postoperative inflammatory response to surgical stress and as a consequence, more efficient immunocompetency against tumor cells might be maintained since the earliest postoperative days [77,78]. All these factors might influence the long-term oncological results of SILS with a potential improvement in survival rates of patients operated on for colorectal cancer.

Author details

Fabio Cianchi[1,2*], Fabio Staderini[1,2] and Benedetta Badii[1,2]

*Address all correspondence to: fabio.cianchi@unifi.it

1 Department of Surgery and Translational Medicine, Center of Oncological Minimally Invasive Surgery, University of Florence, Italy

2 Unit of Endocrine and Minimally Invasive Surgery, AOU Careggi, Florence, Italy

References

[1] Jacob BP, Salky B. Laparoscopic colectomy for colon adenocarcinoma: an 11-year retrospective review with 5-year survival. Surg Endosc 2005;19 (5) 643-649.

[2] Lujan HJ, Plasencia G, Jacobs M, Viamonte M 3rd, Hartmann RF. Long-term survival after laparoscopic colon resection for cancer: complete five-year follow-up. Dis Colon Rectum 2002;45 (4) 491-501.

[3] Guillou PJ, Quirke P, Thorpe H, Walker J, Jayne DG, Smith AM, Heath RM, Brown JM; MRC CLASICC trial group. Short-term end points of conventional versus laparoscopic-assisted surgery in patients with colorectal cancer (MRC CLASSICC trial): multicentre, randomized controlled trial. Lancet 2005;365 (9472) 1718-1726.

[4] Clinical outcomes of surgical therapy (COST) study group. A comparison of laparoscopically assisted and open colectomy for colon cancer. N Engl J Med 2004;350 (20) 2050-2059.

[5] Gumbs AA, Fowler D, Milone L, Evanko JC, Ude AO, Stevens P, Bessler M. Transvaginal natural orifice transluminal endoscopic surgery cholecystectomy: early evolution of the technique. Ann Surg 2009;249 (6) 908-912

[6] Brunner W, Schirnhofer J, Waldstein-Wartenberg N, Frass R, Weiss H. Single incision laparoscopic sigmoid colon resections without visible scar: a novel technique. Colorectal Dis. 2010;12(1) 66-70.

[7] Romanelli JR, Earle DB. Single-port laparoscopic surgery: an overview. Surg Endosc 2009;23 (7) 1419-1427.

[8] Remzi FH, Kirat HT, Kaouk JH, Geisler DP. Single port laparoscopy in colorectal surgery. Colorectal Dis 2008;10 (8) 823-826.

[9] Bucher P, Pugin F, Morel P. Transumbilical single incision laparoscopic sigmoidectomy for benign disease. Colorectal Dis 2009;12 (1) 61-65

[10] Curcillo PG 2nd, Podolsky ER, King SA. The road to reduced port surgery: from single big incisions to single small incisions, and beyond. World J Surg 2011;35 (7) 1526-1531

[11] Pelosi MA, Pelosi MA 3rd. Laparoscopic supracervical hysterectomy using a single-umbilical puncture (mini-laparoscopy). J Reprod Med. 1992;37(9) 777-784.

[12] Bresadola F, Pasqualucci A, Donini A, Chiarandini P, Anania G, Terrosu G, Sistu MA, Pasetto A. Elective transumbilical compared with standard laparoscopic cholecystectomy. Eur J Surg. 1999;165(1) 29-34.

[13] Esposito C. One-trocar appendectomy in pediatric surgery. Surg Endosc. 1998;12(2)177-178.

[14] Bucher P, Pugin F, Morel P. Single port access laparoscopic right hemicolectomy. Int J Colorectal Dis. 2008;23(10) 1013-1016

[15] Islam A, Castellvi AO, Tesfay ST, Castellvi AD, Wright AS, Scott DJ. Early surgeon impressions and technical difficulty associated with laparoendoscopic single-site surgery: a Society of American Gastrointestinal and Endoscopic Surgeons learning center study. Surg Endosc 2011:25 (8) 2597-2603.

[16] Chew MH, Wong MT, Lim BY, Ng KH, Eu KW. Evaluation of current devices in single-incision laparoscopic colorectal surgery: a preliminary experience in 32 consecutive cases. World J Surg. 2011;35(4) 873-880.

[17] Dhumane P, Diana M, Leroy J, Marescaux J. Minimally invasive single-site surgery for the digestive system: a technological review. J Minim Access Surg 2011;7 (1) 40-51.

[18] Makino T, Milsom JW, Lee SW. Feasibility and safety of single-incision laparoscopic colectomy: a systematic review. Ann Surg. 2012;255(4) 667-676.

[19] Fung AK, Aly EH. Systematic review of single-incision laparoscopic colonic surgery. Br J Surg. 2012;99(10) 1353-1364.

[20] Diana M, Dhumane P, Cahill RA, Mortensen N, Leroy J, Marescaux J. Minimal invasive single-site surgery in colorectal procedures: Current state of the art. J Minim Access Surg. 2011;7(1) 52-60.

[21] Bucher P, Pugin F, Morel P. Single-port access laparoscopic radical left colectomy in humans. Dis Colon Rectum 2009;52 (10) 1797–1801.

[22] Brunner W, Schirnhofer J, Waldstein-Wartenberg N, Frass R, Weiss H. Single incision laparoscopic sigmoid colon resections without visible scar: a novel technique. Colorectal Dis 2010;12 (1) 66–70.

[23] Lee SW, Milsom JW, Nash GM. Single-incision versus multiport laparoscopic right and hand-assisted left colectomy: a case-matched comparison. Dis Colon Rectum 2011;54(11) 1355–1361.

[24] Gash KJ, Goede AC, Chambers W, Greenslade GL, Dixon AR. Laparoendoscopic single-site surgery is feasible in complex colorectal resections and could enable day case colectomy. Surg Endosc 2011;25(3) 835–840.

[25] Keshava A, Mackenzie S, Al-Kubati W. Single-port laparoscopic right colonic resection. ANZ J Surg 2010; 80(1-2) 30–32.

[26] Ross H, Steele S, Whiteford M, Lee S, Albert M, Mutch M et al. Early multi-institution experience with single-incision laparoscopic colectomy. Dis Colon Rectum 2011;54 (2) 187–192.

[27] Lu CC, Lin SE, Chung KC, Rau KM. Comparison of clinical outcome of single incision laparoscopic surgery using a simplified access system with conventional laparoscopic surgery for malignant colorectal disease. Colorectal Dis 2012;14 (4) 171–176

[28] Gaujoux S, Bretagnol F, Ferron M, Panis Y. Single-incision laparoscopic colonic surgery. Colorectal Dis 2011;13 (9) 1066–1071

[29] Geisler D, Garrett T. Single incision laparoscopic colorectal surgery: a single surgeon experience of 102 consecutive cases. Tech Coloproctol 2011; 15 (4) 397–401.

[30] Ramos-Valadez DI, Patel CB, Ragupathi M, Bokhari MB, Pickron TB, Haas EM. Single-incision laparoscopic colectomy: outcomes of an emerging minimally invasive technique. Int J Colorectal Dis 2011;26 (6) 761–767.

[31] van den Boezem PB, Sietses C. Single-incision laparoscopic colorectal surgery, experience with 50 consecutive cases. J Gastrointest Surg 2011;15 (11) 1989–1994.

[32] Adair J, Gromski MA, Lim RB, Nagle D. Single-incision laparoscopic right colectomy: experience with 17 consecutive cases and comparison with multiport laparoscopic right colectomy. Dis Colon Rectum 2010;53 (11) 1549–1554.

[33] Boni L, Dionigi G, Cassinotti E, Di Giuseppe M, Diurni M, Rausei S et al. Single incision laparoscopic right colectomy. Surg Endosc 2010;24 (12) 3233–3236.

[34] Keshava A, Young CJ, Mackenzie S. Single-incision laparoscopic right hemicolectomy. Br J Surg 2010;97 (12) 1881–1883.

[35] Lim YK, Ng KH, Eu KW. Single site laparoscopic right hemicolectomy: an oncological feasible option. World J Surg Oncol 2010;8 (8) 79.

[36] Pietrasanta D, Romano N, Prosperi V, Lorenzetti L, Basili G, Goletti O. Single-incision laparoscopic right colectomy for cancer: a single-centre preliminary experience. Updates Surg 2010; 62(2) 111–115.

[37] O'Connor DJ, Feinberg E, Jang J, Vemulapalli P, Camacho D. Single-incision laparoscopic-assisted right colon resection for cancer. JSLS 2010;14 (4) 558–560.

[38] Ramos-Valadez DI, Patel CB, Ragupathi M, Bartley Pickron T, Haas EM. Single-incision laparoscopic right hemicolectomy: safety and feasibility in a series of consecutive cases. Surg Endosc 2010;24 (10) 2613–2616.

[39] Cianchi F, Qirici E, Trallori G, Mallardi B, Badii B, Perigli G. Single-incision laparoscopic colectomy: technical aspects and short-term results. Updates Surg 2011;64(1) 19-23.

[40] Katsuno G, Fukunaga M, Nagakari K, Yoshikawa S, Ouchi M, Hirasaki Y. Single-incision laparoscopic colectomy for colon cancer: early experience with 31 cases. Dis Colon Rectum 2011;54 (6) 705–710.

[41] Papaconstantinou HT, Thomas JS. Single-incision laparoscopic colectomy for cancer: assessment of oncologic resection and short-term outcomes in a case-matched comparison with standard laparoscopy. Surgery 2011;150 (4) 820–807.

[42] Saber AA, El-Ghazaly TH. Single-incision transumbilical laparoscopic right hemicolectomy using SILS port. Am Surg 2011;77 (2) 252–253.

[43] Arezzo A, Morino M. Endoscopic surgery through single-port incision: time for a trial?. Surg Endosc. 2011; 25(6) 1709-1711.

[44] Tsujinaka S, Konishi F, Kawamura YJ, Saito M, Tajima N, Tanaka O et al. Visceral obesity predicts surgical outcomes after laparoscopic colectomy for sigmoid colon cancer. Dis Colon Rectum 2008;51 (12) 1757–1765.

[45] Chen WT, Chang SC, Chiang HC, Lo WY, Jeng LB, Wu C et al. Single-incision laparoscopic versus conventional laparoscopic right hemicolectomy: a comparison of short-term surgical results. Surg Endosc 2011;25 (6) 1887–1892.

[46] Waters JA, Guzman MJ, Fajardo AD, Selzer DJ, Wiebke EA, Robb BW et al. Single-port laparoscopic right hemicolectomy: a safe alternative to conventional laparoscopy. Dis Colon Rectum 2010;53 (11) 1467–1472.

[47] Wong MT, Ng KH, Ho KS, Eu KW. Single-incision laparoscopic surgery for right hemicolectomy: our initial experience with 10 cases. Tech Coloproctol 2010;14 (3) 225–258.

[48] Papaconstantinou HT, Sharp N, Thomas JS. Single-incision laparoscopic right colectomy: a case-matched comparison with standard laparoscopic and hand-assisted laparoscopic techniques. J Am Coll Surg 2011;213 (1) 72–80.

[49] Waters JA, Rapp BM, Guzman MJ, Jester AL, Selzer DJ, Robb BW, Johansen BJ, Tsai BM, Maun DC, George VV. Single-port laparoscopic right hemicolectomy: the first 100 resections. Dis Colon Rectum. 2012;55(2) 134-139

[50] Chew MH, Chang MH, Tan WS, Wong MT, Tang CL. 1.Conventional laparoscopic versus single-incision laparoscopic right hemicolectomy: a case cohort comparison of short-term outcomes in 144 consecutive cases. Surg Endosc. 2012 18. [Epub ahead of print].

[51] Uematsu D, Akiyama G, Magishi A, Nakamura J, Hotta K. Single-access laparoscopic left and right hemicolectomy combined with extracorporeal magnetic retraction. Dis Colon Rectum 2010;53 (6) 944–948.

[52] Takemasa I, Sekimoto M, Ikeda M, Mizushima T, Yamamoto H, Doki Y, Mori M. Video. Transumbilical single-incision laparoscopic surgery for sigmoid colon cancer. Surg Endosc 2010; 24 (1) 2321.

[53] Law WL, Fan JK, Poon JT. Single incision laparoscopic left colectomy for carcinoma of distal transverse colon. Colorectal Dis 2010;12 (7) 698–701.

[54] Uematsu D, Akiyama G, Narita M, Magishi A. Single-access laparoscopic low anterior resection with vertical suspension of the rectum. Dis Colon Rectum 2011;54 (5) 632–637.

[55] Co CS, Cheung HY, Yau KK, Chung CC, Li M. Combined single-port and endoluminal technique for laparoscopic anterior resection. Surg Laparosc Endosc Percutan Tech 2010;20 (4) 253–256.

[56] Kawahara H, Watanabe K, Ushigome T, Noaki R, Kobayashi S, Yanaga K. Umbilical incision laparoscopic surgery with one assist port for anterior resection. Dig Surg 2010;27 (5) 364–366.

[57] Bulut O, Nielsen CB, Jespersen N. Single-port access laparoscopic surgery for rectal cancer: initial experience with 10 cases. Dis Colon Rectum. 2011; 54(7) 803-809

[58] Remzi FH, Kirat HT, Geisler DP. Laparoscopic single-port colectomy for sigmoid cancer. Tech Coloproctol 2010;14 (3) 253–255.

[59] Uematsu D, Akiyama G, Matsuura M, Hotta K. Single-access laparoscopic colectomy with a novel multiport device in sigmoid colectomy for colon cancer. Dis Colon Rectum 2010;53 (4) 496–501.

[60] Ramos-Valadez DI, Ragupathi M, Nieto J, Patel CB, Miller S, Pickron TB et al. Single-incision versus conventional laparoscopic sigmoid colectomy: a case-matched series. Surg Endosc 2012;26 (1) 96–102.

[61] Vestweber B, Galetin T, Lammerting K, Paul C, Giehl J, Straub E, Kaldowski B, Alfes A, Vestweber KH. Single-incision laparoscopic surgery: outcomes from 224 colonic resections performed at a single center using SILS™. Surg Endosc. 2013; 27 (2) 434-442.

[62] Geisler DP, Condon ET, Remzi FH. Single incision laparoscopic total proctocolectomy with ileopouch anal anastomosis. Colorectal Dis 2010;12 (9) 941–943.

[63] Nagpal A, Soni H, Haribhakti S. Single-incision laparoscopic restorative proctocolectomy with ileal pouch anal anastomosis for ulcerative colitis: first Indian experience and literature review. Int J Colorectal Dis 2011;26 (4) 525–526.

[64] Fichera A, Zoccali M, Gullo R. Single incision ('scarless') laparoscopic total abdominal colectomy with end ileostomy for ulcerative colitis. J Gastrointest Surg 2011;15 (7) 1247–1251.

[65] Cahill RA, Lindsey I, Jones O, Guy R, Mortensen N, Cunningham C. Single-port laparoscopic total colectomy for medically uncontrolled colitis. Dis Colon Rectum 2010;53 (8) 1143–1147.

[66] Geisler DP, Kirat HT, Remzi FH. Single-port laparoscopic total proctocolectomy with ileal pouch–anal anastomosis: initial operative experience. Surg Endosc 2011;25 (7) 2175–2178.

[67] Leblanc F, Makhija R, Champagne BJ, Delaney CP. Single incision laparoscopic total colectomy and proctocolectomy for benign disease: initial experience. Colorectal Dis 2011;13 (11) 1290–1293.

[68] Paranjape C, Ojo OJ, Carne D, Guyton D. Single-incision laparoscopic total colectomy. JSLS. 2012;16(1) 27-32.

[69] Huscher CG, Mingoli A, Sgarzini G, Mereu A, Binda B, Brachini G, Trombetta S. Standard laparoscopic versus single-incision laparoscopic colectomy for cancer: early results of a randomized prospective study. Am J Surg. 2012;204(1) 115-120.

[70] Poon JT, Cheung CW, Fan JK, Lo OS, Law WL. Single-incision versus conventional laparoscopic colectomy for colonic neoplasm: a randomized, controlled trial. Surg Endosc. 2012;26(10) 2729-2734.

[71] Zhou YM, Wu LP, Zhao YF, Xu DH, Li B. Single-incision versus conventional laparoscopy for colorectal disease: a meta-analysis. Dig Dis Sci. 2012;57(8) 2103-2112.

[72] Yang TX, Chua TC. Single-incision laparoscopic colectomy versus conventional multiport laparoscopic colectomy: a meta-analysis of comparative studies. Int J Colorectal Dis 2013;28 (1) 89-101.

[73] Kim SJ, Ryu GO, Choi BJ, Kim JG, Lee KJ, Lee SC, Oh ST. The short-term outcomes of conventional and single-port laparoscopic surgery for colorectal cancer. Ann Surg. 2011;254(6) 933-940

[74] Vasilakis V, Clark CE, Liasis L, Papaconstantinou HT. Noncosmetic benefits of single-incision laparoscopic sigmoid colectomy for diverticular disease: A case-matched comparison with multiport laparoscopic technique. J Surg Res 2013; 180 (2) 201-207.

[75] Hassan I, Advani V. Single incision laparoscopic colon surgery. Is the ride worth the curve? Colorectal Dis 2010;12 (9) 847–848.

[76] National Institute for Health and Clinical Excellence (NICE). NICE Implementation Uptake Report: Laparoscopic Surgery for Colorectal Cancer, 2010; http://www.nice.org.uk/ media/B4D/4A/UptakeReportColorectalCancer.pdf

[77] Sammour T, Kahokehr A, Chan S, Booth RJ, Hill AG. The humoral response after laparoscopic versus open colorectal surgery: a meta-analysis J Surg Res. 2010;164(1) 28-37.

[78] Huang C, Huang R, Jiang T, Huang K, Cao J, Qiu Z. Laparoscopic and open resection for colorectal cancer: an evaluation of cellular immunity. BMC Gastroenterol. 2010;28(10) 127.

7

Role of Tumour Markers in Diagnosis and Follow Up of Colorectal Cancer — Potential for Future Research

Robert Partyka

1. Introduction

1.1. Immunodiagnostics of Colorectal cancer — CEA and CA 19-9

Colorectal cancer is the second most common cancer in terms of incidence in men and women. Another concern is the high rate of morbidity and mortality in patients with this cancer. Therefore, researchers are constantly searching for new diagnostic methods that would enable the early detection of recurrent, clinically asymptomatic periods. The development of clinical immunodiagnostics has enriched oncology with the possibility of determining the quantity of glycoproteins and glycolipids in the blood of patients with cancer. These are called neoplastic markers. The usefulness of a neoplastic marker assay has been confirmed in diagnosing alimentary tract neoplasms, mainly in the early post-operative detection of a recurrence of neoplastic disease and in the evaluation of the efficacy of surgery.

According to an account published by The European Group on Tumor Markers (EGTM) of 2003, CEA is the main marker that is used in detecting colorectal cancer. It is important to point out, however, that approximately 10-15 % of patients do not produce CEA at all or that it is secreted in only minimal amounts. In such cases, the normal level of CEA concentration does not exclude the existence of a neoplasm even at an advanced stage. Therefore, the use of CA 19-9 as a tumor marker in diagnostics has been proposed.

1.1.1. Characteristic of CEA tumour marker

Carcinoembryonic antigen is a glycoprotein that contains about 60% carbohydrates. CEAs have epitopes that are specific to the neoplasm and epitopes that connect antibodies against nonspecific cross-reacting antigens (NCA, NCA2, BGP). Its upper normal range is 3 ng/ml [1, 2]

1.1.2. Characteristic of CA 19-9 tumour marker

The CA 19-9 Antigen is associated with gastrointestinal cancers. It occurs in the sialyated Lewis A blood group antigen that is produced in a small amount in the salivary and bronchial glands as well as in the pancreatic and bile ducts. This marker is very useful in the diagnosis of gastrointestinal cancers such as gastric, pancreatic, bile duct cancers and pancreatitis. Its upper normal range is 37 U/ml, but in approximately 1% of healthy people, concentrations reaching 120 U/ml have been detected [1, 2].

1.2. Aim of the study

The purpose of the study was to estimate the usefulness of selected neoplastic markers – conditioned by their location in the pre-operative and post-operative histological evaluations of patients with gastrointestinal cancers.

1.3. Material and methods

256 patients, both won men and women, aged 19-86, in whom colorectal cancer was diagnosed and histopathology was confirmed, were included into the research that was performed between 1991-1998.

Patients were divided into two groups according to the progression of the disease on the TMN scale and patients with a proctologic neoplasm on the Dukes and TMN scales. Neoplasm markers were marked in serum using commercial kits (blood samples were collected from the cubital vein and stored at -20°C after centrifugation). CEA and CA 19-9 were detected using the MEIA method using an Abbott's kit (USA). The upper normal range in healthy subjects is 3 ng/ml for CEA and 37 U/ml for CA 19-9.

The detection of neoplastic markers was performed in the Independent Laboratory of Clinical Immunodiagnostics at State Hospital No. 5 in Sosnowiec, Poland. Blood samples were collected preoperatively, in the first, second and third months after surgery and next after every 3 months for 2-5 years.

1.4. Results

The detection of neoplastic markers was extended about lab tests, abdominal ultrasonography; CT was performed in certain cases. Results were worked out using the t-Student test, the Cochran-Cox test, variance analysis (ANOVA) and the Shapiro-Wilk test for hardly large test.

Table I describes the results of the division of patients according to the stage of the disease on the TNM scale. The pre-operative CEA and CA 19-9 concentrations is presented in Figure 1 and Figure 2.

A pre-operative elevation of the CEA concentration in serum was found in 182 patients (71%). CEA did not exceed the normal range in the Dukes A group. CA 19-9 was increased in 83 (32%) patients in the Dukes C and D groups. The mean concentration of CEA and CA 19-9 changed according to the stage of the disease and were: Dukes A group – CEA ($\bar{x}$=1.82 ng/ml, CA 19-9 $\bar{x}$=12.45 U/ml, Dukes B group – CEA $\bar{x}$=5.97 ng/ml, CA 19-9 $\bar{x}$=15.37 U/ml, Dukes C group – CEA $\bar{x}$=7.42 ng/ml, CA 19-9 $\bar{x}$=55.73 U/ml, Dukes D group – CEA $\bar{x}$=17.97 ng/ml, CA 19-9 70.42 U/ml. In the post-operative follow-up, in which the Dukes D group was excluded, a recurrence was found in 53 patients, an elevation of CEA was found in 47 patients (88.6%) and CA 19-9 was found in 36 patients (67.9%). The recurrence was detected in 100% of the patients when an elevation of CEA CA 19-9 was accepted as a criterion. The results are shown in Figure 3.

Numbers of patients	Dukes scale	TNM scale
8	A	3 – T1N0M0 5 – T2N0M0
61	B	61 – T3N0M0
94	C	37 – T3N1M0 57 – T3N2M0
7	D	2 – T4N2M1 5 – T4N2M1

Table 1. The stages of the disease on the Dukes and TNM scales.

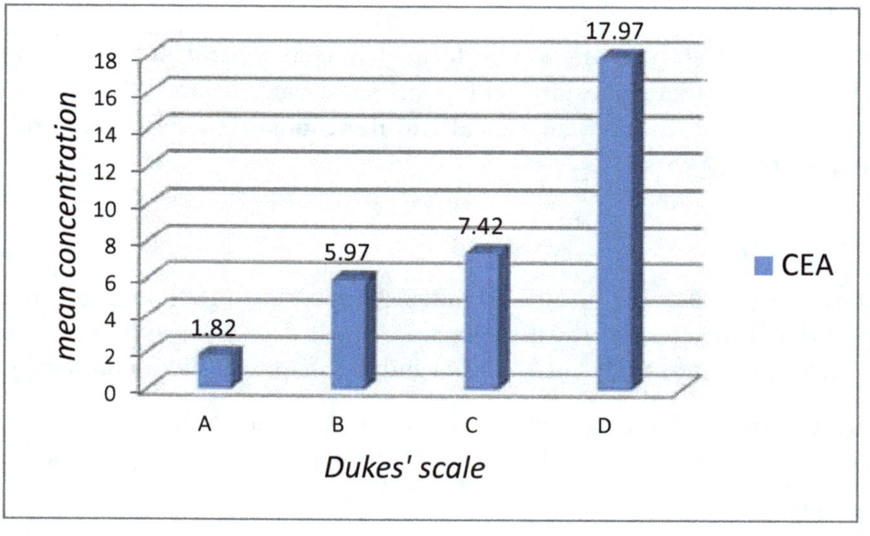

Figure 1. Mean concentration of CEA markers in pre-operative patients.

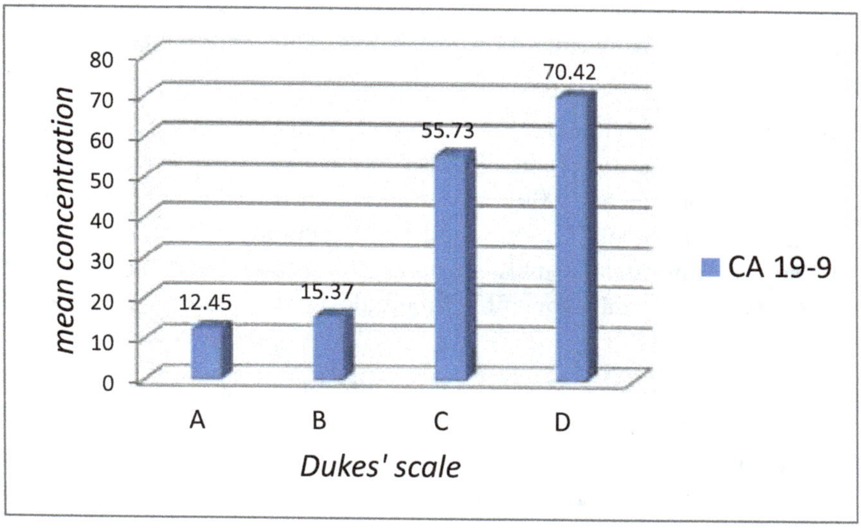

Figure 2. Mean concentration of CA 19-9 markers in pre-operative patients.

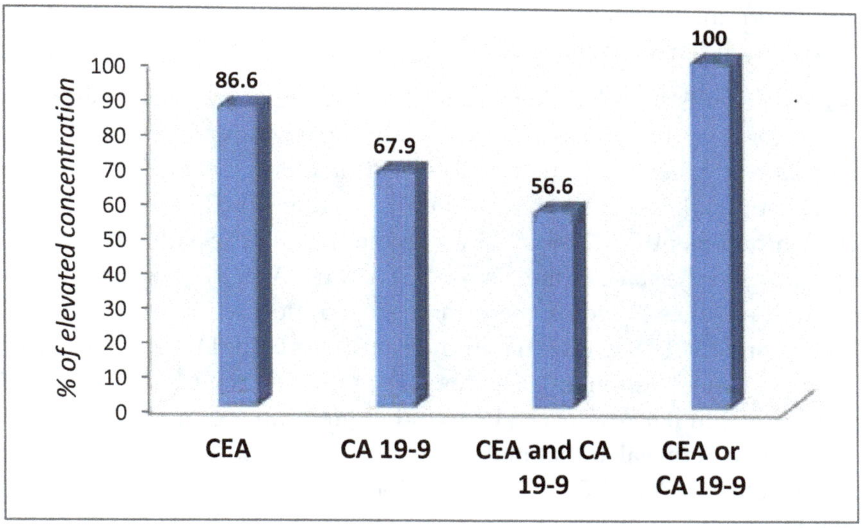

Figure 3. Percentage of CEA and CA 19-9 concentration in patients with a recurrence.

1.5. Discussion

Although the dreams of Bates et al. [3] to find an ideal marker for an active neoplastic process, i.e. that they have a different effect depending on the location of an organ and are absent in healthy people, were frustrated, neoplastic markers are now widely used in clinical diagnostics, usually for patients who have undergone surgery to remove cancerous tissue. Studies that lasted several years revealed that in order to estimate the efficacy of surgery, to detect a recurrence of a neoplastic process in the asymptomatic phase and to estimate the effectiveness of supplementary therapy, a determination of markers in the serum of patients plays a crucial role [1, 2, 4, 5, 6, 7, 8, 9].

Gold and Freedman [10] isolated carcinoembryonic antigen in colon cancer in 1966. They thought that it was specific to colorectal adenocarcinomas. The process of a quantitative determination of CEA in systemic fluids was described shortly thereafter, which indicated that more cancers produce CEA than had been previously thought. Moreover, it was found that its serum concentration may be higher than the normal range in non-neoplastic diseases such as pneumonia, bronchitis, tuberculosis, infections of the urinary tract and also in 30% of smokers [1, 10].

CEA is increased in non-neoplastic diseases of the intestines like colitis ulcerosa and Crohn's disease [1, 4, 11]. This information appeared to reduce the clinical value of a CEA assay; however, the development of monoclonal antibodies against CEA improved the specificity of the assays. This antigen is not present in the serum of all patients, even in a case of a recurrence, which was shown in studies that lasted for several years. Therefore, it is important to enhance clinical immunodiagnostics through the use of other markers (epitopes), which can use the information provided by the assay of CEA. The studies included 256 patients divided according to the stage of the cancer on the Dukes and TNM scales. Two neoplastic cancers CEA and CA 19-9 were determined in all 256 patients. Increased CEA was found in 182 patients (71%) and CA 19-9 was found in 83 patients (32%).

An analysis of the results revealed that in addition to CEA, CA 19-9 is an especially helpful marker. This agrees with the reports of Dienst et al. [12], who found increased concentrations of CEA in 49-58.5% of patients and increased concentrations of CA 19-9 in 21-67% of patients. However, Filela et al. [5] observed increased concentrations of CEA in 61% of patients and increased concentrations of CA 19-9 in 35% of patients. The concentration of both markers changed depending on the stage of the disease. CEA and CA 19-9 concentrations were within normal limits in the Dukes A group; the mean concentration of CEA was above the normal limits, 5.97 ng/ml, and CA 19-9 was within the normal limits in the Dukes B group. In the Dukes C group, the mean concentration of CEA was 7.42 ng/ml and the mean concentration of CA 19-9 was 55.73 U/ml. Similar results can be found in literature. Szymendera [2], Nowacki [7] and Lindmark et al. [13] revealed that in the advanced stages of colon cancer, a percentage of patients have elevated CEA and CEA concentrations. However, about 10-15% of patients do not secrete CEA.

The literature reveals that about 11-13% of patients with histopathologically confirmed colorectal cancer do not "produce" CEA and that an assay of these markers can lead to false negative results [2, 4, 9]. In these cases, the presence of advanced cancer is not excluded by a CEA concentration within the normal limits. CA 19-9 is the marker of first choice in this group of patients. The addition of CA 19-9 to an assay of CEA increased the sensitivity from 71% to 83.6% in our studies; however, 12.5% of patients with CEA within the normal limits had elevated CA 19-9. A positive correlation of CEA, CA 19-9 and the Dukes scale was revealed. Similar results were obtained by other authors. Fillela et al. [5] revealed that multifactoral analysis indicates the prognostic significance of CA 19-9 independent of the Dukes scale. New information about the CA 19-9 antigen has been revealed in recent years. CA 19-9 is sialofucololactotetraosyl and is included in the group of E-selectines. E-selectines enable a rise of remote metastases that is caused by the adhesion of neoplastic cells to epithelial cells in macrocirculation vessels. A pre-operative statistical analysis showed that the probability of recurrence is higher in cases where there is a higher CEA concentration before a treatment. However, Filela et al. [5] revealed that the risk of recurrence is 2.95 times greater in pre-operative patients with an increased concentration of CA 19-9 than in patients with a normal concentration of CA 19-9. 170 of 256 the patients who underwent surgery were tested in the follow-up phase. Patients in the Dukes D group were not tested. A recurrence was observed in 53 of the 170 patients (31%). The mean concentration of CEA was 20.71 ng/ml in the Dukes B group and 20.55 ng/ml in the Dukes C group. The mean concentration of CA 19-9 was 61.61 U/ml and 197.18 U/ml, respectively. A recurrence was detected in 100% of the patients when an increased concentration of CEA or CA 19-9 was used as a criterion. A recurrence was detected in 88.6% of patients when only CEA was estimated and 67.9% of patients when only CA 19-9 was estimated. The differentiation of a local neoplasm and remote metastases is difficult. Szymendera [2] reported that a concentration of CEA that is greater than 20 indicates metastases in the liver, while a small concentration of CEA or CA 19-9 might indicate metastases in the bones or lymph nodes.

1.6. Conclusions

1. Simultaneous detection of CEA and CA 19-9 should be the first immunodiagnostic test in patients suspected of having colorectal cancer.
2. The use of carcinoembryonic antigen is advisable in order to monitor the course of the disease in the case of an increased serum concentration of CEA and CA 19-9.
3. An increased concentration of CA 19-9 along with a normal lack of CEA in the serum of patients with colorectal adenocarcinomas is unfavorable prognostically.

The continuous development of immunodiagnostic methods and the production of monoclonal antibodies can bring new neoplastic markers into diagnostics. One of these is the TPS (Tissue Polipeptide Specific Antigen). Its structure is similar to the TPA (Tissue Polipeptide Antigen). Reports in the last 2-3 years suggest the great value of the determination of TPS in the serum of patients, including patients with gastrointestinal cancers, especially for the early detection of release and estimation of therapy effectiveness. TPS is a marker of cell proliferation and an increase in its concentration in serum often precedes the markers of a tumor

2. Scientific literature indicates interest of a cellular proliferation marker — TPS

A review of medical reports from recent years shows an increasing interest in estimating TPS levels mainly in oncologic diagnostics. Estimating TPS- concentration (which is a marker connected with the proliferation of neoplastic cells) is very important for monitoring patients who have undergone cancer surgery (esp. of the digestive tract, but also for breast and ovarian cancer) proceeding the clinical symptoms of metastasis for 2-7 months.

2.1. Characteristic of tissue polypeptide specific antigen (TPS) — Soluble fragments of cytokeratine 18

TPS (tissue polypeptide specific antigen) is a new marker of cellular proliferation. The antibody directed against TPS enables the determination of the concentration of the soluble fragments of cytokeratin 18 [14]. TPS was introduced into oncological immunodiagnostics by Bjorklund. It has one of the two active epitopes of TPA (tissue polypeptide antigen) that are detectable by the monoclonal antibody M3. TPS is a singular conjugated polypeptide chain that is created in the S and G2 phases of the cellular cycle and is released immediately after mitosis. It has 33 antigen determiners, two of which are connected with the activity of a tumor. TPS is strictly connected with the proliferation of neoplastic cells and is a function of the velocity of cell divisions [15].

2.2. Clinical results of serum concentration of TPS in patients with colorectal cancer

2.2.1. Aim of the study

1. To estimate pre-operative CEA and TPS concentrations in the blood serum of patients with colorectal cancer and rectal carcinomas depending on the advancement of their disease.

2. To attempt to determine whether TPS provides additional information that cannot be obtained from CEA tests only.

2.2.2. Material and methods

178 patients (101 men and 77 women) aged 22-86 years who had been diagnosed with colorectal cancer and had undergone surgery in the years 1991-2002 were included in the study. The patients were being treated at the Department of General Surgery and Coloproctology of the Medical University of Silesia in Sosnowiec. The CEA concentration was determined in the patients' blood serum using the MEIA method and commercial sets from Abbott (USA). TPS was determined using the enzyme-immunological method (EIA) and sets from BEKI (Sweden). The normal concentration of CEA was determined as 3 ng/ml and in the case of TPS – 90 U/l.

The criteria for choosing patients for the research: 178 patients whose pre-operative diagnostics confirmed the existence of a colon or rectal adenocarcinoma in a histopathological examination.

The criteria for excluding patients from the research. The research excluded patients who were diagnosed with:

- an inflammation of the large intestine (colitis ulcerosa, Leśniowski-Crohn disease),
- chronic kidney diseases,

- chronic liver diseases,
- an inflammation of the rheumatoid joints,
- autoimmunological diseases caused by autoimmunity (Hashimoto, Graves-Basedov, thyroid cysts),
- diabetes, or
- chronic infections.

The largest number of patients in the research was in the Dukes C group – 89 patients (50%). The fewest number of patients was in the Dukes A group – 8 patients (10.11%)(Table II)

Numbers of patients	Dukes scale	TNM scale
8	A	3 – T1N0M0 5 – T2N0M0
62	B	62 – T3N0M0
89	C	53 – T3N1M0 36 – T3N2M0
19	D	11 – T4N2M1 8 – T4N2M1

Table 2. The degree of the clinical advancement of colon and rectal carcinomas according to Dukes.

2.2.2.1. Statistical methods

All results were statistically measured using the Statistica 6.0 program from StatSoft Inc.

2.2.3. Results

No increased abnormal CEA concentration was found in any patient in the Dukes A subgroup. An increased amount of CEA was found in 37 cases (59.7%) in the Dukes B subgroup, in 75 patients (83.9%) in the Dukes C subgroup and in 17 cases (89.57%) in the Dukes D subgroup.

Another profile was observed when determining TPS. An increased concentration was found in 3 patients (37.5%) in the Dukes A subgroup. An increased concentration was found in 48 cases (77.4%) in the Dukes B subgroup, in 59 cases (65.5%) in the Dukes C subgroup and in 6 cases (31.6%) in the Dukes D subgroup. (Table III)

Dukes	CEA [%]	TPS [%]
A	0,00	37,5
B	59,68	77,41935
C	83,91	65,51724
D	89,47	31,57895

Table 3. The percentage of patients with an increased abnormal concentration of CEA and TPS in relation to the Dukes scale.

In cases where the division according to the degree of advancement in the whole group of 178 patients was not taken into account, the sensitivity for pre-operative CEA concentration was 72.5% and for TPS – 65.2%. When only cases with increased levels of CEA and TPS concentrations were taken into account, the sensitivity of the test increased to 82.6%.

The concentration of CEA was: 2.34 ng/ml in the Dukes A subgroup, 5.71 ng/ml in the Dukes B subgroup, 8.66 ng/ml in the Dukes C subgroup and 19.97 ng/ml in the Dukes D subgroup, respectively. (Table IV)

Dukes	Number of patients	Average amount	Standard deviation	Standard error	-95% CI	+95% CI
A	8	2,34	0,362284	0,128087	2,03462	2,64038
B	62	5,71	4,385849	0,557003	4,59636	6,82396
C	89	8,66	7,035047	0,745713	7,17906	10,14296
D	19	19,97	9,826148	2,254273	15,23553	24,70763

Table 4. CEA concentration in patients before surgery in relation to the degree of the advancement of the cancer according to Dukes.

Another characteristic was observed in the case of the determination of TPS concentration. The highest average pre-operative TPS concentration was found in the Dukes C subgroup – 226.7 U/l. It was 107.4 U/l in the Dukes A subgroup and 181.2 U/l in the Dukes B subgroup. However, the average amount measured in the Dukes D subgroup was 167.37 U/l, which may be connected with a decrease in proliferation. (Table V)

Dukes	Number of patients	Average amount	Standard deviation	Standard error	-95% CI	+95% CI
A	8	107,41	60,0221	21,22102	57,2328	157,5922
B	62	181,20	75,9138	9,64106	161,9283	200,4853
C	89	226,71	126,6201	13,42170	200,0392	253,3848
D	19	167,37	145,3267	33,34024	97,3295	237,4200

Table 5. TPS concentration in patients before operation in relation to the degree of the advancement of the cancer according to Dukes.

A recurrence of the disease was detected in 47 patients (Dukes B and C). When the concentration of CEA was used, recurrence was detected in 89.4% of patients and when the concentration of TPS was used, recurrence was detected in 80.85% of patients. If the criterion was an elevated concentration of CEA or TPS, recurrence was detected in of 100% patients. The concentration of CEA in patients with a recurrence was $\bar{x}$=12.82 ± 4.73 ng/ml in the Dukes B group and $\bar{x}$=13.5 ± 7.69 ng/ml in the Dukes C group. The concentration of TPS was $\bar{x}$=282.95 ± 56.08 U/l in the Dukes B group and C $\bar{x}$= 313.77 ± 116.62 U/l in the Dukes C group.

2.2.4. Discussion

In diagnosing carcinomas of the digestive system, particularly in the case of colon and rectal carcinomas, the carcinoembryonic antigen (CEA) still remains the "gold standard" [16, 17, 18]. However, great expectations are connected with the introduction of the soluble fragments of cytokeratin 18 (TPS) into the immunodiagnostics of colorectal cancer because TPS reflects the velocity of cell divisions [19].

Our results of pre-operative CEA concentrations are similar to those that have been reported by other researchers. Treska et al. obtained the highest sensitivity of CEA assessment from 45% to 80% depending on the degree of the progression of cancer [20]. Similar results were reported by Turoldo et al. and Marchena et al. [21, 22].

The main aim of the presented research was to estimate the usefulness of determining TPS concentration. The TPS sensitivity was 65.17% in our own clinical research. The highest pre-operative sensitivity equaling 70% was reported by Plebani et al. [23].

We also observed that the sensitivity of the test increased when the results of the determination of TPS and CEA were combined. An abnormal pre-operative CEA concentration was recorded in 129 patients (72.47%). When determining TPS concentration, 116 patients were found to have increased abnormal levels (65.17%). When the established criterion was an increased level of TPS or CEA, then the sensitivity of the test increased to 82.31%. Lindmark et al. using the CEA, CA 19-9, CA 50 and TPS tests proved their correlation with one another; however, only the TPS concentration test had the highest diagnostic sensitivity [18].

It is important to stress that adding TPS determination to the standard tests used for detecting and monitoring colon and rectal carcinomas has recently been approved by the European Group of Tumor Markers. According to the EGTM tests, adding TPS determination to the list of "mass tumor" markers enables an increase in sensitivity, particularly in the earlier stages of colorectal cancer [24].

2.2.5. Conclusions

1. The profile of the activity of pre-operative TPS concentration in the blood serum of patients with colorectal cancer in relation to the degree of the advancement of the cancer is different from that observed for CEA.

2. Determination of TPS concentration in patients with colorectal cancer provides essential information necessary to confirm the cancer, particularly at the earliest stages of its advancement.

3. Apoptosis and proliferation – Bcl-2

The mechanism of malignancy is considered to be an imbalance between apoptosis and the processes of proliferation. A phenotype that is resistant to apoptosis is one of the major features of cancer cells. Recently, attention has been drawn to the function of a number of proteins that inhibit the process of apoptosis within a tumor. To date, only a few works connected with the assessment of apoptosis proteins serum concentrations have been published. Most of the works about apoptosis concern immunohistochemistry studies.

This study attempts to find an answer to the question of whether the serum concentration of antiapoptotic the Bcl-2 protein provides additional information for the post-operative monitoring of patients with colorectal cancer.

3.1. Material and methods

The research was conducted on 46 patients (21 with a B Astler-Coller's stage cancer and 25 with a C Astler-Coller's stage cancer) was it colon cancer, who underwent surgery (resection RO). Their ages ranged from 47 to 85 (average age 67); sex (19 women, 27 men). The patients were divided into 2 groups: I –patients with a recurrence of cancer and II – patients without a recurrence of cancer. The control group consisted of 20 healthy people, mainly medical staff. The average CEA concentration in this group was 1.6 ng/ml+/- 0.43; TPS: 48.67U/l+/- 9.1; Bcl2: 0.31ng/ml+/- 0.13. The period of the observation of the patients and conducting the research was 1-5 years. The recurrence of the disease or the lack of a recurrence was confirmed using a physical examination and additional examinations during the oncological follow-up. Ten ml of venous shunt blood was collected from each patient. The serum was frozen at -20°C after centrifuging-. The blood for testing was collected one day before the surgery and 1, 3, 6 and 12 months after the surgery. CEA was measured using MEIA method and a commercial set from ABBOT (USA). The standard concentration for a healthy person was adopted as 3ng/ml. TPS was measured using the EIA method and sets from Beki Diagnostic Bromma (Sweden). The standard for a healthy person does not exceed 90 U/I. Bcl-2 concentration was labeled using the ELISA method using SORIN-BIOMEDICA tests (Italy). A standard for healthy people is 0.5 ng/ml. The results obtained were analyzed statistically. Calculations were done using Microsoft Excel 2003. The Ethical Committee at the Silesian Medical University approved the studies.

3.2. Results

Of the 46 patients who underwent surgery, a recurrence was detected in 14 patients including 6 with an initial stage of a tumor – B according to the Dukes classification as modified by Astler-Coller and 8 – degree C. The detection time of the recurrence was from 6 to 23 months. Most of the recurrences were distant metastases: 9 in the liver and 2 in the lungs. A local recurrence was observed in the intestinal stapling or retroperitoneal space in 3 patients. (Table VI) and (Figures 4, 5 and 6)

It was established that the Bcl-2 concentration was statistically significantly higher in the recurrence group than in the non-recurrence group when examined 1, 3, 6 and 12 months after the surgery. The TPS concentration was statistically significantly higher in the recurrence group than in the non-recurrence group when examined before and 3, 6 and 12 months after the surgery. The concentration of the antigen, i.e. CEA, was statistically significantly higher in the recurrence group in relation to the non-recurrence group, as was TPS in the pre-operative determinations and 3, 6 and 12 months after the surgery. Bcl-2, TPS and CEA serum concentrations were unrelated to the Astler-Coller stage of colorectal cancer. However, insignificantly higher concentrations of CEA at degree C than at degree B were observed. There was also no dependence related to the sex, the age of a patient, the original location of the tumor and the recurrence. Correlations between the concentrations of the determined parameters in all patients (with a recurrence and without a recurrence) were also noticed. A strong correlation between the concentrations of Bcl-2 and TPS proteins occurred 12 months after the surgery in the recurrence group.

Feature	No recurrence				Recurrence			
	Average	SD	Min.	Max.	Average	SD	Min.	Max.
Bcl2_0	8,09	6,82	0,41	24,39	10,39	6,78	0,57	23,02
Bcl2_1	7,34	6,07	1,74	28,41	8,87	3,17	4,09	14,61
Bcl2_3	7,40	6,58	0,50	29,79	12,15	8,14	0,55	30,00
Bcl2_6	6,97	6,99	0,41	26,40	17,50	7,98	1,98	29,74
Bcl2_12	8,38	7,67	1,47	25,09	20,52	7,03	12,14	29,81
CEA_0	5,26	7,22	1,70	42,60	5,75	2,60	2,30	11,90
CEA_1	2,61	1,00	1,10	6,30	2,46	0,53	1,70	3,00
CEA_3	1,87	0,90	0,40	3,70	4,94	3,88	1,20	17,40
CEA_6	2,21	2,19	0,30	11,90	10,72	5,74	3,70	20,30
CEA_12	2,57	2,97	0,40	14,60	14,86	13,92	1,30	41,00
TPS_0	98,9	19,1	60,4	160,3	118,1	31,1	60,7	168,9
TPS_1	92,8	16,8	64,6	143,7	101,6	17,7	80,3	144,1
TPS_3	95,9	27,0	64,7	188,3	125,2	31,0	90,7	193,7
TPS_6	96,8	35,7	70,3	197,6	152,0	49,0	80,4	279,1
TPS_12	96,6	37,9	70,4	207,4	152,4	34,2	100,0	190,4
Age	66,2	10,9	47,0	85,0	70,4	4,0	64,0	77,0

Table 6. Values of the basic description parameters (0 – preoperative results and 1-, 3-, 6-, and 12 months after the surgery.

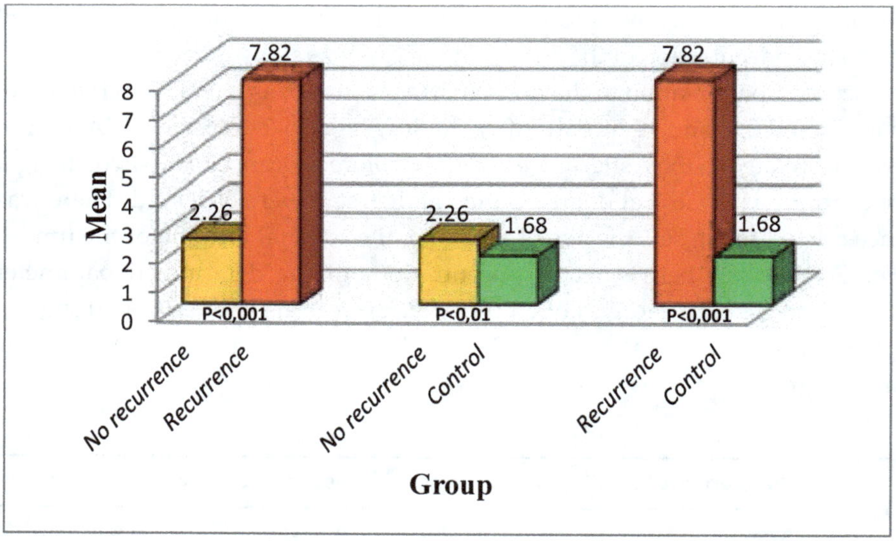

Figure 4. Results of the evaluation of post-operative CEA levels in the group without recurrence, with recurrence and the control group.

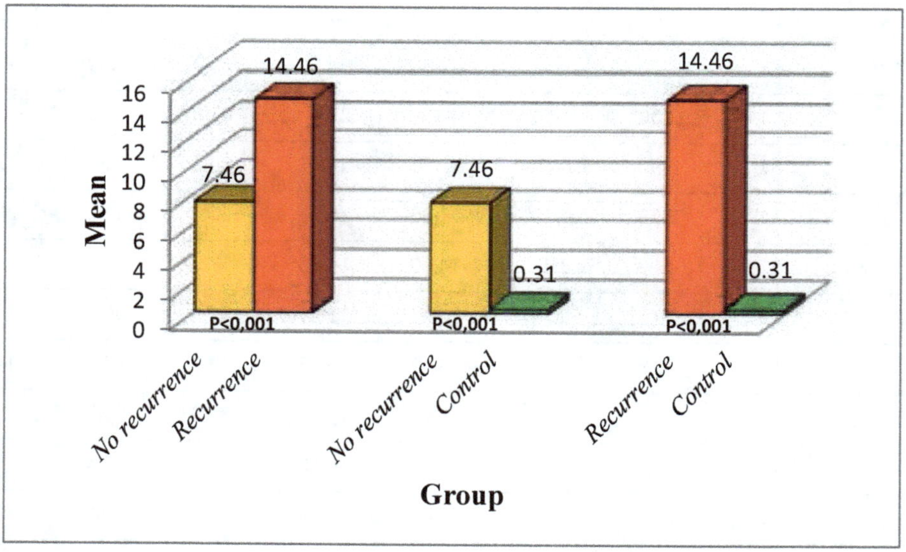

Figure 5. Results of the evaluation of post-operative Bcl-2 levels in the group without recurrence, the recurrence and the control group.

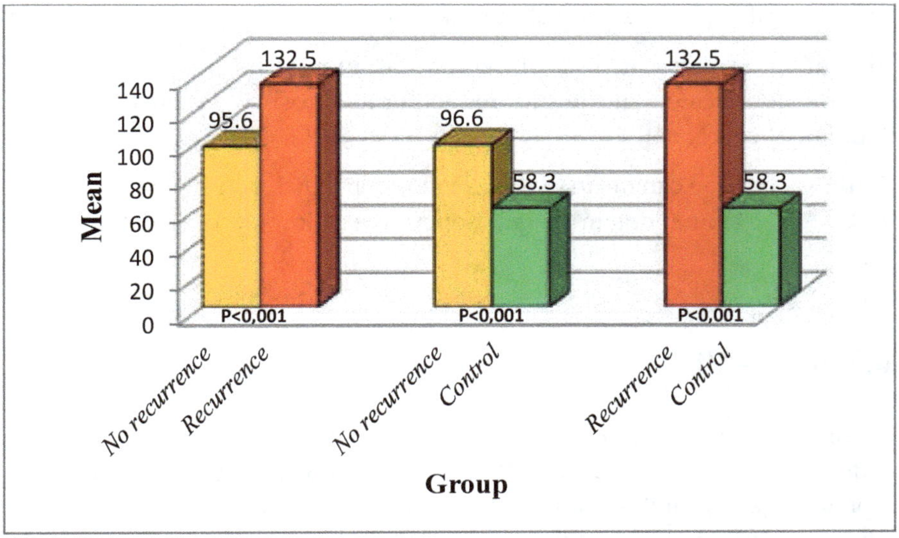

Figure 6. Results of the evaluation of post-operative TPS levels in the group without recurrence, the recurrence and the control group.

3.3. Discussion

The European Tumor Markers Association recommended CEA as a useful clinical marker in the diagnosis and monitoring of patients with colorectal cancer in 2003. To date, many scientific researchers have been shown that the addition of tumor markers in the diagnosis of patients with colorectal cancer is necessary. Colorectal cancer, like breast and lung cancer, reveals a high expression of the antiapoptotic proteins: Bcl-2, Bcl-XL, PED, Il-4, which are secreted by tumor cells, strengthens that expression and protects neoplastic cells by environmental death signals.

A low expression of BAX expression correlates with disease recurrence of the disease in preoperatively irradiated rectal carcinomas and is connected with a worse response. A decrease in the expression of BAX indicates the worst response to chemotherapy and reduces the life expectancy of patients [25, 26, 27].

Our results show that an increase of Bcl-2 in the serum of patients with colorectal cancer is bad prognostically. A high concentration ($\bar{x}$=14.46 ng/ml) was observed in the group with a recurrence of the disease. The concentration of the Bcl-2 protein has been correlated with TPS – a marker of cell proliferation. A high correlation in 12th month after surgery may confirm that the suppression of the apoptosis of cancer cells increases their proliferation.

At the present time the apoptotic process and the process of cell proliferation are the targets of many researchers in different areas of specialization.

3.4. Conclusions

1. A statistically significant excess of Bcl-2 in patients who have a recurrence of colorectal cancer makes information saying about the suppression of cancer cells apoptosis.
2. A statistically significant increase of the concentration of TPS in the group with a recurrence seems to indicate that the suppression of apoptosis is conductive to an excessive proliferation of cancer cells.
3. The findings obtained can mean that the evaluation of Bcl-2 and TPS may be complementary to CEA determinations in the post-operative follow-up of patients with colorectal cancer.

4. Angiogenesis – VEGF

The process of angiogenesis, which is the creation of new blood vessels, plays an important role in the development and metastasis of cancer. It can be initiated by tumor cell hypoxia, tumor suppressor gene mutations and oncogenes. As a result of the accumulation of these processes, tumor cells activate the angiogenic factors. The main factor involved in angiogenesis is VEGF-A. Blocking angiogenesis is one of the ways of preventing the development and metastasis of cancer and is the future of cancer therapy.

4.1. Aim of the study

1. An assessment of the concentration of VEGF-A in the blood serum of patients with colorectal cancer.
2. An attempt to answer the question of whether the determination of VEGF-A provides clinically meaningful information in the post-operative monitoring of patients.

4.2. Material and methods

117 patients underwent surgery for colorectal cancer in the years 2004-2009. Patients were divided according to the Dukes and TNM classifications. The control group consisted of 20 healthy volunteers. A recurrence was detected in 35 patients in the period of 623 months after the surgery, including 11 patients in the Dukes B group and 24 patients in the Dukes C group. Patients with a recurrence were grouped together, while the remaining 71 patients made up the group without a recurrence.

The concentration of CEA and VEGF-A was determined in all of the patients before the surgery and 1, 3, 6 and 12 months after the surgery. CEA was determined by MEIA using Abbott kits (USA); the standard concentration in healthy people is 3 ng/ml. VEGF-A was determined by ELISA using BIOMEDICA Sorin kits (Italy); the standard concentration in healthy people is 350 pg/ml.

The results were analyzed statistically. ROC curves were marked for the diagnostic parameters studied.

4.3. Results

The pre-operative mean CEA concentrations differed significantly in all three degrees of the severity of the disease (p<0.01). In the post-operative control, patients demonstrated statistically significant differences in CEA concentrations 3, 6 and 12 months after surgery with the largest concentration at the month follow-up (p<0,001). (Figure 7).

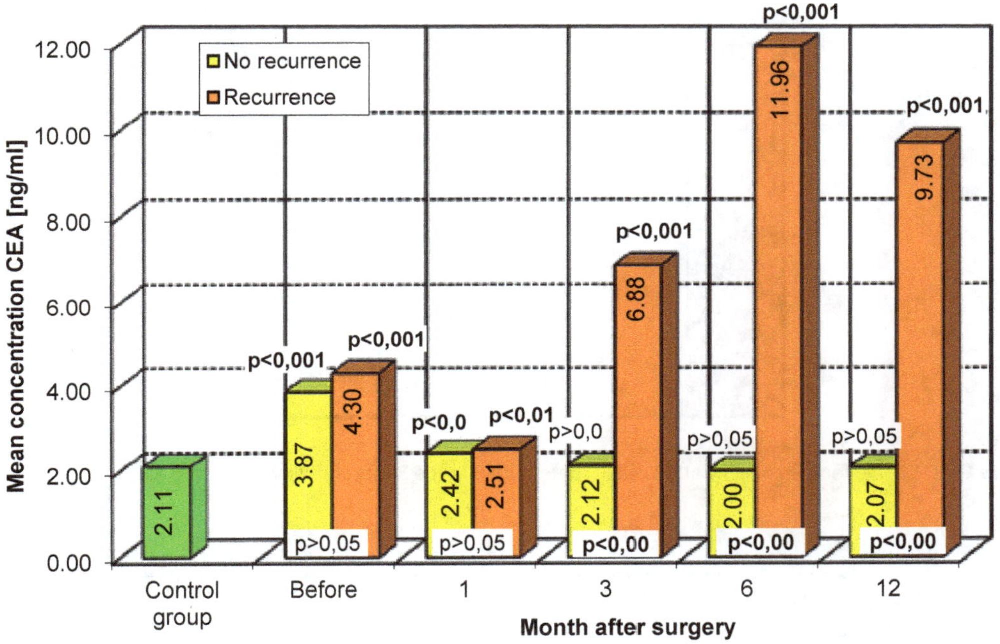

Figure 7. Evaluation of the concentration of CEA in the control group and in the groups of patients with and without a recurrence of a tumor in the subsequent stages of observation.

Most recurrences were detected during this period. The average concentrations of CEA in patients without a recurrence was 2.18 ng/ml and in patients with a recurrence 7.58 ng/ml. The ROC curves analysis showed a concentration of CEA of 3.1 ng/ml as early as 3 months after the surgery, which confirms the recurrence of the cancer (Figure 8).

Pre-operatively, a high concentration of VEGF-A was found in each stage of the disease; however, it showed no difference in levels of statistical significance. Throughout the period of post-operative observation, patients demonstrated a very high statistical significance between the group without a recurrence and those with a recurrence of the neoplastic process (p<0,001). (Figure 9)

The average concentration in patients without a recurrence was 294.24 pg/ml, while in patients with a recurrence it was 501.89 pg/ml. ROC curves showed the usefulness of VEGF-A in detecting a recurrence a month after surgery and a concentration of 412 pg/ml, it is confirmed (Figure 10).

In addition, a high, statistically significant correlation between VEGF-A and CEA was demonstrated 3, 6 and 12 months after surgery (Figure 11 and 12).

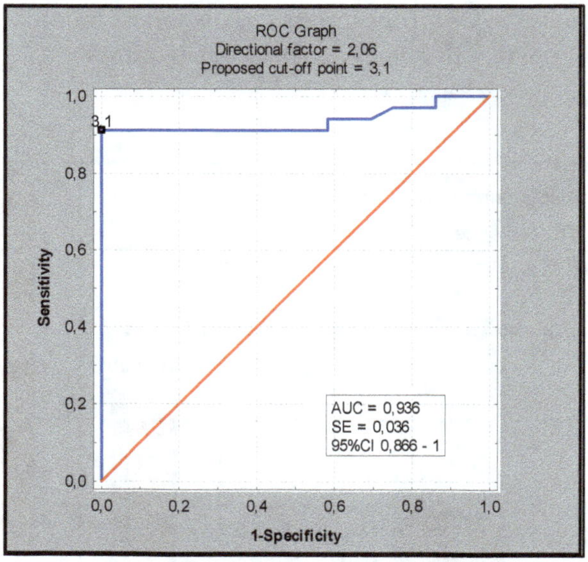

Figure 8. ROC curve for the concentration of CEA determined at the 3-month follow-up.

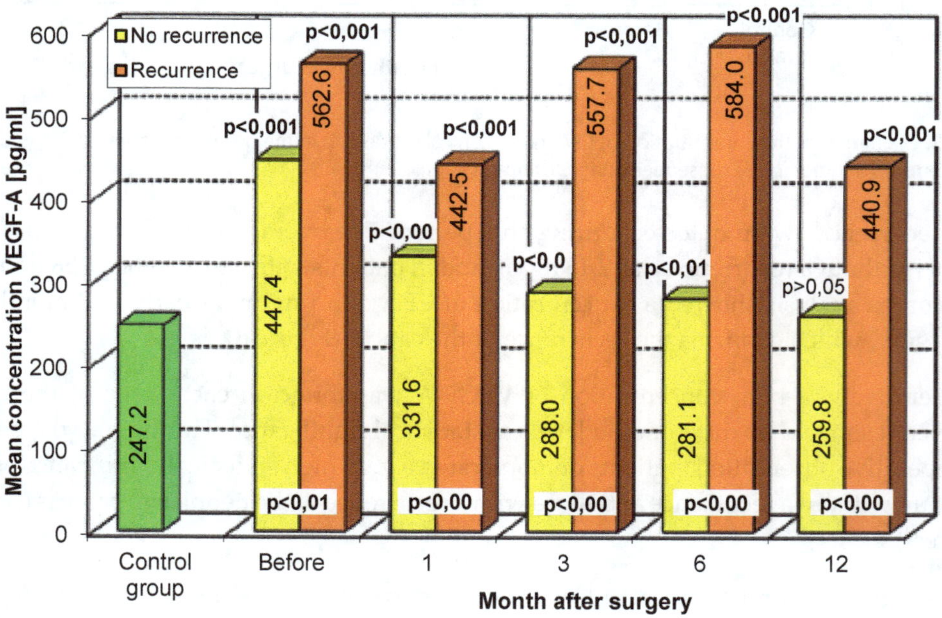

Figure 9. Evaluation of the concentration of VEGF-A in the control group and in the group of patients with and without a recurrence of a tumor in the subsequent stages of observation.

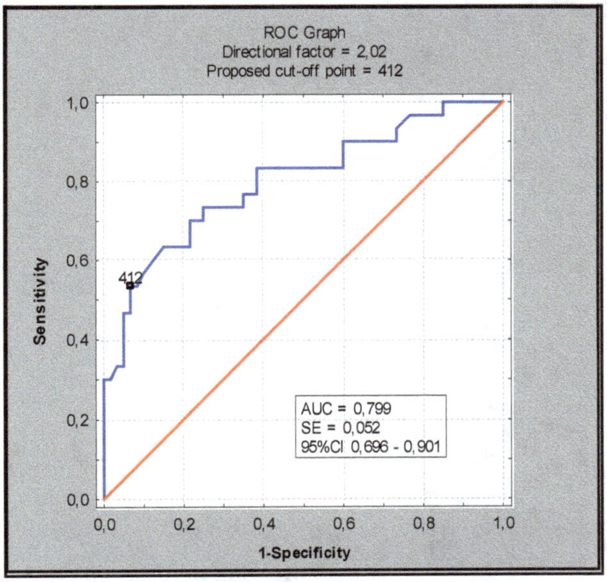

Figure 10. ROC curve for the concentration of CEA determined at a one-month follow-up.

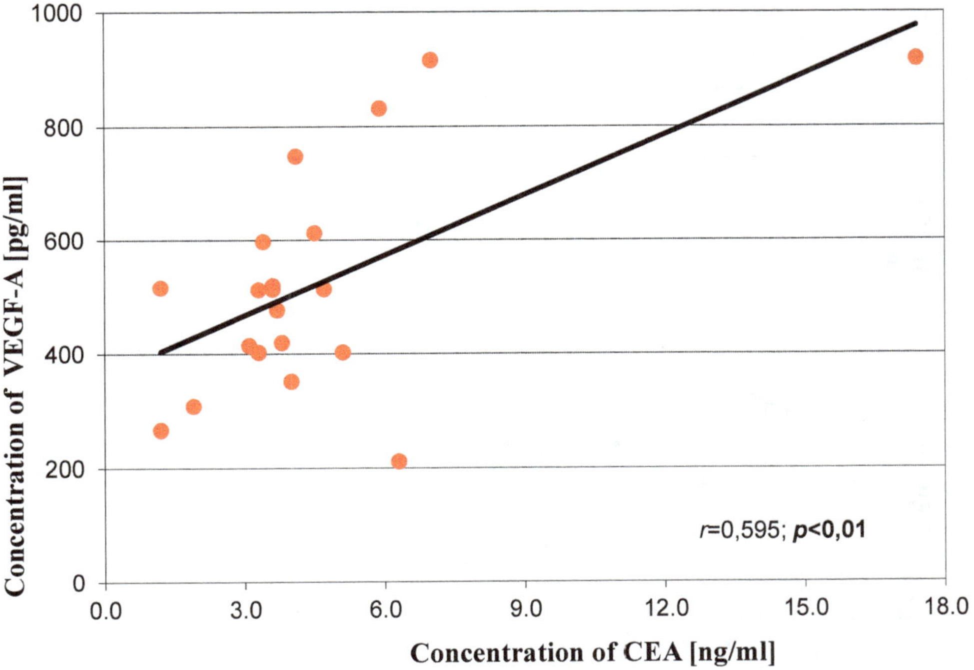

Figure 11. Correlation between the concentrations of CEA and VEGF-A in patients with a recurrence of a tumor 3 months after surgery.

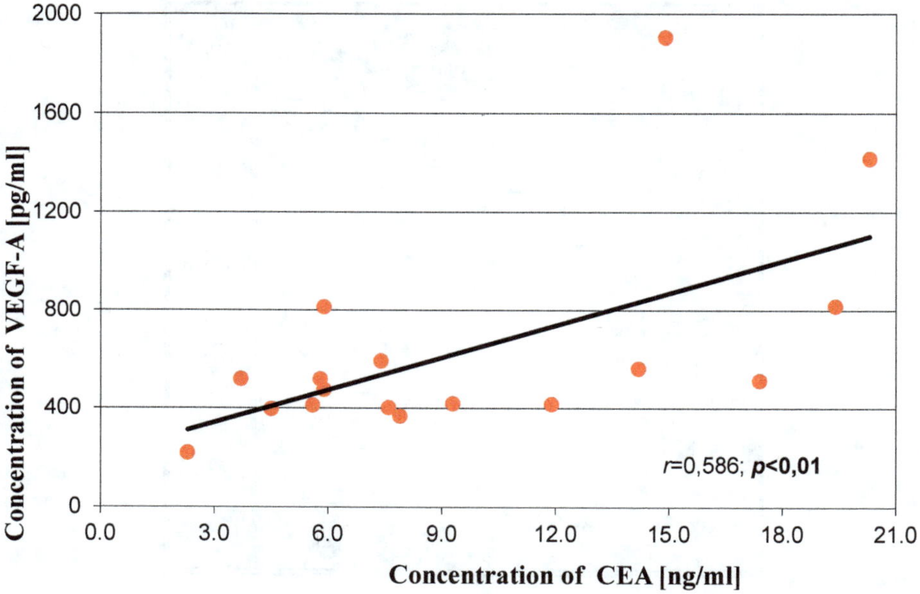

Figure 12. Correlation between the concentrations of CEA and VEGF-A in patients with a recurrence of a tumor 6 months after surgery.

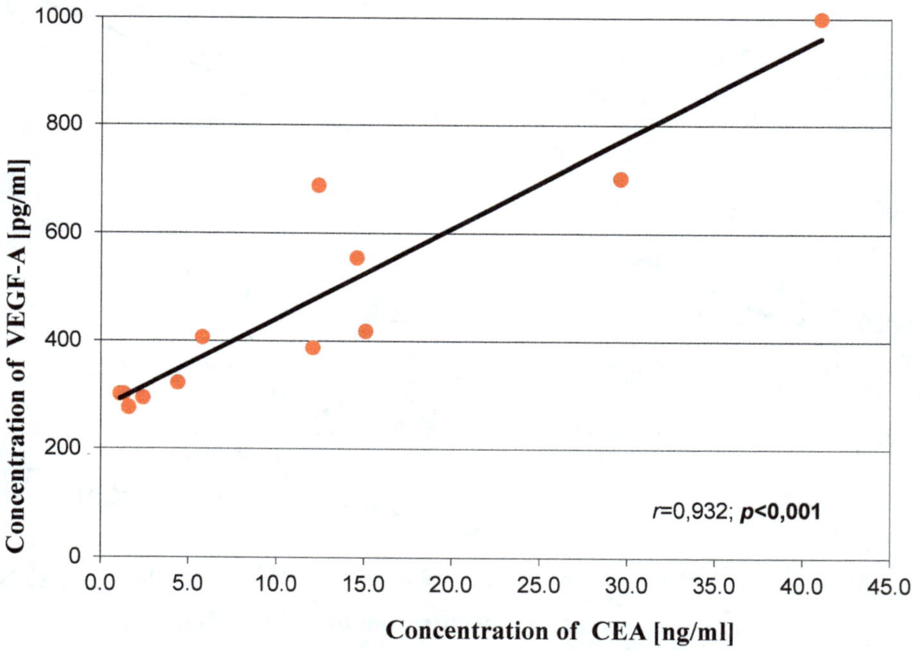

Figure 13. Correlation between the concentrations of CEA and VEGF-A in patients with a recurrence of a tumor 12 months after surgery.

4.4. Discussion

Our results are similar to the results shown by Bombardieri [28], Treska [29], Kokocińska [30] and many others. CEA was discussed in the first part of this chapter. VEGF-A was examined in the blood of patients after the surgery.

We did not find any statistically significant differences between the Dukes classification. In contrast, Fujisaki et al. [31] and Fuhrmann-Benzakein et al. [32] observed such a correlation. The highest concentration of VEGF was observed in patients with a liver metastasis.

Chung et al. [33] and Ohta et al. [34] reported that VEGF may be considered as a proliferation and prognostic factor. A high expression or concentration of VEGF indicates the possibility of the recurrence of a disease in a relatively short time.

Afify et al. [35] also indicated that the concentration of VEGF is very useful in detecting a recurrence of the disease and a metastasis to the liver.

However, Werther et al. and Karatzas et al. [36] reported that A high pre-operative concentration of VEGF suggests liver metastasis in the post-surgery period. Our results confirm those of Afify, Werther and Chung.

The results of our researches show a statistically significantly correlation between VEGF-A and CEA. It is possible that VEGF-A may stimulate the proliferation of tumor cells. To date, only Chung et al. and Ohta et al. have confirmed a connection of VEGF with the proliferation of tumor cells and with the development of cancer [33, 34].

All researches suggest that VEGF-A be added to the immunodiagnostics of CEA in patients with colorectal cancer.

5. Conclusions

1. A statistically significant increase in VEGF-A in patients with a recurrence of a tumor in the early post-operative period supports the usefulness of the inclusion of this marker for monitoring patients, especially in planning their antiangiogenic therapy.
2. The high correlation between CEA and VEGF-A seems to indicate that the concentration of VEGF-A has a close relationship with the proliferation of cells and the development of cancer.

6. Summary

A review of the scientific literature on colorectal diseases over the last 20 years indicates the continued development of Clinical Immunodiagnostics and the "gold standard", which is CEA, but also showed the usefulness and necessity of adding new markers: TPS, Bcl-2, VEGF and their receptors.

In the future, proteins, gene products, phenotyping of patients (determining the phenotype of patients) and molecular cytology should also be added.

Author details

Robert Partyka

Department of Anesthesiology, Intensive Treatment and Emergency Medicine, Medical University of Silesia, Katowice, Poland

The chapter was prepared based on results of research at the Institute of Tumor Markers, which were then compared to the results obtained by other researchers.

References

[1] Kokocińska D.: Przygotowanie składników testu radioimmunologicznego i enzymoimmunologicznego dla oznaczeń progesteronu, oczyszczanie i frakcjonowanie przeciwciał: IgG, F(ab)'2 przeciw progesteronowi i przeciw ferrytynie dla potrzeb diagnostyki klinicznej. Rozprawa habilitacyjna, Katowice, Śl. AM 1993; XVI: 234.

[2] Szymendera JJ, Góźdź S: Rola krążących markerów nowotworowych w diagnostyce I monitorowaniu leczenia chorych na nowotwory. Nowotwory 1995; 45: 369-383.

[3] Bates SH, Longo DL: Use of serum tumor markers in cancer diagnosis and management. Semin Onkol 1987; 14: 102-138.

[4] Dusza D: Dobór oznaczeń markerów nowotworowych u chorych na raka jelita grubego i odbytnicy. Rozprawa doktorska. Śląska AM 1996.

[5] Fillela X, Molina MD, Gran MD et al.: Prognostic value of CA 19-9 levels in colorectal cancer. Ann Surg 1992; 210: 55-59.

[6] Kokocińska D, Kuśmierski S: Antygen CA 72-4 – nowy marker choroby nowotworowej układu pokarmowego. Medycyna 2000 1994; 45(46): 46-47.

[7] Nowacki M: Przydatność kliniczna badań antygenu karcinoembrionalnego (CEA) w surowicy, określenie stopnia zaawansowania, rokowania, leczenia chirurgicznego nowotworów jelita grubego. Nowotwory 1983;1: 13.

[8] Staab HJ, Brummendorf T, Hornung A et al.: The clinical validity of circulating tumor associated antigens CEA and CA 19-9 in primary diagnosis and follow-up patients with gastrointestinal malignancies. Klin Wschr 1985; 63: 106-115.

[9] Wilson MS, Schofieln PF: Markers to study human colonic cell proliferation. Gut 1995; 36(1): 152.

[10] Gold P, Freedman SO: Specific carcinoembryonic antigens in the human digestive system. J Exp Med 1965; 122: 439-462.

[11] Ogata S, Ho J, Chen A et al.: Tumor associated sialylated antigens are constitutively expressed in normal human colonic mucosa. Cancer Res 1995; 1; 36: 1869-1874.

[12] Dienst C, Clodius T, Oldorp T: CA 19-9, CA 50 and CEA bei Pankreas und Gastrointestinaltumoren vergleichende Untersuchungen. Bred Klein 1987; 82: 49-50.

[13] Lindmark G, Bergensrom R, Pahlman I et al.: The association of preoperative serum tumor markers with Dukes' stage and surival in colorectal cancer. Br J Cancer 1995; 71: 1090-1094.

[14] Bonfrer J, Groenveled E, Korse C, Van Dalen A, Oomen LC, Ivanyi D. (1994). Monoclonal antibody M3 used in tissue polypeptide-specific antigen assay for the quantification if tissue polypeptide antigen recognizes keratin 18. Tumor Biol; 15(4): 210-222.

[15] Barak V, Goike H, Panaretakis KW, Einarsson R. Clinical utility of cytokeratins as tumor markers. Clin Biochem 2004; 37(7): 529-540.

[16] Lucsaite R, Sauer-Eppel M, Oremek GM. Value of biomarkers in diagnosis of gastric carcinoma. Clin Exp Med Let 2009; 50(1): 1-4.

[17] Takagawa R, Fujii S, Ohta M, Nagano Y, Kunisaki C, Yamagishi S, Osada S, Ichikawa Y, Shimada H. Preoperative serum carcinoembryonic antigen level as a predictive factor of recurrence after curative resection of colorectal cancer. Ann Surg Oncol 2008; 15(12): 3433-3439.

[18] Lindmark G, Bergstrom R, Pahlman L, Grimelius B. The association of preoperative serum tumor markers with Dukes's stage and survival in colorectal cancer. Brit J of Cancer 1995; 71: 1090-1094.

[19] Barak V, Goike H, Panaretakis KW, Einarsson R. Clinical utility of cytokeratins as tumor markers. Clin Biochem 2004; 37(7): 529-540.

[20] Treska V, Topolcan O, Stanislav K i wsp. Preoperative tumor markers as prognostic factors of colorectal liver metastases. Hepato-Gastroenterology 2009; 56(90): 317-320.

[21] Turoldo A, Balani A, Scaramucci M, Pistan V, Roseano M, Liguori G. Preoperative CEA: prognostic significance in colorectal carcinoma. Tumori 2003; 89(4): 95-97.

[22] Marchena J, Acosta MA, Garcia-Anguiano F, Simpson H, Cruz F. Use of the preoperative levels of CEA in patients with colorectal cancer. Hepatogastroenterology 2003; 50(52): 1017-1020.

[23] Plebani M, De Paoli M, Basso D, Roveroni G, Giacomini A, Galeotti F, Corsini A. Serum tumor markers in colorectal cancer staging, grading, and follow-up. J Surg Oncol 1996; 62(4): 239-244.

[24] Duffy MJ, van Dalen A, Haglund C, Hansson L, Klapdor R, Lamerz R, Nilsson O, Sturgeon C, Topolcan O. Clinical utility of biochemical markers in colorectal cancer:

European Group on Tumor Markers (EGTM) guidelines. Eur J Cancer 2003; 39(6): 718-727.

[25] Paul-Samojedny M, Kokocińska D, Samojedny A i wsp. Expression of cell survival/ death genes: bcl-2 and bax at the rate of colon cancer prognosis. Biochimica et Biophisica Acta 2005; 1741: 25 – 29.

[26] Schelwies K, Sturm I, Grabowski P et al.: Analysis of p53/BAX in primary colorectal carcinoma: low BAX protein expression is a negative prognostic factor In UICC stage III tumors. Int J Cancer 2002; 99 (4): 589-596.

[27] Nehls O, Okech T, Hsieh CJ et al.: Low BAX protein expression correlates with disease recurrence in preoperatively irradited rectal carcinoma. Int J Radiat Oncol Biol Phys 2005; 61(1): 85-91.

[28] Bombardieri E, Saccani JG, Cocciolo MG, Mori M, Rusca M, Seregni E, Becchi G, Fontanesi M, Tardini A et al. Tissue polypeptide antigen and carcinoembryonic antigen in colon tumors: serum levels and immunohistochemical localization. Cancer Detect Prev 1985; 8: 219-226.

[29] Treska V, Topolcan O, Stanislav K, Liska V, Holubec L. Preoperative tumor markers as prognostic factors of colorectal liver metastates. Hepatogastroenterology 2009; 56(90): 317-320.

[30] Kokocińska D, Jarząb B, Kawecki M, Donocik J, Kusmierski S. Antygeny CA 19-9, CEA, CA 50 I ferrytyna w nowotworach przewodu pokarmowego. Pol Przegl Chir 1993; 65: 237-243.

[31] Fujisaki K, Mitsuyama K, Toyonaga A, Matsuo K, Tanikawa K. Circulationg vascular endothelial growth factor in patients with colorectal cancer. Am J Gastroenterol 1998; 93(2): 249-252.

[32] Fuhfmann-Benzakein E, Ma MN, Rubia-Brandt L et al. Elevated levels of angiogenic cytokinez in the plasma of cancer patients. Int J Cancer 2000; 85: 40-45.

[33] Chung Y.S, Maeda K, Sowa M. Prognostic value of angiogenesis in gastrointestinal tumors. Eur J Cancer 1996; 32A(14): 2501-2505.

[34] Ohta Y, Endo Y, Tanaka M, Shimizu J, Oda M, Hayashi Y, Watanabe Y, Sasaki T. Sagnificance of vascular endothelial growth factor messenger RNA expression in primary lung cancer. Clin Cancer Res 1996; 2: 1411-1416.

[35] Afify M, Samy N, Hashim M, Essam T. Clinical significance of vascular endothelial growth factor in Egyptian colorectal cancer patients. Int J Integf Biol 2008; 4(2): 100-107.

[36] Karatzas G. Clinical significance of preoperative serum vascular endothelial growth factor levels in patients with colorectal cancer and effect of tumor surgery. Surgery 2002; 131(5) 548-555.

8

Robotic Colorectal Cancer Surgery

Ray Swayamjyoti, Jim Khan and Amjad Parvaiz

1. Introduction

A robot is a mechanical or virtual agent, usually an electro-mechanical machine that is guided by a computer program or electronic circuitry. Robots have been linked with the future and modern civilization but have been around for more than 2000 years since ancient Greek automata. Their real surgical application has been in the last 20 years [1, 2].

Robots were first used in medicine to help people with disabilities to aid in their rehabilitation process. The Edinburgh Modular Arm System [3] was one of the first bionic arm which was engineered by Dr. David Gow in the early eighties.

The National Aeronautics and Space Administration (NASA) developed the first telemanipulator robot in 1985 at the behest of the Defense Department of the United States of America with the aim to decrease war casualties using telerobotic surgery [4].

It was believed that robots could have prevented more than a third of the soldiers from dying during the Vietnam War secondary to haemorrhage [5].

Robotic colorectal operations have gained considerable interest after successful implementation in the field of urology and gynaecology. The advantages of a stable platform, better vision and better access has made this an attractive tool in many specialities. [6] Pelvic and rectal resections are best suited for robotic operations [6].

2. The Da Vinci surgical robotic system

The Federal Drug and Administration approved the use of the da Vinci robotic system for surgical treatment in 2000 and it was first used at the Ohio State University Hospital for oesophageal and pancreatic surgery [22].

Year	Milestones
1985	• PUMA 560 was used under computerised tomography guidance to orient a needle for brain biopsy [7]
1992	• PROBOT - developed at Imperial College, London and was used to perform prostatic surgery at Guy's and St Thomas' Hospital, London [8] • The ROBODOC developed by Integrated Surgical Systems was used to curve out accurate fittings in the femur for hip replacement [8]
1998	• Zeus robotic surgical system – used for reconstruction of the Fallopian tube performed at the Ohio State University Medical Center [9]
1999	• Robotics assisted closed chest bypass on a beating heart was performed at the London Health Sciences Centre [10]
2000	• **FDA approval of da Vinci robotic system**[11]
2002	• Robotic cholecystectomy [12] • **Robotic Right Hemicolectomy** [13] • Robotic bowel resections [14]
2006	• Unassisted robotic surgery using artificial intelligence to correct atrial fibrillation at a hospital in Milan [15]
2007	• Denervation of spermatic cord for testicular pain using robotic assisted microsurgery performed at Winter Haven Hospital and University of Florida [16]
2008	• Magnetic Resonance guided neurosurgical procedure performed at University of Calgary [17] • Microsurge developed by German Aerospace Center [18]
2010	• Sophie Surgical System developed by Eindhoven University of Technology [19] • Femoral reconstruction [20] • World's first all robotic operation i.e. prostatectomy using the da Vinci robot along with McSleepy robot used for anaesthesia at McGill University Hospital, Canada [21]

Table 1. Development of Robotics to aid in Surgical Procedures.

At present it is extensively used throughout the world and has sold over 2000 units worldwide in 2013. It is estimated then more than 200,000 operations have been performed in 2012 [23, 24].

The initial model of da Vinci was released in the year 1999, later this was updated to "S" in 2007 and in 2009 Si was released with improved functions and better performance. The author uses the da Vinci "Si" robotic system for his colorectal operations.

The da Vinci system consists of a surgeon's console and four interactive robotic arms attached to the robotic cart controlled by the surgeon from the console. One of the arms carries an endoscopic camera via a 12mm port. The camera has two lenses, which gives a 3D image with stereoscopic vision when the surgeon looks through the eyepiece in the console. The three other arms are used to hold tools and tissues i.e. scissors, bovies, electrocautery. The arms are maneuvered using two-foot pedals and two hand controllers.

Unlike laparoscopy the da Vinci system allows the surgeon to perform operation seated at the console, with the hands and eyes positioned in line with the instruments. The operating surgeon is able to control the movements of the camera using the foot pedal rather than relying on an assistant. The system is able to filter and decipher surgeon's hand movements into steady and precise micro movements.

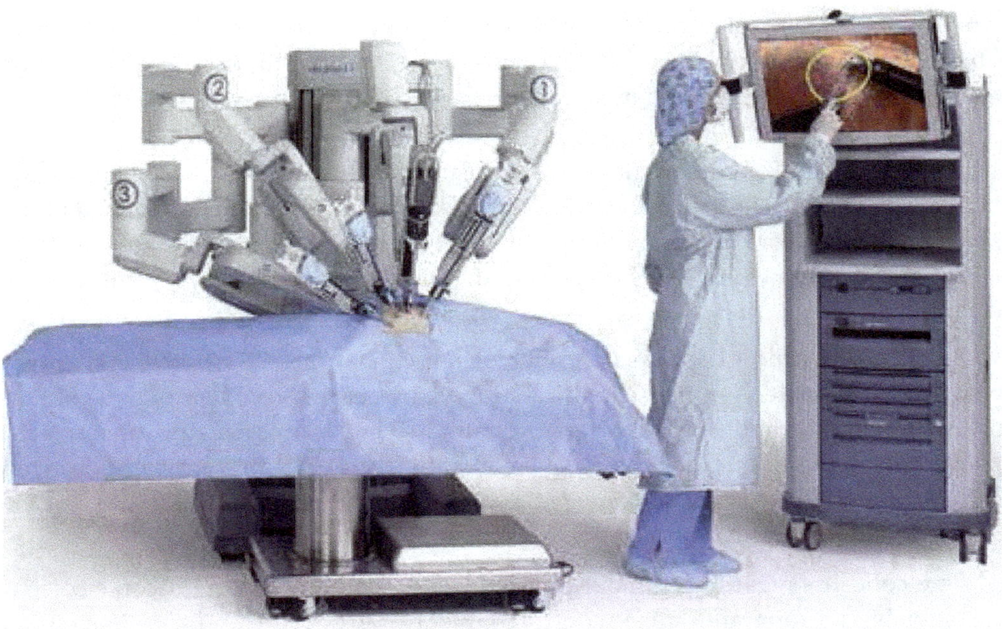

Figure 1. [25]: showing the robotic stack/cart and the monitor used by the assistant to follow the operation

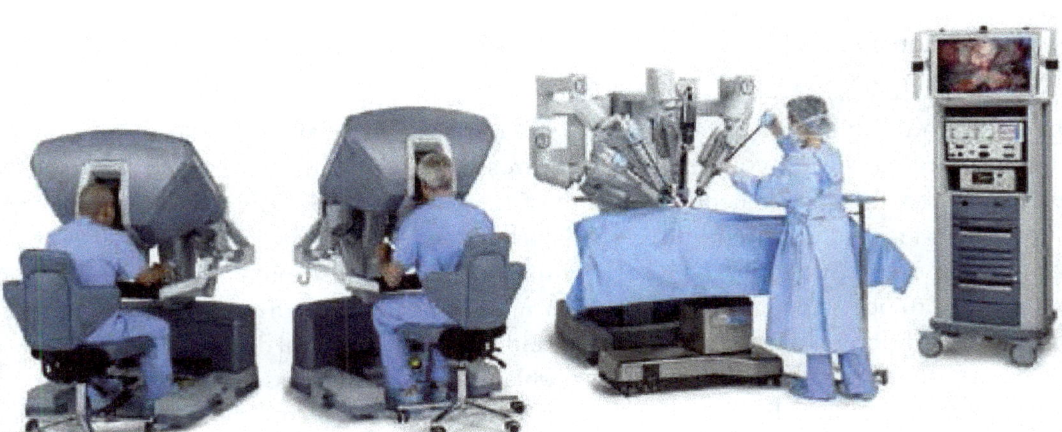

Figure 2. [26] : showing robotic and vision carts and the surgeon's console with an additional teaching console

3. Evidence of robotics in colorectal surgery

Robotic colorectal surgery is gaining widespread interest worldwide and in the continent. Data collected in 2012 suggests that most of the reported or published data shows that majority of the robotic colorectal operations have been performed in the United States (32%) followed by South Korea (20%), Italy (15%), Canada, Germany and Netherlands accounted for 5% and the rest of the world less than 2% [13].

The first colorectal surgical publication was published by Weber et al in 2002 [27] and since then there has been a tenfold rise in publication in colorectal surgery [13]. The important landmark studies are summarized in table 2.

Laparoscopic colorectal operations have many advantages over conventional open operations. The benefits in terms of short term outcomes are well established and include shorter hospital stay, faster return to work, better cosmesis, less post operative pain, less risk of bleeding and ileus. Long term outcomes including cancer specific and disease free survival have been subject of many well-designed trials.

The COLOR (COlon cancer Laparoscopic or Open resection) trial (330 stated that laparoscopic colectomy was associated with less significant blood loss, earlier recovery of bowel function, use of fewer analgesics and with a shorter hospital stay when compared with open colectomy. It however took half an hour longer than open operations and had 19% chances of converting to open operation. The reasons for conversion were mainly attributed to tumour size of more than 6cms and in patients who had involvement of adjacent structures.

There were concerns regarding tumour recurrence associated with laparoscopic colectomy. The meta-analysis of four randomized control trials (CLASICC trial, COST trial, Barcelona trial and COLOR trial) where patients with colonic cancers were randomised to either open or laparoscopically assisted colectomy concluded that the positive margins were found in specimens after open operations were 2.1% as compared to 1.3% after laparoscopic operation. The overall disease free survival at three years was 83.5% for open operations and 82.2% for laparoscopic operations [34]. Hence, the evidence shows that laparoscopic colonic operation is oncologically safe and viable with comparable outcomes to open surgery [34, 35].

The safety and viability for rectal cancers is still less clear especially with the higher circumferential margin (CRM) involvement with laparoscopic rectal operations when compared to open rectal operations as mentioned in the CLASSIC trial [34]. There was however, no difference in local recurrence at three years [36]. There was a higher conversion rate in the laparoscopic rectal subgroup (34%) in comparison to laparoscopic colonic group (25%). Conversions to open operations led to higher mortality and morbidity [34, 37]. Conversions were mainly attributed to bulky tumours [33] and increased technical difficulty [37]. The robot promises to abolish some of these technical problems faced during dissection of rectal tumours using laparoscopy and the ROLARR (RObotic versus LAparoscopic Resection for Rectal cancer) trial results are awaited. It is an international, multicentre, prospective, randomised, and controlled, unblinded, parallel-group trial of robotic-assisted versus laparoscopic surgery for the curative treatment of rectal cancer [37].

Year	Reference	Country	Study type	Number of patients
2002	Weber et al.	USA	Case series	2,
				3,
	Hashizume et al.	Japan		18
	Talamini et al.	USA		
2003	Vibert et al.	France	Case series	3,
	Giulianotti et al.	Italy		16
2004	Hubens et al.	Belgium	Case series,	8,
	Anvari et al.	Canada	Prospective Comparative	10,
	D'Annibale	Italy	Comparative	53
2005	Woeste et al.	Germany	Comparative,	6,
	Bonder et al.	Austria	Case series,	14,
	Ruurda et al.	Holland	Case series	23
2007	Heemskerk et al.	Netherlands	Comparative	19
2008	Baik et al.	Korea,	Randomized trial,	18,
	Spinoglio	Italy,	Comparative,	50,
	Huettner et al.	USA,	Comparative,	70,
	Soravia et al.	Switzerland	Case series	40
2009	Baik et al.	Korea	Comparative,	56,
	DeHoog et al.	Netherlands	Case control	20
2010	Tsoraides et al.	USA,	Retrospective,	102,
	Kim and kang	Korea,	Comparative,	100,
	Bianchi et al.	Italy,	Comparative,	56,
	Pernazza and Morpurgo	Italy,	Case series,	50,
	DeSouza et al.	USA,	Case control,	40,
	Zimmern et al.	USA,	Case series,	131,
	Popescu et al.	Romania	Comparative	122
2011	Kang and kim	Korea	Retrospective	204
2012	Antoniou SA et al [28]	Germany	Case series	39
2013	Casillas MA Jr et al [29]	USA	Case series	344
	Germain A et al [30]	France	Case Series	77
	Barrie J et al [31]	UK	Comparative	34
	Wormer BA et al [32]	USA	Comparative	1809

Table 2. [13]

The skills required for laparoscopic operations are different to open operations.

Limitations of laparoscopic surgery include loss of depth perception, reduced tactile feedback and a declined range of motion [33]. The author believes that limited space in the pelvis, with two-dimensional visions and a bulky specimen can make laparoscopic operations very difficult.

Laparoscopic TME rectal resections have a steep learning curve [38], requiring precise pelvic dissection with preservation of autonomic nerves. There is higher incidence of male sexual dysfunction due to inadvertent injury to the nerves following TME resections [39]. It is estimated that 50% of colorectal surgeons perform laparoscopic colorectal operations in the UK and only a quarter of them perform laparoscopic TME resections [40]. Approximately 50-70 cases are needed to surmount the laparoscopic colorectal learning curve [35, 38, 41].

The COREAN trail [42] trial compared open surgery with laparoscopic surgery for mid or low rectal cancer after neoadjuvant chemoradiotherapy. There was a conversion rate of 1.2% in the COREAN trial as compared to 34% in the CLASSIC trial. The low conversion rate in the COREAN trial was attributed to greater experience of the surgeons who has performed an average of seventy laparoscopic operations as compared to twenty per average surgeon in the CLASSIC trial [43].

The learning curve for performing robotic colorectal operations is shorter and is achieved after 15-20 cases [37, 38]. There are three phases that has been identified in the learning curve for robotic colorectal operations [44, 45, 46]

- Phase 1 – initial learning (1-15 cases)
- Phase 2 – increased competence (15-25 cases)
- Phase 3 – period of highest skill (>25 cases)

The other advantages of robotic colorectal resections are that

- It is superior in narrow areas like the pelvis and it's safe and feasible [47] with good three dimensional view and zoom magnification [37]
- It has 7 degrees of freedom of movement [37]
- It is associated with lower conversion rates to open operation [48]
- It has better pathologic and functional outcomes. It is associated with less complication rates, shorter duration of hospital stay, time to recover to normal bowel function or first flatus and time to start diet. It also causes less postoperative pain [49].
- Hospitals who perform high-volume robotic colorectal operations have significantly lower rates of postoperative bleeding and ileus [50]
- the double console that comes with the robotic cart allow trainees to take part actively at the surgical procedure and learn from it [51]
- simulators are available than can be attached to the console which provides a platform for surgical trainees to practice their skills before actually performing the procedures

There are however some limitations of the da Vinci system. In particular

- there is a definite learning curve for this technique
- loss of tactile feedback although partly compensated by better vision, still can have its effects on the performance and outcomes
- Hospitals that perform less robotic colorectal operations had more complications with longer length of hospital stay causing higher cost for the hospital. [19]
- High cost of purchasing as well as maintaining the robotic system [22]

	LNs (mean N)			Distal margin(mean, cm)			Positive CRM (%)		
	ROB	LAP	*p*	ROB	LAP	*p*	ROB	LAP	*p*
Park et al, 2010	17.3	14.2	*0.06*	2.1	2.3	ns	4.9	3.7	0.5
Kim et al, 2010	14.7	16.6	*ns*	2.7	2.6	0.09	3	2	ns
Kwak et al, 2011	20	21	*0.7*	2.2	2.0	0.8	1.7	0	>0.9
Baek et al, 2011	13	16	*0.07*	3.6	3.8	0.6	2.4	4.9	1
Bianchi et al, 2010	18	17	*0.7*	2	2	1.0	0	4	0.9
Baik et al, 2009	18.4	18.7	*0.8*	4	3.6	0.4	7	8	0.7
Patriti et al, 2009	10.3	11.2	*>0.05*	2.1	4.5	>0.05	0	0	ns

(LNs: lymph nodes, CRM: circumferential resection margin, ns: not significant, ROB: robotic procedure, LAP: laparoscopic procedure.)

Table 3. Oncologic results of robotic and laparoscopic surgery for rectal cancer [52].

	LNs (mean)			Distal margin (mean, cm)			Positive CRM (%)		
	ROB	OPEN	*p*	ROB	OPEN	*p*	ROB	OPEN	*p*
De Souza et al], 2011	15	16.8	0.26	na	na		0	3	0.25
Kim et al, 2012	20	19.6	0.7	2.7	1.9	0.001	1	1	1
Park et al, 2011	19.4	18.5	0.06	2.8	2.3	0.002	1	2	0.9

(LN: lymph nodes, CRM: circumferential resection margin, na: not assessed, ROB: robotic procedure, OPEN: laparoscopic procedure.)

Table 4. Oncologic results of open and robotic surgery for rectal cancer [52].

4. Patient selection

Patient selection is the key especially in the early stages of the learning curve. The author would recommend choosing patients with

- ASA grade 1-3
- BMI <30
- Age <75 years
- No previous pelvic or intra-abdominal surgery
- T1/T2 tumours
- Tumors that are at or just above the peritoneal reflection of the rectum
- Avoid patients who received neo-adjuvant chemo-radiotherapy and
- Avoid patients who for medical reasons will not be able to tolerate Trendelenburg position

5. Patient preparation

- Bowel preparation – phosphate enema for left sided operations. Bowel preparation not necessary for right sided colonic operations.

Bowel preparation is controversial in colorectal surgery. Surgeons differ in their approach. Mechanical bowel preparation results in a colon that is clear of feces. However, it can leave liquid stool in the bowel that is more likely to contaminate the operative field and the pelvis in the event of an anastomotic leak. In our experience, bowel preparation also results in small bowel distension that can make operations more difficult. The authors do not use bowel preparation for right-sided colonic resections. Two-phosphate enemas are used for left sided colorectal resections.

- low residue diet 3-4 days before operation
- 4 high calorie drinks to be taken the night before operation
- Eating and drinking normally up to 6 hours before operation
- 2 high calorie drinks to be taken up to 2 hours before operation
- Intra-operative fluids are restricted to 500 mL per hour as tolerated by the patient. This minimizes the risk of edema of the face and neck that can occur due to the steep Trendelenburg position and excessive fluids. Goal directed therapy is the standard approach using esophageal Doppler.

6. Operating room configuration

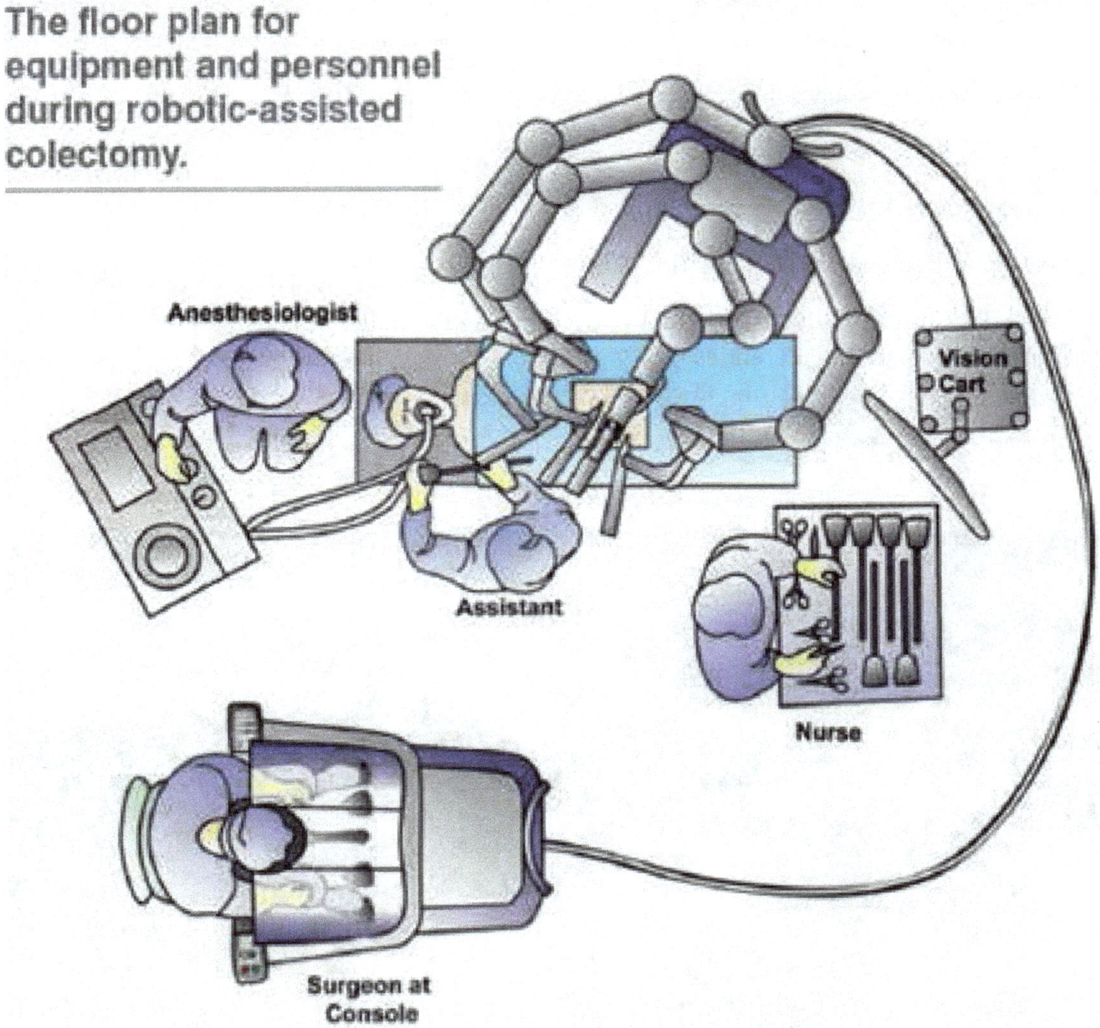

Figure 3. [53]: showing operating room set up during colectomy

7. Positioning

- Patient is positioned supine in a modified lithotomy position with legs wrapped around adjustable stirrups
- Legs are abducted and slightly flexed at the knees

- Patient's arms are wrapped alongside the body to reduce possibility of shoulder injury and additional shoulder harness can be placed to support Trendelburg's position
- Pressure points and bony prominences are padded and the body position is secured with vacuum-mattress device, especially lateral on the right side.
- Secure the patient to the table to avoid any shifting with the Trendelenburg position.
- Patient is tilted right side down and adjust the angle during initial exposure
- A body warmer (bear hugger) is applied to prevent patient hypothermia.
- Sequential compression devices (Flowtrons) are applied to the legs for DVT prophylaxis.
- After positioning, padding, securing and preparing the patient in the supine position, the table is then placed in a Trendelenburg position, whereby the steepness should be adjusted as per exposure needs during the initial exposure step.

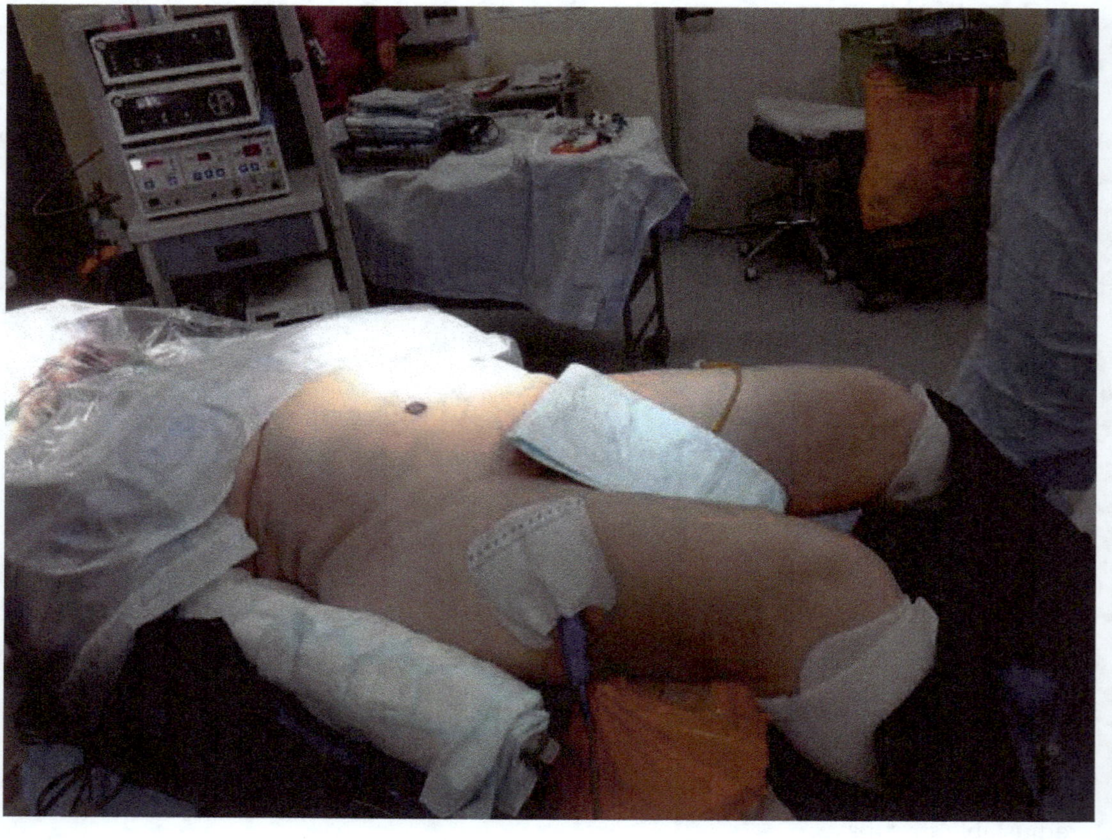

Image 1. Showing positioning of patient

8. Right-sided operations

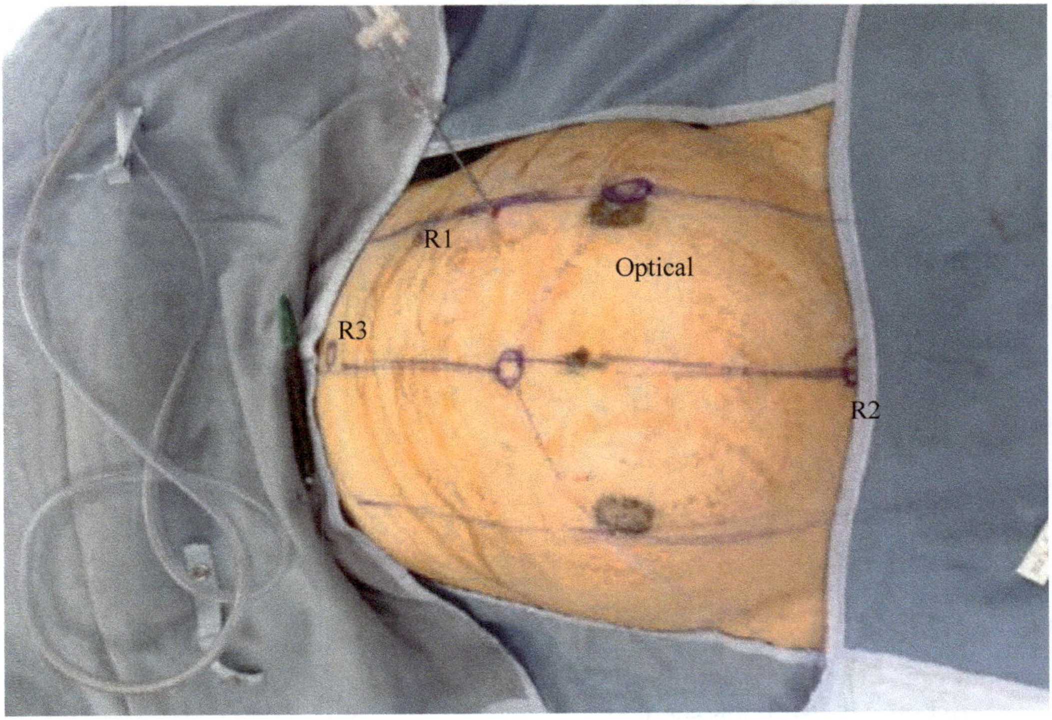

Image 2. Showing marking for Right Colonic resections. Insufflation via Veress needle at LUQ.

9. Port placements

9.1. Preparing for port placement

- Port placement is the key for a successful robotic procedure. Narrow space between the ports will result in clashing of the arms and poor ergonomics. We recommend marking of the abdomen for port placement after CO2 insufflation.
- The initial pneumopertioneum can be established with a Veress needle or Hassan's technique at LUQ or at camera port site.
- Initial assessment of entire anatomy of the abdomen focusing on adhesions, peritoneal seedlings and liver metastasis is carried out once the camera port is inserted. Place remaining ports under endoscopic vision avoiding injury to the inferior epigastric vessels.

9.2. Instrument port placements for left sided colorectal operations [54]

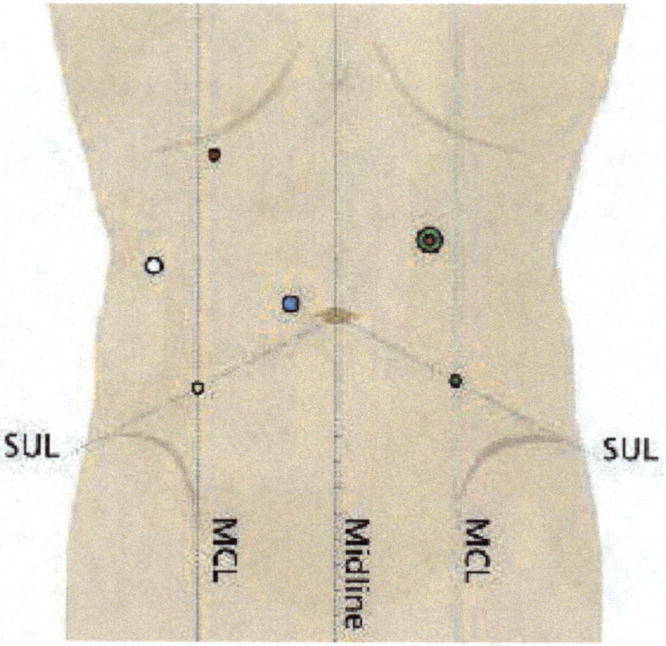

Diagram 1 Showing post placements for left sided colorectal operations

- **Robotic camera port, 12 mm (Blue):** Place the port 3-4 cm right and 3-4 cm above umbilicus. Distance to symphysis pubis should be ~22-24 cm.

- **Robotic instrument arm port, 8 mm (Yellow):** Place the port a minimum of 8 cm from the camera port, on the right spinoumbilical line (SUL) at the crossing of the mid-clavicular line (MCL). Distance to symphysis pubis should be ~14-16 cm. Linear stapler can be used from this port.

- **Robotic instrument arm port, 8 mm (Green):** Place the port a minimum of 8 cm from the camera port, on the left spinoumbilical line (SUL) at the crossing of the mid-clavicular line (MCL). The distance to the symphysis pubis should be ~14-16 cm.

- **Robotic instrument arm port, 8 mm (Red):** Place the port ~ 3 cm sub-xyphoid and ~ 2 cm medial to the right MCL

- **Robotic instrument arm port, 8 mm (Green-Red):** Place the port 7-8 cm below the left costal margin, slightly medial to the left MCL. Place the port a minimum of 8 cm from the other instrument ports and the camera port.

- **Assistant port, 5 mm (White):** Place the port 8-10 cm cephalad to the instrument arm port and ~ 4 cm lateral to the right MCL (a minimum of 8 cm from the camera port). This port is used for suction/irrigation, ligation and retraction.

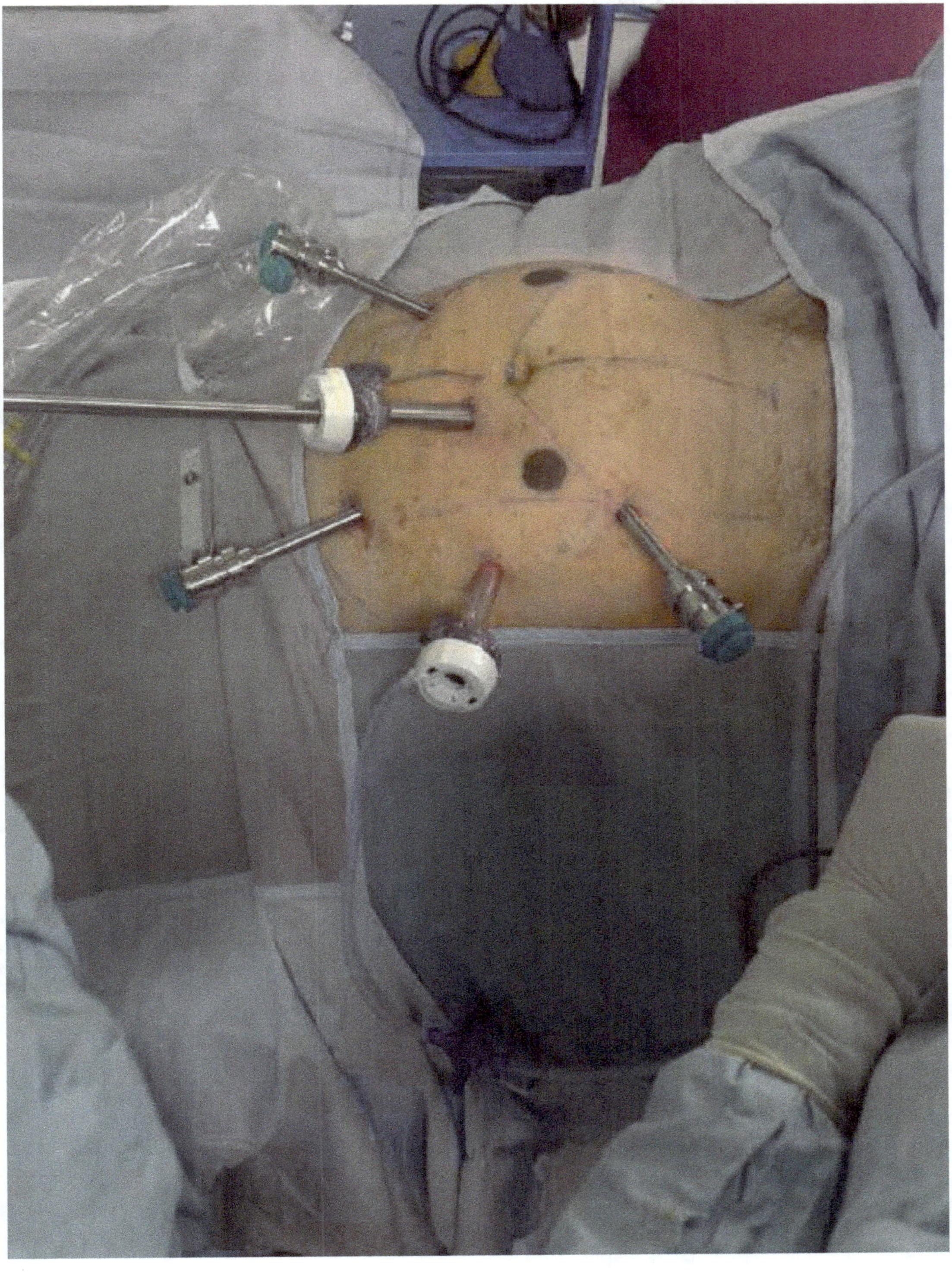

Image 3. Showing port placements for left sided colorectal operations

9.3. Port placement for right sided colonic resections

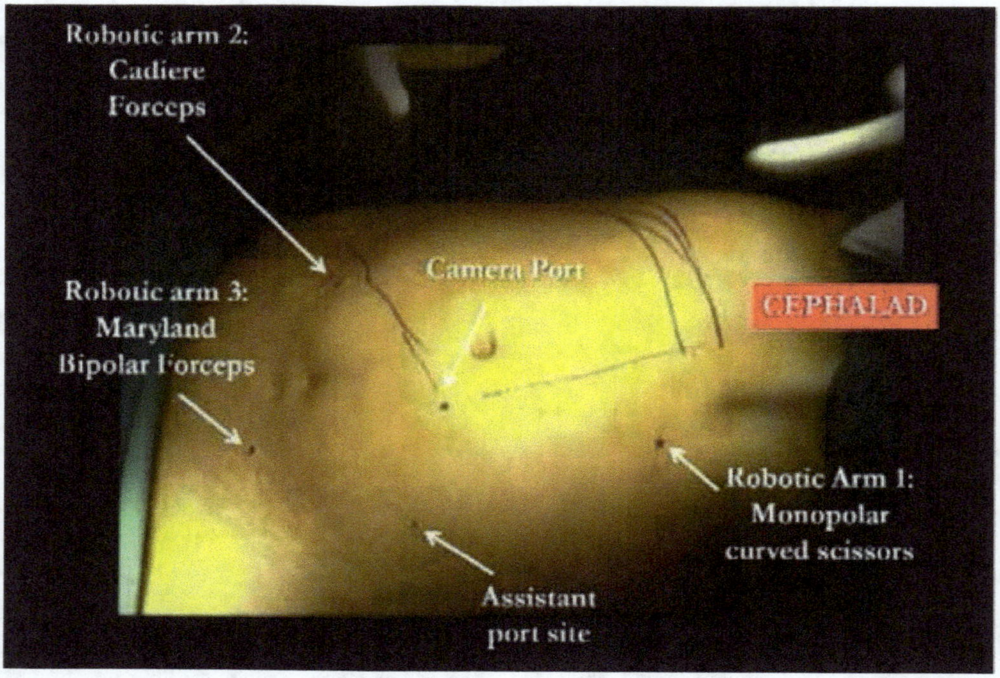

Image 4. [74]: showing port placements for right sided colonic resections

9.4. Instrument port placements for right sided colorectal operations

- Camera port 12mm, at left spinoumbilical line (SUL)
- Robotic arm port 1, 8mm, at left mid-clavicular line (MCL) 8cms below costal margin
- Robotic arm port 2, 8mm, is placed in at right SUL 2cms lateral to right MCL
- Robotic arm port 3, 8mm, is placed in midline 3 cms from pubic symphysis
- Assistant port, 5mm, place at LIF lateral to left MCL

9.5. Operative steps for left sided colorectal operations

- Initial exposure is acquired by cephalad retraction of the omentum to expose the transverse colon and by moving the small bowel out of the pelvis. Loops of small bowel can be stacked in the right upper quadrant to expose the Inferior Mesenteric Vein (IMV). A small swab placed against the small bowel loops can sometimes help by preventing the bowel from slipping into the operative area.
- Primary vascular control is achieved by ligating the Inferior Mesenteric Artery (IMA) and IMV earlier in the operation. Disposable locking clips are used to secure these vessels before division.

- Medial to lateral mobilization of sigmoid and descending colon is carried out towards the left sidewall and superiorly towards the spleen. The plane between mesocolon and Gerota's fascia is developed. Left ureter and gonadal vesssels should be identified at this stage.
- Splenic flexure mobilization (SFM) is not mandatory. However, if the anastomosis is likely to be at tension, SFM is strongly recommended. If SFM is needed, IMV is divided high and the plane above the pancreas is developed which can lead the surgeon into the lesser sac. Gastrocolic omental division from above can complete this step safely.
- Rectal dissection and division – Total Mesorectal Excision (TME) is carried out to the pelvic floor for a mid to low rectal cancer or to the peritoneal reflection for an upper rectal cancer. Great care is taken to avoid injury to the parasympathetic nerves.
- Anastomosis - Rectal division and anastomosis is performed using surgical staplers. Care should be taken not to damage the pelvic floor at this stage. For rectal division, stapler can be inserted through the assistant port or the R1 can be disabled and undocked and the port changed to a 12 mm port to allow the stapler to pass through. In patients with a very narrow pelvis, a supra-pubic port can be used to divide the rectum anteroposteriorly. We perform a routine flexible sigmoidoscopy to check for anastomotic bleeding, viability of the colon and rectum and at the same time perform a leak test to check for anastomotic leak.

9.6. Operative steps for right sided colonic resections

- The patient is positioned in modified Lloyd –Davis position with slight Trendelenberg tilt. The ileocolic and Superior Mesenteric Artery (SMA) pedicles are exposed by retraction of the small bowel and appropriate traction and counter traction on the mesentry. Dissection along the Superior Mesenteric Vein (SMV) will expose the ileocolic vein and artery that are then divided after clipping. Duodenum is identified early and dissection carried out towards the liver to enter the lesser sac.
- Lateral to medial mobilization allows the right colon to be freed up. Sub ileal dissection completes this dissection allowing the whole specimen to come to the midline. Gastrocolic omental division results in complete mobilization of the heaptic flexure.
- Ileocolic anastomosis can be performed intra or extra corporeally depending upon the surgeons preference. Specimen is extracted either through a midline or suprapubic incision.

9.7. Post-operative management — (Enhanced Recovery Programme [55])

Day of operation:

- Pain management with epidural followed by PCA and then oral/IV/IM analgesia
- Post-operatively the patients are transferred to Surgical High Care for close monitoring
- All patients should have DVT (unless contraindicated) and antibiotic prophylaxis
- Patients encouraged to sit out of bed and encouraged to drink straight after the operation including 2 protein drinks

First post-operative day:

- The patient will have an epidural and urinary catheter
- Will be encouraged to drink 2 litres of fluid and drink 4 high protein drinks
- Will be encouraged to eat normal food
- Will be encouraged out of bed for 8 hours and take 3 walks of 50 meters each with help from the physiotherapists

Second post-operative day:

- Epidural and urinary catheter removed. Pain management using PCA.
- Will be encouraged to drink 2 litres of fluid and drink 4 high protein drinks
- Will be encouraged to eat normal food
- Will be encouraged out of bed for 8 hours and take 3 walks of 50 meters each with help from the physiotherapists

Post-operative days 3-5:

- The patient is discharged from the hospital if stable in three to five days i.e. passed flatus and or opening bowels
- Pain controlled with oral medications
- Able to mobilize and physiotherapists happy with progress

Outpatient follow-up:

- Follow up at OPD 2-3 weeks post-operatively
- All Cancer patients are discussed at Multidisciplinary Team Meeting, regarding additional therapy or adjuvant radiation with or without chemotherapy as indicated.

10. Future developments

10.1. Role of ICG in bowel anastomosis and lymph node mapping using da Vinci robot

Indocyanine green (ICG) is a cyanine fluorescent dye that absorbs near infrared wavelengths of light. It binds to plasma proteins and travels in the vascular system [56]. ICG emits an infrared signal when excited by laser light *in situ*, which can be detected with near-infrared fluorescence camera system (NIRF) [57].

The image from NIRF gives visual assessment of blood vessels, blood flow, and tissue perfusion. ICG has been widely used by the ophthalmologists to visualise retinal blood vessels [58] and the technique has been amalgamated into the da Vinci Si robotic system.

Water soluble ICG can be given intravenously during surgical procedure. The surgeon is able switch into fluorescence imaging modes from normal white light mode by pressing pedals in the console and is able to view infrared images of blood flow in the microvasculature as well as tissue perfusion in real time. This is particularly useful during bowel anastomosis and improving patient outcomes [59].

Lymph nodes harvesting can be a difficult procedure to perform in cancer surgery.

The use of ICG is an attractive method to facilitate visualisation of lymphatic vessels, sentinel nodes, and metastatic lymph nodes. It was first introduced by Lim and Soter [60].

ICG has been used in the recent past to harvest lymphnodes for cutaneous rectal carcinoma metastasis [61] and cutaneous Kaposi's sarcoma [62] with successful outcome.

It has also been used in transcutaneous Sentinel Lymph Node detection in vulvar cancer patients [63] and for identification of lymphatic pathway involved in the spreading of prostate cancer [64].

10.2. Robotic Single Incision Laparoscopic Surgery (SILS) or Colectomy (SILC)

Single incision laparoscopic colectomy (SILC) is well established. SILC is associated with shorter post-operative length of hospital stay and smaller skin incision. There is no difference in operating time or in conversion rate when compared to multiport laparoscopic colorectal operations [65]. The main drawback with SILC is exposure, conflict of instruments, ease of instrumentation, camera operation and ergonomics [66].

Robotic single incision laparoscopic surgery may be the answer to some of the problems associated with SILC. The author believes that robotic single incision colectomy will result in less abdominal wall trauma, less pain, needing fewer analgesics, early mobilisation and decreased length of hospital stay. It will have better cosmetic result due to fewer numbers of incisions. There is good evidence to suggest that multiple laparoscopic port incisions can cause port site hernias even with 5mm ports [67, 68].

Early experience with robotic SILC performing right hemicolectomy is safe and feasible [69]. We need more studies to validate robotic SILC for left sided operations.

Other surgical specialties where robotic SILS is gaining interest are listed below:

- Spinioglio G et al mentioned that it took them less time to perform robotic single port laparoscopic cholecystecomies than laparoscopic SILS [70].
- Robotic single-port trans-umbilical total hysterectomy is technically feasible in selected patients with gynaecological disease [71].
- Hahn Tran et al have successfully performed robotic single-port inguinal hernia repair without any complications [72].
- The authors believe that robots will also play a role in natural orifice endoscopic surgery and specimen retrieval via the natural orifice in the near future

The perfect robotic platform should have a low external profile, which can be deployed through a single access site. It should be able to restore intra-abdominal triangulation while maintaining the maximum degree of freedom for accurate maneuvers and strength for reliable traction. Several purpose-built robotic prototypes for single-port surgery are being tested [73].

The author believes that robots will also play a role in natural orifice endoscopic surgery and specimen retrieval via the natural orifice in the near future.

11. Summary

In summary the developments of surgical robotics over the last decade has been very exciting. The technology is improving rapidly. Robots certainly allow the surgeons to perform better operations with improved safety. In colorectal surgery robotics will find its place in pelvic and rectal cancer surgery. The cost of instruments and the system are the biggest barrier to the widespread uptake of robotic surgery by the surgical community. The future applications of this technology may result in further benefits that will offset the cost issue.

Author details

Ray Swayamjyoti, Jim Khan and Amjad Parvaiz

Portsmouth Hospitals NHS Trust, Queen Alexandra Hospital, Portsmouth, UK

References

[1] Ewing DR, Pigazzi A, Wang Y, Ballantyne GH. Robots in the operating room--the history. *Semin Laparosc Surg.* 2004 Jun;11(2):63-71.

[2] Valero R, Ko YH et al Robotic surgery: history and teaching impact. *Actas Urol Esp.* 2011 Oct;35(9):540-5. doi: 10.1016/j.acuro.2011.04.005. Epub 2011 Jun 22.

[3] Dharia SP, Falcone T. Robotics in reproductive medicine. Fertil Steril 2005; 84: 1–11. 4)

[4] Prem N Kakar, Jyotirmoy Das, Preeti Mittal Roy, and Vijaya Pant Robotic invasion of operation theatre and associated anaesthetic issues: A review Indian J Anaesth. 2011 Jan-Feb; 55(1): 18–25. doi: 10.4103/0019-5049.76577

[5] Satava R, Richard M. Surgical robotics: The early chronicles: A personal historical perspective. Surg Laparosc Endosc Percutan Tech. 2002;12:6–16.

[6] Robot-assisted right colectomy: surgical technique and review of the literature Wojciech Witkiewicz, Marek Zawadzki, Marek Rząca, Zbigniew Obuszko, Videosurgery Miniinv 2013; 8 (3): 253–257 DOI:10.5114/wiitm.2011.33761

[7] Kwoh YS, Hou J, Jonckheere EA, Hayati S. A robot with improved absolute positioning accuracy for CT guided stereotactic brain surgery. IEEE Trans Biomed Eng 1988; 35: 153–60.

[8] http://www.robot.md/publications/robodoc-surgical-robot-sucess-story.pdf

[9] McConnell, PI; Schneeberger, EW; Michler, RE (2003). "History and development of robotic cardiac surgery". Problems in General Surgery 20 (2): 20–30.

[10] http://biomed.brown.edu/Courses/BI108/BI108_2000_Groups/Heart_Surgery/Robotics.html Biomed.brown.edu. Retrieved 13/11/2013

[11] http://en.wikipedia.org/wiki/Da_Vinci_Surgical_System

[12] Marescaux J, Smith MK, Foelscher D, Jamali F, Malassagne B, Leroy J. Telerobotic laparoscopic cholecystectomy: initial clinical experience with 25 patients. Ann Surg 2001;234:1-7.

[13] Robotic Colorectal Surgery: A Systematic Review, Sami AlAsari and Byung Soh Min, *ISRN Surg.* 2012; 2012: 293894. Published online 2012 May 13. doi: 10.5402/2012/293894

[14] Robotic gastrointestinal surgery: early experience and system description. Talamini M, Campbell K, Stanfield C. *J Laparoendosc Adv Surg Tech A.* 2002 Aug;12(4):225-32.

[15] http://www.engadget.com/2006/05/19/robot-surgeon-performs-worlds-first-unassisted-operation/

[16] http://www.roboticinfertility.com/main.html

[17] http://www.ucalgary.ca/news/may2008/neuroArm

[18] Hagn, U., Nickl, M., Jörg, S., Tobergte, A., Kübler, B., Passig, G., Gröger, M., Fröhlich, F., Seibold, U., Konietschke, R., Le-Tien, L., Albu-Schäffer, A., Grebenstein, M., Ortmaier, T. & Hirzinger, G. (2008). "DLR MiroSurge – towards versatility in surgical robotics". Proceedings of CURAC 7: 143–146.

[19] http://w3.wtb.tue.nl/nl/nieuws/artikel/?tx_ttnews%5Btt_news%5D=10041&tx_ttnews%5BbackPid%5D=465&cHash=ebb243e7ff

[20] http://med.over.net/clanek/php?full=1&id=25545&title=V_UKC_Ljubljana_prvi___na_svetu_uporabili___ilnega_robota_za_posege_na_femoralnem___ilju#.UoN3TaWc9MI

[21] http://www.smartplanet.com/blog/smart-takes/worlds-first-all-robotic-surgery-performed-in-canada/

[22] Melvin, W. S.; Needleman, B. J.; Krause, K. R.; Ellison, E. C. (February 2003). "Robotic Resection of Pancreatic Neuroendocrine Tumor". Journal of Laparoendoscopic & Advanced Surgical Techniques 13 (1): 33–36. doi:10.1089/109264203321235449.

[23] Babbage Science and technology (18 January 2012). "Surgical robots: The kindness of strangers" (http://www.economist.com/blogs/babbage/2012/01/surgical-robots). *The Economist*. Retrieved 21 February 2013.

[24] "da Vinci Products FAQ" (http://www.intuitivesurgical.com/products/products_faq.html#18). Intuitive Surgical. Retrieved 21 February 2013.

[25] http://intuitivesurgical.com/company/media/images/davinci_si_images.html

[26] http://intuitivesurgical.com/company/media/images/systems-si/Si_0185_%20two_male_surgeons_lookin_in_sm.jpg

[27] Weber PA, Merola S, Wasielewski A, Ballantyne GH, Delaney CP. Telerobotic-assisted laparoscopic right and sigmoid colectomies for benign disease. *Diseases of the Colon and Rectum*. 2002; 45(12):1689–1696.

[28] Robot-assisted laparoscopic surgery of the colon and rectum. Antoniou SA, Antoniou GA, Koch OO, Pointner R, Granderath FA. Surg Endosc. 2012 Jan;26(1):1-11. doi: 10.1007/s00464-011-1867-y. Epub 2011 Aug 20.

[29] Improved perioperative and short-term outcomes of robotic versus conventional laparoscopic colorectal operations. Casillas MA Jr, Leichtle SW, Wahl WL, Lampman RM, Welch KB, Wellock T, Madden EB, Cleary RK. *Am J Surg*. 2013 Oct 23. pii: S0002-9610(13)00608-9. doi: 10.1016/j.amjsurg.2013.08.028.

[30] Long-term outcome of robotic assisted laparoscopic rectopexy for full-thickness rectal prolapse in elderly patients. Germain A, Perrenot C, Scherrer ML, Ayav C, Brunaud L, Ayav A, Bresler L. Colorectal Dis. 2013 Dec 5. doi: 10.1111/codi.12513.

[31] Attaining Surgical Competency and Its Implications in Surgical Clinical Trial Design: A Systematic Review of the Learning Curve in Laparoscopic and Robot-Assisted Laparoscopic Colorectal Cancer Surgery. Barrie J, Jayne DG, Wright J, Murray CJ, Collinson FJ, Pavitt SH. Ann Surg Oncol. 2013 Nov 12.

[32] The first nationwide evaluation of robotic general surgery: a regionalized, small but safe start. Wormer BA, Dacey KT, Williams KB, Bradley JF 3rd, Walters AL, Augenstein VA, Stefanidis D, Heniford BT. Surg Endosc. 2013 Nov 7.

[33] Wittich P, Kazemier G, Schouten WR, Jeekel J, Lange JF, Bonjer HJ. The 'Colon cancer laparoscopic or open resection' (COLOR) trial. *Ned Tijdschr Geneeskd*. 1997 Sep 27;141(39):1870-1. 34)

[34] Bonjer, H. J., et al. "Laparoscopically assisted versus open colectomy for colon cancer: a meta-analysis." *Arch Surg* 142 (2007): 298-303.

[35] Nelson H, Sargent DJ, Wieand HS, et al. A comparison of laparoscopically assisted and open colectomy for colon cancer. *New England Journal of Medicine*. 2004;350(20): 2050–2059.

[36] Jayne DG et al. J Clin Oncol 2007; 25: 3061-8.

[37] ttp://www.eme.ac.uk/projectfiles/085201protocol.pdf

[38] Jayne DG, Guillou PJ, Thorpe H, et al. Randomized trial of laparoscopic-assisted resection of colorectal carcinoma: 3-Year results of the UK MRC CLASICC trial group. *Journal of Clinical Oncology*. 2007;25(21):3061–3068.

[39] 8. Jayne DG et al. Br J Surg. 2005; 92: 1124-32.

[40] Schwab KE, Dowson HM, Van Dellen J, Marks CG, Rockall TA. The uptake of laparoscopic colorectal surgery in Great Britain and Ireland: a questionnaire survey of consultant members of the ACPGBI. *Colorectal Disease*. 2009;11(3):318–322.

[41] Neutel CI, Gao RN, Wai E, Gaudette LA. Trends in in-patient hospital utilization and surgical procedures for breast, prostate, lung and colorectal cancers in Canada. *Cancer Causes and Control*. 2005;16(10):1261–1270.

[42] Sung-Bum Kang, et al. Open versus laparoscopic surgery for mid or low rectal cancer after neoadjuvant chemoradiotherapy (COREAN trial): short-term outcomes of an open-label randomised controlled trial. Lancet Oncol. 2010;11:637–45. doi: 10.1016/S1470-2045(10)70131-5.

[43] Paolo Pietro Bianchi, Fabrizio Luca, Wanda Petz, Manuela Valvo, Sabine Cenciarelli, Massimiliano Zuccaro, and Roberto Biffi, The role of the robotic technique in minimally invasive surgery in rectal cancer, *Ecancermedicalscience*. 2013; 7: 357. Published online 2013 September 26. doi: 10.3332/ecancer.2013.357

[44] Malak B. Bokhari, Chirag B. Patel, Diego I. Ramos-Valadez, Madhu Ragupathi, and Eric M. Haas, Learning curve for robotic-assisted laparoscopic colorectal surgery, *Surg Endosc*. 2011 March; 25(3): 855–860. Published online 2010 August 24. doi: 10.1007/s00464-010-1281-x

[45] Jiménez-Rodríguez RM, Díaz-Pavón JM, de la Portilla de Juan F, Prendes-Sillero E, Dussort HC, Padillo J. Learning curve for robotic-assisted laparoscopic rectal cancer surgery. Int J Colorectal Dis. 2013 Jun;28(6):815-21. doi: 10.1007/s00384-012-1620-6. Epub 2012 Dec 15.

[46] Sng KK, Hara M, Shin JW, Yoo BE, Yang KS, Kim SH. The multiphasic learning curve for robot-assisted rectal surgery. Surg Endosc. 2013 Sep;27(9):3297-307. doi: 10.1007/s00464-013-2909-4. Epub 2013 Mar 19.

[47] Halabi WJ,Kang CY,Jafari MD,Nguyen VQ,Carmichael JC,Mills S,Stamos MJ,Pigazzi A, Robot-assisted laparoscopic colorectal surgery. Alimoglu O, Atak I, Orhun K, Eren

T, Minerva Chirurgica, October 2013, vol./is. 68/5(471-8), 0026-4733;0026-4733 (2013 Oct)

[48] Robotic-assisted Colorectal Surgery in the United States: A Nationwide Analysis of Trends and Outcomes. World Journal of Surgery, 12 2013, vol./is. 37/12(2782-90), 0364-2313;1432-2323 (2013 Dec)

[49] Kim CW, Baik SH, Robotic rectal surgery: what are the benefits?. Minerva Chirurgica, October 2013, vol./is. 68/5(457-69), 0026-4733;0026-4733 (2013 Oct)

[50] Deborah S. Keller, Lobat Hashemi, Minyi Lu, and Conor P. Delaney, Short-Term Outcomes for Robotic Colorectal Surgery by Provider Volume, Journal of the American College of Surgeons, 2013-12-01, Volume 217, Issue 6, Pages 1063-1069.e1

[51] Bertani E, Chiappa A, Ubiali P, Cossu ML, Arnone P, Andreoni B, Robotic colectomy: is it necessary?, Minerva Chirurgica, October 2013, vol./is. 68/5(445-56), 0026-4733;0026-4733 (2013 Oct)

[52] http://www.gastroendonews.com/ViewArticle.aspx?d_id=187&a_id=13617

[53] https://www.davincisurgerycommunity.com/

[54] http://www.colorectal-surgeon.com/enhanced-recovery-programme.htm

[55] http://www.cancer.gov/

[56] Jarmo T. Alander, Ilkka Kaartinen, Aki Laakso, Tommi Pätilä, Thomas Spillmann, Valery V. Tuchin, Maarit Venermo, and Petri Välisuo, A Review of Indocyanine Green Fluorescent Imaging in Surgery. Int J Biomed Imaging. 2012; 2012: 940585. Published online 2012 April 22. doi: 10.1155/2012/940585

[57] Flower RW. Injection technique for indocyanine green and sodium fluorescein dye angiography of the eye. Investigative Ophthalmology. 1973;12(12):881–895.

[58] Bae, Se Jin Baek, Hyuk Hur, Seung Hyuk Baik, Nam Kyu Kim, and Byung Soh Min, Intraoperative Near Infrared Fluorescence Imaging in Robotic Low Anterior Resection: Three Case Reports Sung Uk, Yonsei Med J. 2013 July 1; 54(4): 1066–1069. Published online 2013 May 14. doi: 10.3349/ymj.2013.54.4.1066

[59] Lim H, Soter N. *Clinical Photomedicine*. New York, NY, USA: Marcel Dekker Inc.; 1993.

[60] Karrer S, Abels C, Bäumler W, Steinbauer M, Landthaler M, Szeimies RM. Photochemotherapie von kutanen Rektumkarzinom- Metastasen mit Indocyaningrun [photochemotherapy with indocyanine green in cutaneous metastases of rectal carcinoma] *Deutsche medizinische Wochenschrift*. 1997;122(37):1111–1114.

[61] Abels C, Karrer S, Bäumler W, Goetz AE, Landthaler M, Szeimies R-M. Indocyanine green and laser light for the treatment of AIDS-associated cutaneous Kaposi's sarcoma. *British Journal of Cancer*. 1998;77(6):1021–1024.

[62] Crane LMA, Themelis G, Arts HJG, et al. Intraoperative near-infrared fluorescence imaging for sentinel lymph node detection in vulvar cancer: first clinical results. *Gynecologic Oncology*. 2011;120(2):291–295.

[63] Inoue S, Shiina H, Arichi N, et al. Identification of lymphatic pathway involved in the spreading of prostate cancer by fluorescence navigation approach with intraoperatively injected indocyanine green. *Journal of the Canadian Urological Association*. 2011;5(4):254–259.

[64] Maggiori L, Gaujoux S, Tribillon E, Bretagnol F, Panis Y., Single-incision laparoscopy for colorectal resection: a systematic review and meta-analysis of more than a thousand procedures. Colorectal Dis. 2012 Oct;14(10):e643-54. doi: 10.1111/j.1463-1318.2012.03105.x.

[65] Ross H, Steele S, Whiteford M, Lee S, Albert M, Mutch M, Rivadeneira D, Marcello P. Early multi-institution experience with single-incision laparoscopic colectomy. Dis Colon Rectum. 2011 Feb;54(2):187-92. doi: 10.1007/DCR.0b013e3181f8d972.

[66] Khurshid N, Chung M, Horrigan T, Manahan K, Geisler JP., 5-millimeter trocar-site bowel herniation following laparoscopic surgery. JSLS. 2012 Apr-Jun;16(2):306-10.

[67] Yamamoto M, Minikel L, Zaritsky E., Laparoscopic 5-mm trocar site herniation and literature review. JSLS. 2011 Jan-Mar;15(1):122-6. doi: 10.4293/108680811X13022985131697.

[68] Ostrowitz MB, Eschete D, Zemon H, DeNoto G., Robotic-assisted single-incision right colectomy: early experience. Int J Med Robot. 2009 Dec;5(4):465-70. doi: 10.1002/rcs.281.

[69] Spinoglio G, Lenti LM, Maglione V, Lucido FS, Priora F, Bianchi PP, Single-site robotic cholecystectomy (SSRC) versus single-incision laparoscopic cholecystectomy (SILC): comparison of learning curves. First European experience., Grosso F, Quarati R. Surg Endosc. 2012 Jun;26(6):1648-55. doi: 10.1007/s00464-011-2087-1. Epub 2011 Dec 17.

[70] Eun Ji Nam, Sang Wun Kim, Maria Lee, Ga Won Yim et al, Robotic single-port transumbilical total hysterectomy: a pilot study, *Gynecol Oncol.* 2011 June 30; 22(2): 120–126. Published online 2011 June 30. doi: 10.3802/jgo.2011.22.2.120. *PMCID:* PMC3152752

[71] Hanh Tran, Robotic Single-Port Hernia Surgery, F *JSLS.* 2011 Jul-Sep; 15(3): 309–314. doi: 10.4293/108680811X13125733356198. *PMCID:* PMC3183567

[72] Autorino R, Kaouk JH, Stolzenburg JU, Gill IS, Mottrie A, Tewari A, Cadeddu JA.Current status and future directions of robotic single-site surgery: a systematic review. *Eur Urol.* 2013 Feb;63(2):266-80. doi: 10.1016/j.eururo.2012.08.028. Epub 2012 Aug 23.

[73] Mathew R, Kim SH. Robotic right hemicolectomy with D3 lymphadenectomy and complete mesocolic excision: Technical detail. OA Robotic Surgery 2013 Jun 01;1(1):6. http://www.oapublishinglondon.com/article/710,

9

Laparoscopy in the Management of Colorectal Cancer

Anton Tonev, Nikola Kolev, Valentin Ignatov,
Vasil Bojkov, Tanya Kirilova and Krassimir Ivanov

1. Introduction

Since the introduction of laparoscopic surgery, minimally invasive techniques have been widely used for benign and malignant diseases. [1, 2] Although many surgeons perform laparoscopic colectomy for benign diseases, its application for colorectal malignancy had slow progress because of oncological considerations. [3] Over time, many randomized controlled trials have been published comparing open to laparoscopic surgery for colorectal cancer, which show that in experienced hands, competent oncology resections can be performed the results are equivalent to open surgery [4-7]. However, the results of the minimally invasive surgery for rectal cancer have not been thoroughly investigated and large multicenter randomized trials are underway.

Large number of randomized controlled trials comparing laparoscopic to open surgery for colon cancer have established better short-term results - less pain, shorter length of stay, faster return of bowel function and equivalent oncological outcomes [2-5]. Laparoscopic rectal surgery is still developing with promising short-term benefit, although depending on the skills and techniques of the surgeon [6]. Surgery of rectal cancer requires more technical skills (total mesorectal excision, low pelvic anastomosis), many fear that the oncological principles could be compromised during laparoscopic resection. In addition to oncological concerns, the widespread of laparoscopic surgery for colorectal cancer is impeded by the significant learning curve.

Hand-assisted techniques introduced in the 1990s were an attempt to overcome some of these limitations and provide an overlap between open and laparoscopic techniques and the transition from open to minimally invasive surgery for many surgeons [1, 8]. Acceptance of minimally invasive procedures by patients and surgeons led to the developent of new technologies to ease the laparoscopic approach. The introduction of single incision laparoscopic surgery (SILS) devices has allowed fewer cuts. [9] The clinical application of endoscopic natural orifice transluminal surgery (NOTES) in colorectal disease is not yet fully accepted, but it was possible great advances in instrumentation and improving techniques for specimen extraction after laparoscopic colectomy [12].

2. Systemic benefits

Basic science studies have demonstrated the better preservation of oncological and immunological functions after laparoscopic surgery before trials on humans [7-9], thus giving hope for better long-term oncologic outcome. Tumor cells are found in systemic blood circulation and in the peritoneal fluid immediately after surgery and if they survive may avoid the immunological defense of the organism. The surgical trauma causes immunological alterations and the organism might be vulnerable during the postoperative period [7-9]. Laparoscopic surgery causes lesser trauma and therefore less effect on the immune system, decreases the proliferation stimuli for cancer cells and neoangiogenesis [7-9, 11]. The changes can last shortly after the operation, but some are observed after months or longer [11]. These potential advantages do not provide better long-term outcomes in human trials, although some report better oncological results after laparoscopic surgery in terms of longer cancer-related survival and less tumor recurrences [10-14].

The rate of conversion to open surgery is still very high, as demonstrated by three multicenter prospective trials - the NCI Clinical Outcomes of Surgical Therapies (COST; 21%), Colon Cancer Laparoscopic or Open Resection (COLOR; 17%), and the Conventional versus Laparoscopic-Assisted Surgery in Colorectal Cancer (CLASICC; 29%) [15, 16]. This could be due to more precautious behavior of the surgeons and their inexperience.

A meta-analysis from 2006 demonstrated intriguing results. It includes 1134 patients after colectomy in two periods – 1996-2000 and 2000-2004. Laparoscopic colectomy was introduced as an option only in the second period. The authors found that 3-year overall survival decreased in the latter, while the overall survival of patients after open colectomy remained the same over the two periods. [17]

Intracorporeal anastomosis for right laparoscopic colectomy improved patient outcome compared with patients who underwent extracorporeal anastomosis. There is found faster recovery of nutrition, faster recovery of intestinal function, and shorter hospitalization. However, there was no difference in average surgery time between the two groups.

According to the differences in age, gender, BMI, ASA class, or abdominal surgical history, in laparoscopic colectomy with extracorporeal anastomosis (laparoscopic-assisted colectomy), the bowel is externalized through a lateral mini-incision. With this approach, bowel mobilization and ligation of vessels is usually laparoscopic, whereas resection of the specimen and creation of the anastomosis is extracorporeal. On the other hand, in laparoscopic right colectomy with intracorporeal anastomosis (totally laparoscopic colectomy), bowel mobilization, ligation of vessels, resection of the specimen, and creation of the anastomosis are totally intracorporeal.

Regarding oncological radicality, there are significant differences in the number of lymph nodes removed. An average of 19 lymph nodes from the intracorporeal group and 14 lymph nodes from the extracorporeal group are reported to be removed. In the literature, some authors have reported no differences in safety, whereas others noted that the only advantage was a smaller incision. On the other hand, other studies affirmed the safety of intracorporeal anastomosis, with the same complication rate as for extracorporeal anastomosis. Because intracorporeal anastomosis is considered more difficult, only a few surgeons have used this kind of technique; however less mobilization is required, and less tension is applied to the bowel and mesentery because the bowel does not need to reach the anterior abdominal wall for externalization. [11] Furthermore, the excessive tension on the mesentery during the mobilization is associated with an increased risk of mesenteric or portal vein thrombosis. Concerning surgical times, there is not a significant difference in surgical time between the two groups. Patients in the intracorporeal group had a shorter hospitalization duration. In some cases, the hospitalization duration was longer possibly because of age (43.2% of patients in the intracorporeal group and 33.4% in the extracorporeal group were over 80 years old). Our results showed a significantly shorter average hospitalization stay in the intracorporeal group. These data agree with a recent Spanish study, although this difference was not significant ($P = 0.5424$) because hospitalization duration is influenced by many patient factors. On the other hand, we found that 71.4% of patients in the intracorporeal group went home within 7 d, and 54.7% of patients in the extracorporeal group went home within this period. [20, 21] Patients in the intracorporeal group and extracorporeal group went home within 7 d. Concerning the recovery of intestinal function, our results found significantly shorter average times for resumption of gas evacuation after 3 d in the intracorporeal group compared to after 3.8 d in the extracorporeal group. Bowel movements occurred after an average of 4.9 d in the intracorporeal group. In the intracorporeal group, the nasogastric tube was removed after 1.8 d, whereas it was removed after 3 d in the extracorporeal group. This difference can be explained by an increased percentage of paralytic ileus in the second group, which is due to the traction of the right colon and terminal ileum through the mini-incision on the pancreas and duodenum. This approach allowed a more rapid recovery of liquid and solid nutrition consumption. [25-27] There are met some major complications, which included severe anemia, occlusion, anastomotic dehisces, and enterocutaneous fistulae. There were no significant differences between the two groups.

In conclusion, our study clearly shows that laparoscopic right colectomy with intracorporeal anastomosis improves patient outcome. Intracorporeal anastomosis resulted in faster recovery of nutrition consumption, faster recovery of intestinal function, and shorter hospitalization duration. The higher number of lymph nodes removed seems to be related to vascular division as the first surgical step as a rule. This confirms that a mini invasive approach improves patient outcome.

3. Port site metastasis

The early trials of laparoscopic colectomy have established high rate of tumor recurrence near the port wounds, which was considered a serious drawback of the new approach. The etiology is unclear, although some authors suggest poor surgical technique and tumor biology as a probable cause. The reported rate in the early trials reached 21%. Recent trials (Hughes et al., 1603 patients, [15] found the rate to be 0.68%. Fleshman et al. [5] reported results based on the NCI COST trial, which demonstrated comparable rates for open and laparoscopic surgery after 5- and 8-year follow up (0.5% and 0.9%, respectively). The Barcelona trials had similar outcome after a median follow-up of 95 months [7]. The European randomized controlled study, the Colon Cancer Laparoscopic or Open Resection (COLOR) trial (2009) established after 53-month median follow-up that the port site metastasis rate was 0.4% after open (n=542) and 1.3% after laparoscopic colectomy (n=534). [19] The location of the recurrences was near the extraction port (n=2) and near the trocar sites (n=5) [5]. Recent studies do not report such high recurrence rates.

Proper training and the use of safe oncologic techniques are essential in the prevention of port site metastases. Such safe techniques are the routing use of wound protectors, less instrument exchange, avoidance of direct trauma to the tumor, avoidance of inadvertent desufflation.

4. Enhanced recovery after surgery

The approach employs a multimodal perioperative care pathway with the aim of attenuating the stress response to surgery and accelerating recovery [21]. Implementation of enhanced recovery protocols has led to improved outcomes across a range of different specialties including reductions in postoperative morbidity and hospital stay [61-65]. The fundamental premise of ERAS is the incorporation of evidence-based practice. It would seem to follow therefore that the evolution of enhanced recovery guidelines should be dynamic, allowing modifications of certain aspects of the program as new data becomes available. Some authors have advocated a rigid adherence to the ERAS protocol, citing study data that demonstrates a proportional relationship between deviation from the protocol and increased morbidity [61]. However, as evidence for components of the ERAS protocol change, it may be that a more flexible and individualised approach should be considered.

5. Perioperative fluid administration

Traditionally, patients undergoing major colorectal surgery have received liberal volumes of intravenous fluids [49]. Excess intravenous fluid during and after surgery has been associated with delayed gut function and increased complication rates [50, 51]. Fluid restriction has been proposed as a possible method of improving recovery and reducing postoperative complications. Brandstrup *et al* [58] found that randomising patients undergoing elective colorectal surgery resection to a restricted fluid protocol reduced cardiopulmonary and wound morbidity. MacKay *et al* [59] found no difference in recovery of gastrointestinal function or time to discharge with postoperative fluid restriction while using a conservative intra-operative protocol. Goal directed fluid therapy *via* oesophageal Doppler (OD) monitoring offers an opportunity to individualise peri-operative fluid administration. OD provides a real time representation of haemodynamic function, and has been shown to be comparable with other methods for estimating cardiac output such as LIDCO. A number of studies have shown that goal-directed fluids reduce morbidity, critical care admissions, and hospital stay [62]. It is not clear however whether these benefits are still significant within an enhanced recovery protocol. Other goal-directed techniques employ central venous oxygen saturation ($ScvO_2$) as a surrogate for mixed venous oxygen saturation. $ScvO_2$ is related to tissue oxygenation and so can be used to titrate oxygen and fluid therapy, particularly in the immediate postoperative period. This approach requires central venous access which is not always available as some groups have developed a less invasive approach to monitoring. While a number of different fluid protocols have been proposed, the optimal approach is still unclear.

6. Evolving postoperative analgesia

Epidural analgesia was considered central to early ERAS protocols, since it reduces the endocrine-mediated stress response [53, 54], and improves postoperative intestinal function [55]. Epidural analgesia also provides superior pain control to systemic opiates, particularly in the first 24-36 h after surgery [56]. Data on the effect of epidural analgesia come predominantly from studies in open surgery while the benefits in laparoscopic surgery are less clear. Levy *et al* [65, 66] performed a meta-analysis to address this question but concluded that there was a paucity of quality data. The authors subsequently performed a study in which patients were randomised to receive epidural, spinal or patient-controlled opiate analgesia following elective laparoscopic colorectal resection. They demonstrated a significantly longer hospital stay, time to return of bowel function and duration of nausea in the epidural group. Intrathecal morphine has been proposed as an alternative [67]. A meta-analysis provides encouraging results in patients undergoing abdominal surgery; reduced post-operative pain in the first 48 h and significantly reduced opiate consumption compared with systemic opiates [68]. Transversus abdominus plane blocks have also been gaining in popularity although comparative data is still lacking [69]. Epidurals can cause vasodilatation and hypotension [70], resulting in excess fluid challenges, third space shift and fluid overload. As studies emerge demonstrating benefits of alternative analgesic techniques, it does raise the question: Should epidural analgesia be the standard technique for all colorectal resections? Perhaps a more individualised approach dependent on the procedure, use of laparoscopy and placement of incisions should be considered. In this way more patients may be able to avoid potential complications while maintaining adequate analgesia and facilitating early mobilisation.

7. Laparoscopic and open surgery in enhanced recovery

The adoption of laparoscopic techniques within colorectal surgery came at a similar time to the introduction of "fast-track" surgery. Early studies examining the effect of laparoscopic surgery showed clear superiority in short term outcomes when compared with open surgery using traditional recovery technique [63, 64]. Patients undergoing laparoscopic surgery have reduced in-patient stays, less morbidity and improved postoperative pain [65, 66]. What is less clear is how much of the benefit is attributable to laparoscopy and how much is an effect of differing perioperative care pathways. Since these early trials there have been a number of small trials comparing laparoscopic and open colorectal surgery within an enhanced recovery setting with conflicting results [55-61]. Most recently a four-armed randomised study of patients undergoing either open or laparoscopic surgery, in an enhanced recovery or standard recovery programme was performed. They demonstrated a significantly faster recovery time following colonic surgery in those patients undergoing laparoscopic procedures within an ERAS programme. What is clear is that there are still a number of areas within the enhanced recovery protocol where the evidence-base continues to change. The relative contributions of different facets of the protocol also remain to be determined. While this is the case we should accept a flexible approach to facilitate the adoption of techniques supported by randomised data. There may also be scope for a degree of individualisation to reflect the wide range of patients and procedures to which enhanced recovery is now being applied. [70]

8. Laparoscopic colectomy

After the initial description in 1991, several reports of laparoscopic colectomy (LC) for colorectal cancer were described. Significant concerns regarding this approach surfaced when minimally invasive techniques applied to colorectal malignancy lead to increased surgical complications and worse cancer outcomes compared to conventional open approaches. An early report, using minimally invasive techniques for benign colorectal disease, showed a significantly high rate of serious complications (18%), including inadvertent enterotomies, intraoperative hemorrhage, anastomotic leaks, and pelvic abscesses. When LC was used to treat colorectal cancer, several papers noted early wound or trocar site recurrences, including one case series documenting a 21% rate. With a less than 1 percent wound implantation rate for open surgery, serious concerns were raised as to the possibility that poor oncologic results were due to a combination of poor technique and abnormal distribution of malignant cells secondary to pneumoperitoneum. Further concerns that laparoscopic techniques may be problematic to cancer patients arose when some studies demonstrated statistically significant worse cancer-specific survival in patients who had conversion from laparoscopic to open surgery. Moloo et al. described decreased survival at 2 years of 76% from 87% for all stages ($P = 0.02$) of colorectal cancer collected from a prospective database of 377 consecutive laparoscopic patients. In the same cohort, at 5 year followup, there was a trend toward decreased overall survival in converted patients (61.9% versus 69.7%, $P = 0.077$). Chan et al. showed an increased local recurrence rate at 3 year followup of 9.8% in the laparoscopically converted group as compared to 2.8% in open patients ($P = 0.03$). The oncological concerns raised in early reports provided a compelling argument to study the question of oncologic equivalence between the open and laparoscopic approach to colorectal cancer in a controlled fashion.

In the early 1990s, several multicenter prospective randomized controlled trials comparing laparoscopic and open surgery for colorectal cancer were initiated. Ultimately, seven large-scale trials compared laparoscopic and open colectomy for colon carcinoma and examined short-term and long-term outcomes. These trials included the Clinical Outcomes of Surgical Therapies (COST) trial funded by the National Cancer Institute in the United States, the Conventional versus Laparoscopic-Assisted Surgery in Colorectal Cancer (CLASICC) trial in the United Kingdom, the Colon Cancer Laparoscopic or Open Resection (COLOR), a multi-center European trial, the Barcelona trial, and several others [20–26]. The main focus of these trials was oncologic outcomes, but short-term outcomes, quality of life, and safety were also evaluated. The CLASICC trial was the only large trial that also evaluated MIS in rectal cancer. Though modest in early studies, the short-term patient-related advantages of laparoscopic surgery have now been confirmed and are significant over the open approach. The Minimally Invasive Colorectal Resection Outcomes (MICRO) review identified 22 randomized controlled trials and 66 cohort series for benign and malignant colorectal disease [27]. Laparoscopic colectomy results in significantly lower pain scores and analgesia requirements, estimated blood loss, return of bowel function, and length of stay. Numerous other trials, including the COST, COLOR, and CLASICC trials, examining short-term outcomes following laparoscopic colectomy for colorectal cancer have confirmed these findings [20–26, 28]. Several studies have also identified a decreased rate of postoperative morbidity including fewer wound infections [21, 23, 27, 29]; this was recently reinforced by a large trial from the National Surgical Quality Improvement Program (NSQIP) database of over 10, 000 patients identifying decreased incidence of wound infection following laparoscopic colectomy (9.5% versus 16.1%, $P < 0.001$) [30]. Quality of life has been assessed in several trials and results varied from no difference to favoring improved quality of life in laparoscopic colectomy [31].

The initially cited oncologic concerns of laparoscopic colectomy for colorectal cancer were later dispelled when surgeons trained in appropriate laparoscopic oncologic resection performed operations in the trial setting. Major trials, including the COST, CLASICC, and COLOR trials, examined tumor specimens and reported long-term data on recurrence and survival. The surgical specimens were evaluated, and parameters such as lymph node yield, circumferential resection margins, and longitudinal margins were quantified. No trial identified statistically significant differences in lymph node yield [20–26] or resection margins [20, 22, 26]. This initial evidence allayed some concerns regarding oncologic resections, but the long-term measures for recurrence and survival were still unknown. Trial data matured, and more evidence accumulated confirming similar recurrence patterns and rates between laparoscopic and open colectomy. Local recurrence, distant recurrence, and wound or port site metastases were the same between groups [4, 5, 7, 24, 32–34]. Disease-free and overall survival in long-term follow-up (up to 7 years) is equivalent [4, 5, 7, 32–34]. The concern that conversion from laparoscopic to open surgery in patients with colon cancer may lead to worse oncologic outcomes was not seen when 5-year COST trial data showed no statistical difference in these two groups.

Despite evidence demonstrating improved short-term outcomes of laparoscopic colectomy and oncologic equivalence, widespread implementation of this technique was slow. The lack of formalized training, outside single-day laparoscopic training courses, and the significant learning curve for straight laparoscopic techniques likely represented significant barriers to adoption. As hand-assisted laparoscopic surgery grew in popularity, a more widespread adaptation with fewer conversions to open surgery occurred in part due to a shorter learning curve with this technique. Three randomized controlled trials have been performed to compare a hand-assisted technique to a laparoscopic technique including patients with both benign and malignant disease, all demonstrating decreased rates of conversion to open surgery [35–37]. A recent meta-analysis compiling 13 studies demonstrated decreased operative times and decreased open conversion rates with a hand-assisted approach [38]. There were no differences in short-term clinical outcomes or oncologic resection results. A recent study by the Mayo Clinic prospectively analyzed the use of hand-assisted surgery in a minimally invasive colorectal practice and found that when applied to a center performing large volumes of laparoscopic surgery, hand-assisted techniques were responsible for more complex procedures to be done laparoscopically [39]. This technique is a minimally invasive approach that has been helpful for surgeons to transition from open to laparoscopic colectomy, especially if they have had little previous laparoscopic experience. Moreover, this technique has allowed a MIS approach in patients otherwise not previously considered candidates (obese, adhesions).

As surgeon experience increased and as more studies demonstrated that laparoscopic colectomy for benign and malignant disease is an acceptable alternative to open surgery, the overall ratio of laparoscopic to open colectomies in the United States has increased. A recent analysis from 2000 through 2004 demonstrated an increasing incidence of laparoscopic colectomy from 3% to 6.5% nationally with increased rates of laparoscopic approaches in urban centers and teaching hospitals [40]. A separate study and database of patients from 2004 through 2006 identified over 32, 000 patients, of which 34% underwent laparoscopic colectomy [41]. This trend toward increased laparoscopy has also been influenced by public knowledge and patient demand for this approach, as well as improved and formalized laparoscopic training in residency programs.

The short-term advantages of laparoscopic surgery over the open approach are confirmed. The minimally invasive approach is characterized by lower pain score and analgesia requirement, estimated blood loss; earlier return of bowel function and shorter length of stay (Minimally Invasive Colorectal Resection Outcomes (MICRO), [20]. The postoperative recovery of pulmonary function is quicker after laparoscopic colectomy. None of the randomized trials have observed significant increase in the anastomotic leakage rate [2-5]. Several studies demonstrated the decreased rate of postoperative morbidity and less wound infections [2-7]. Quality of life after laparoscopic surgery has been evaluated in several trials and the results varied from similar to better QoL than after open surgery [21].

In 2008 Lacy et al. reported the long-term outcomes of Barcelona trial (median follow-up 95 months). The overall survival rate was higher in the laparoscopic (64%) group when compared with the open group (51%) with no statistically significant difference ($p<0.07$). Laparoscopic group demonstrated higher cancer-related survival and lower cancer recurrence in ($p<0.07$ for both). The differences in survival and recurrences between the open and laparoscopic groups were observed for III stage tumors, with significantly better results in terms of overall-survival, cancer-related survival and chances of being free of recurrence. Results for stage I and II did not show any statistical difference. The conclusion is that in a dedicated laparoscopic center, LAC may result in a long-term survival benefit compared with OC, particularly in advanced cases". This oncological advantage can be explained by a preserved cellular immunity, attenuated stress and inflammatory response. [7]

These results seem encouraging and lead the way for laparoscopic surgery, although in a 2007 study by Fleshman (5-year follow-up, COST trial) the data did not demonstrate significant difference in the 5-year overall survival, 5-year disease-free survival, and recurrence rates between the two groups. The pattern of recurrence is also similar. [5] In 2007 Bonjer et al. reported meta-analysis, based on 3-year follow-up data from Barcelona, COST, COLOR and CLASSIC trials. No significant difference in 3-year survival, 3-year disease free survival or tumor recurrence rates between study groups was observed. Analysis by stages did not show any statistical difference in survival between both groups [16].

The hand-assisted laparoscopic surgery is a potential way to decrease operative time and maintain the benefits of the minimally invasive approach. The type of laparoscopic surgery allows introducing a hand through special device in the abdominal cavity, while preserving pneumoperitoneum. This provides proprioception and tactile feedback and ability to perform manual dissection and retraction. A study by Marcell [8] reported the results after multicenter randomized trial. The hand assisted sigmoidectomy group had significantly shorter operative time by 30-minutes when compared with straight laparoscopic group. Both groups had similar short-term outcomes. There were no differences in time to bowel function, pain scores, narcotic use, or time to bowel function. Conversion to open surgery was also significantly less for the hand-assisted group. Incision length was significantly longer for the hand-assisted group, but the difference was small. The authors concluded that hand-assisted surgery results in significantly shorter operative time, while maintaining similar outcomes as straight laparoscopic surgery [17]. Hand-assisted surgery allows to perform more complex procedures and to operate on patients with adhesion or obesity.

9. Laparoscopy for rectal cancer

The use of laparoscopic approach in the treatment of rectal cancer has led to increase of surgical complications and worse cancer outcomes in comparison to the open surgery [6] strong statement to make, may be phrase it differently. Several papers reported increased rate of port-site recurrences, reaching up to 21% [3]. The same parameter for the open approach is 1%. Those results might be explained by poor surgical technique and abnormal distribution of cancer cell due to the pneumoperitoneum [7]. The cancer-specific survival was significantly lower after conversion to open surgery [8, 9].

Based on the data of a prospective trial, including 377 laparoscopic patients [22] the survival decreased from 87% to 76% at 2 years for all stages of colorectal cancer. After a 5-year follow-up the overall survival decreased in converted patients. The local recurrence also proved to be higher: 9.8% and 2.8% for the laparoscopic and open groups, respectively. Several large trials were initiated in the 1990 (Clinical Outcomes of Surgical Therapies (COST) [21]in the

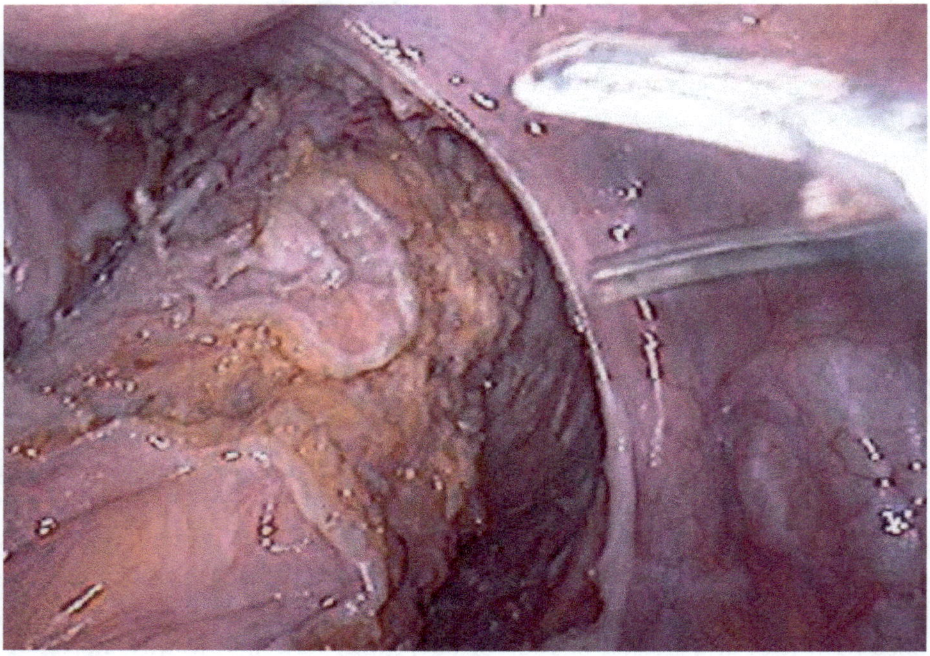

Figure 1. Laparoscopic resection of rectal cancer –anterior mobilization of the rectum

USA, the Conventional versus Laparoscopic-Assisted Surgery in Colorectal Cancer (CLASICC) [6] in the United Kingdom, Colon Cancer Laparoscopic or Open Resection (COLOR) in Europe and the Barcelona trial) [15]. Those trials evaluated laparoscopic and open colectomy for colon carcinoma and examined short-term and long-term outcomes, as well as short-term outcomes, quality of life and safety. Only the CLASSIC trials evaluated minimally invasive surgery for rectal cancer.

The potential benefits of laparoscopic rectal surgery are known and were proven by meta-analysis of studies of non-randomized trials – shorter time of bowel function restoration, shorter length of stay [22]. A characteristic advantage of the laparoscopic surgery is that it provides unobstructed view to the entire surgical team and magnified view of the operating field, thus allowing more accurate dissection. The pneumoperitoneum helps to open the planes of dissection of the mesorectum. The limitations of the laparoscopic rectal surgery are the unsure data on oncological safety [2-5], the concerns about inadequate oncological distant dissection, anastomotic leakage, technical challenges [23, 24].

Significant difficulty poses the obtaining of adequate exposure of the rectum. The narrow pelvis in some patients may cause clashing of the instruments and poor dissection. An experience assistant is required in such cases. The CLASSIC trial reported increased rate of positive circumferential margin after laparoscopic rectal surgery (12%) in comparison to the open group (6%). The distant margin of the tumor is difficult to be identified, as it cannot be palpated. This may cause inadequate distal resection.

The use of laparoscopic stapler requires multiple firings to complete distal rectal resection. In the case of low rectal anastomoses, this increases the anastomotic leakage rate (17% below 12cm from the anal verge [11], 20% below 15cm [23]. The leakage rate after open total mesorectal dissection varies from 4% to 11% [25, 26]. Future improvement of the stapler technology is required.

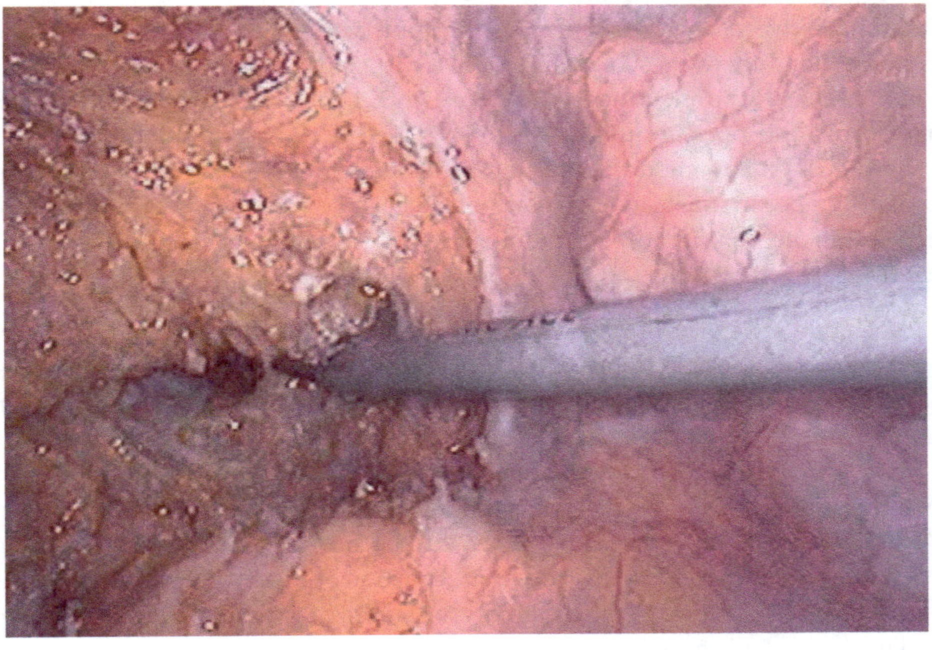

Figure 2. Lymph node dissection in laparoscopic rectal cancer resection

The proven benefits of laparoscopy noted in colon cancer surgery including decreased intraoperative blood loss, smaller length of incision, less postoperative pain, faster recovery of intestinal function, and shorter length of hospital stay likely also apply to rectal cancer surgery [37]. In RCTs the mean operative time for open surgical resection of rectal cancer ranged from 106 to 284 min compared to 120 to 245 min for laparoscopic resection. As expected, duration of operation was significantly longer in the laparoscopic group compared to the open group in 6 of the 8 RCTs [7, 22, 31, 38-40]. Similar results were reported in RCTs of open *vs* laparoscopic resection for colon cancer. Zhou *et al* [24] reported both shorter open and laparoscopic operative times compared to other trials with no significant difference between the two operative approaches (120 min *vs* 106 min for laparoscopic *vs* open resection respectively, P= 0.051). However, no details were provided on tumor stage, conversion rate, or whether the analysis was performed on an intent-to-treat basis. Araujo *et al* [25] was the only RCT to demonstrate significantly shorter operative times with laparoscopic compared to open resection (228 min *vs* 284 min respectively, $P = 0.04$). However, they attributed these results to fact that the surgical team performing laparoscopic APR was the same whereas open APR was often performed by different surgical teams. In addition, extraction of the specimen from the perineum likely decreased operative time because there was not an abdominal incision to close. Two meta-analyses included operative time as an outcome of interest. Aziz *et al* [17] included 22 studies comparing laparoscopic *vs* open rectal cancer resection in 2071 patients and found that operative time was significantly increased with the laparoscopic group as compared to the open group with a weighted mean difference (WMD) of 40.18 (95% CI, 26.46-56.13). Gao *et al* [26] performed a meta-analysis of short-term outcomes after laparoscopic resection for rectal cancer based on 11 studies and included 643 patients which reported no difference in operating time between open and laparoscopic approaches with a WMD of 1.59 [1.2-1.98]. Intraoperative blood loss was significantly less for the laparoscopic group compared to the open group in 4 of 6 RCTs and ranged from 20 mL to 321.7 mL and from 92 mL to 555.6 mL in the laparoscopic and open groups respectively [31, 35, 38, 40]. Araujo *et al* [25] did not specifically report on the amount of intraoperative blood loss but there was no statistically significant difference in the need for blood transfusions between the two groups which was attributed to the fact that in an APR the majority of blood loss occurs during the perineal portion of the case which is the same regardless of surgical access.

A recent Cochrane review by Breukink *et al* [41] evaluating the safety and efficacy of elective laparoscopic TME for the resection of rectal cancer found that in the majority of studies blood loss was reduced with the laparoscopic approach although this did not translate to fewer blood transfusions. Length of incision was measured in 3 of 8 RCTs and ranged from an average of 5 cm to 10 cm with the laparoscopic approach compared to an average of 19.1 cm to 22 cm with the open approach [7, 38, 40]. Seven of the 8 trials reported a conversion rate which ranged from 0%-34% [7, 38-40]. Conversion to the open approach was commonly defined as length of incision greater than the size needed for tumor extraction or premature abdominal incision to allow improved mobilization. In the majority of studies conversion to open surgery was required because of local tumor invasion or difficult dissection in a narrow pelvis although bulky tumor, dilated small bowel, dense adhesions, bleeding, rectal perforation, difficulty mobilizing the splenic flexure, failure to identify or injury to the ureter, ischemia of the descending colon, and anastomotic failure were also cited. Breukink *et al* [41] reported that 36 of 48 studies assessed conversion and showed a highly variable rate ranging from 0% to 33%. However, they report that the lack of consensus in the definition made results difficult to interpret. In addition, surgeon experience and patient selection criteria were often not mentioned. Two trials reported particularly high rates of conversion. Ng *et al* [37] had a conversion rate of 30.3% but they did not routinely perform preoperative staging with computed tomography scans and therefore frequently converted after diagnostic laparoscopy. Twelve of the 23 patients randomized to laparoscopic surgery were converted to open due to local tumor invasion, bulky tumor, or dilated small bowel which may have been recognized by preoperative imaging. In the CLASICC trial the conversion rate for laparoscopic resection of rectal cancer was reported at 34% and attributed to excessive tumor fixation and uncertainty of tumor clearance [6]. Surgeon learning curve may account for this high rate of conversion as evidenced by the fact that the overall rate of conversion dropped by year of study from 38% in year one to 16% in year six. However, consistent with several non-randomized reports, in the CLASICC trial patients converted to open resection had a higher operative mortality compared to patients in the laparoscopic or open groups (9% *vs* 1% *vs* 5% respectively) [6].

Conversion was also associated with worse oncologic outcomes in nonrandomized comparative and descriptive studies [46].

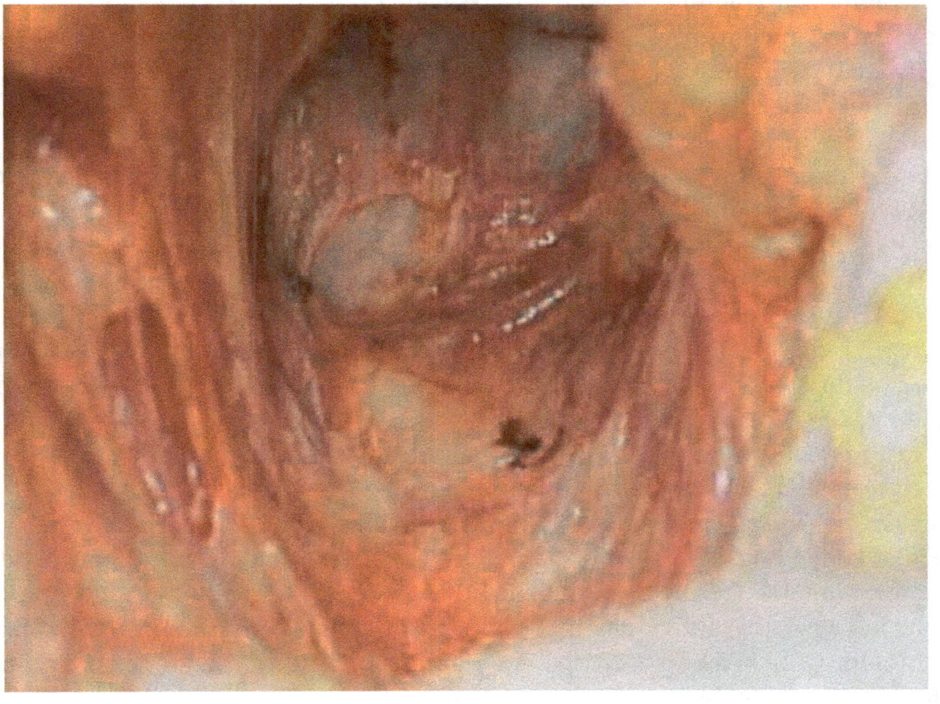

Figure 3. Total mesorectal excision after laparoscopic rectal resection

10. Short-term oncologic outcomes

While the number of lymph nodes retrieved can vary based on age, gender, tumor site, use of pre-operative radiation, and tumor grade, the extent and quality of surgical resection can also have an impact on the number of nodes collected and is therefore often considered a surrogate marker of the oncologic completeness of the resection [37]. The American Joint Committee on Cancer recommends that at least 12 lymph nodes be examined in patients with rectal cancer to confirm the absence of nodal involvement by the tumor [34]. In addition, a number of studies have reported that the number of lymph nodes examined may be associated with patient outcome [25, 26]. Six of the 8 RCTs reported the mean number of lymph nodes retrieved with a range of 5.5 to 17 nodes in the laparoscopic group compared to 11.6 to 18 nodes in the open group [22, 31, 34]. In 4 of the 6 trials the number of lymph nodes isolated was not significantly different based on surgical approach. Araujo *et al* [25] reported a significantly lower yield of lymph nodes with laparoscopic rectal resection compared to open resection (5.5 *vs* 11.9 respectively, $P = 0.04$). They suggested that laparoscopy offered better dissection and accuracy due to better visualization and exposure of structures with less manipulation of the mesorectum especially in a narrow pelvis. Four of the 8 RCTs reported the use of pre-operative chemoradiation. In these trials, the mean number of lymph nodes retrieved ranged from 5.5 to 17 nodes in the laparoscopic group and from 11.6 to 18 nodes in the open group [31, 34, 38, 40]. Some authors [37] found that in the 17 trials that reported the number of lymph nodes retrieved, the mean number of nodes was 10 for the laparoscopic group and 12 for the open group ($P = 0.001$) with the majority of trials reporting a median of 11 or fewer nodes obtained. In 9 of these 17 trials, both groups were treated with preoperative radiation therapy and reported a mean of 10 lymph nodes harvested in the laparoscopic group and 11 in the open group. One of the greatest concerns of laparoscopic TME is that obtaining a complete oncologic resection will be more difficult. Involvement of the circumferential or distal margin is one of the most important prognostic factors in rectal resection with TME and can lead to an increase in local recurrence and a reduction in survival. Radial margins of less than 2 mm are associated with a local recurrence rate of 16% compared to a significantly reduced local recurrence rate of 6% with margins greater than 2 mm [27]. Six of the 8 RCTs reported the involvement of the CRM and no difference was found by surgical approach [7, 31, 38-40, 45]. In the majority of trials the rate of CRM involvement was less than 5%. Patients with positive radial margins often had tumor invading the pelvic side wall or adjacent structure and were frequently converted from a laparoscopic to an open procedure [39]. In the CLASICC study, the only multicenter trial, a positive CRM was identified in 14 of 97 (14%) patients with open surgery and in 30 of 193 (16%) patients with laparoscopic rectal resection [6]. Of patients undergoing anterior resection, the CRM was positive in 16 of 129 (12%) individuals in the laparoscopic group and in 4 of 64 (6%) individuals in the open group. While there is a non-significant higher positivity of the CRM in the laparoscopic anterior resection group, this is once again likely due to the fact that the learning curve was not completed before the start of this study. Two RCTs reported on distal margin status and the incidence of distal margin positivity was not significantly different between the two surgical approaches and in fact was 0% [3, 31]. All 3 meta-analyses and the Cochrane review by Breukink *et al* [41] found no difference in positive margins based on surgical access.

11. Postoperative course

Less postoperative pain, faster recovery of intestinal function, and shorter length of stay are important benefits of laparoscopic colorectal surgery. Only 3 of 8 RCTs compared the exact amount of post-operative pain medication and 2 of these studies reported a significant reduction in analgesic use in the laparoscopic group [39, 40, 45]. Zhou et al [24] did not quantify the exact usage of pain medication, but found no significant difference in the number of days parental analgesics were necessary (4.1 *vs* 3.9 in the open and laparoscopic groups respectively). Resumption of bowel function was usually reported on post-operative days 3 to 5 and ability to tolerate a solid food diet was reported on post-operative days 3 to 6 [7, 31, 35, 39, 40, 45]. In the majority of RCTs earlier bowel movements and diet advancement was reported with the laparoscopic approach. The return of bowel function and reduction in wound pain was thought to contribute to earlier discharge after laparoscopic surgery. While in a majority of trials, the length of stay was not significantly different between surgical approaches, there was a trend toward decreased length of stay with laparoscopic rectal surgery. Breukink *et al* [41] found that laparoscopic TME resulted in earlier return of normal diet, less pain, less narcotic use and a shorter hospital stay.

12. Complications

Rectal cancer surgery is associated with a high rate of morbidity and mortality. Post-operative mortality in RCTs ranged from 1%-4% and demonstrated no statistically significant difference based on surgical approach. The rate of post-operative complications ranged from 6% to 69% and with the exception of Zhou et al [24] did not differ significantly between laparoscopic and open groups. Wound infection and urinary tract infection accounted for the majority of perioperative complications in both groups. There was a higher incidence of wound infection with the open approach however this did not reach statistical significance. Breukink *et al* [41] found no difference in morbidity between the laparoscopic and open groups although there was a trend toward lower morbidity with laparoscopic TME. Aziz *et al* [17] found no difference in perioperative morbidity between the 2 groups while Gao *et al* [26] found that the overall morbidity rate of the laparoscopic group was significantly lower than that of the open group. Anastomotic leak is the most serious complication after sphincter sparing rectal cancer resection especially with neoadjuvant chemoradiation. In addition, development of an anastomotic leak is reported to be associated with decreased long-term survival and higher rates of local recurrence after curative resection for colorectal cancer [39-43]. Operative expertise and selective diversion in high risk patients has resulted in a anastomotic leak rate of 1%-17% in most published series studying laparoscopic resection for rectal cancer [29, 30]. Consistent with reports from non-randomized comparative trials, RCTs demonstrated no significant difference in the incidence of anastomotic leak between the laparoscopic and open technique for the resection of rectal cancer. While the incidence of perioperative morbidity was not different based on surgical access, fewer patients had long-term complications with laparoscopic rectal cancer resection compared to the open approach. Adhesion related bowel obstruction was the most common longterm morbidity. With a median follow-up of greater than 9 years, Ng *et al* [37] found that adhesion-related obstruction requiring hospitalization (18.9% *vs* 2.7%) and reoperation (6.8% *vs* 0%) was higher in the open group. They report a cumulative probability of adhesion-related bowel obstruction at 10 years of 20.5% in the open group and 3.9% in the laparoscopic group. [45] Data on long-term complications was not separated by site of disease but the overall occurrence of incisional hernia (7.9% *vs* 10.9%, P = 0.32) and reoperation for adhesions (1.1% *vs* 2.5%, P = 0.30) was not statistically difference between laparoscopic and open resection. Long-term studies need to be done to determine if laparoscopy decreases the incidence of intra-abdominal adhesion formation by reduced surgical trauma, less tissue handling, and smaller incisions.

13. Long-term outcomes

The initial reports of the long-term outcomes after laparoscopic surgery for rectal cancer were discouraging. Several randomized trials report of the rate of positive circumferential radial margin in the laparoscopic group in comparison to the open group (12-5.9% and 6-4.2%, respectively). The 3-year follow-up did not establish higher local recurrence rate – 7.0% and 7.8%, respectively. The local recurrence rate after laparoscopic and open abdomino-perineal resection were 15.1% and 21.1%, respectively. The overall disease-free survival rate was also similar after laparoscopic and open anterior resection 70.9% and 70.4% and APR – 49.8% and 46.9%. Other data demonstrated 5-year disease survival reaching 83.7% for laparoscopic and 80.4% for open surgery. According to a meta-analysis of 20 laparoscopic rectal cancer studies between 1993 and 2004, including over 2000 patients, there is no significant difference in the number of harvested lymph nodes [22]. Despite the encouraging results, the laparoscopic rectal surgery could be fully evaluated only after long-term results are available. The ongoing studies are the American College of Surgeons Oncology Group (ACOSOG) Z6051 trial from the U.S.; the COLOR II trial from Europe, Canada, and Asia; and the Japanese Japan Clinical Oncology Group (JCOG) 0040 trial.

A number of the clinical trials were performed to determine the safety and feasibility of the laparoscopic approach for rectal adenocarcinoma and therefore the data we have for long-term outcomes is limited [5]. Braga *et al [48]* found no difference in local recurrence (4.0% in the laparoscopic group vs 5.2% in the open group, P= 0.97), overall five-year survival, or disease free five-year survival based on surgical approach. With a median follow-up of 87.2 mo in the laparoscopic group and 90.1 mo in the open group, Ng et al [45] demonstrated that after curative resection, the probability of five-year survival was 75.2% vs 76.5% for laparoscopic vs open APR respectively (P = 0.20). In addition, stage-by-stage comparison for the two groups showed no statistical difference. There were no port site recurrences and overall recurrence rates were not significantly different between the two groups (laparoscopic 20% vs open 25%, P = 0.60). Despite the higher rate of circumferential margin positivity in patients undergoing laparoscopic anterior resection in the CLASICC trial, there was no difference in local recurrence, three- year overall or three-year disease free survival between the two approaches (open OS 66.7% and laparoscopic OS 74.6%, P = 0.17; open DFS 70.4% and laparoscopic DFS 70.9%, P = 0.72; open LR 7.0% and laparoscopic LR 7.98%, P = 0.70) [6]. In addition, there was no significant difference in the rates of local recurrence, three-year overall survival, or three-year disease-free survival in patients undergoing laparoscopic vs open APR [12]. However, the sample size is small and therefore larger studies are needed for conclusive results. Ng et al [37] published results of a randomized trial of laparoscopic vs open anterior resection for upper rectal cancer with a median follow-up of 9 years. No difference in local recurrence, overall survival, or disease-free survival was reported. Although these studies suggest comparative oncologic outcomes between laparoscopic and open rectal cancer resection, they include small sample sizes and are almost all are single institution studies, highlighting the need for large, multi-center RCTs to provide confirmatory data. With a mean follow-up of 35 mo for both groups, overall local recurrence was not statistically different between the 2 groups (laparoscopic 7% vs open 8%, P = NS). Eleven studies provided sufficient data to compare overall survival. Overall survival was 72% for patients undergoing laparoscopic rectal cancer resection and 65% for open resection at an average of 4.4 years (P = 0.5). Subset analysis by [36] demonstrated no significant difference between laparoscopic and open rectal cancer resection in terms of local recurrence (laparoscopic 7.2% vs open 7.8%, P = 0.46), development of distant metastases (laparoscopic 13.5% vs open 9.1%, P = 0.60), or cancer-related mortality (laparoscopic 9% vs open 10%, P = 0.16). While, this data is encouraging, it is no conclusive.

14. Hybrid and hand-assisted laparoscopic rectal surgery

Some authors have introduced a new method of hybrid rectal surgery, aiming to combine the benefits of open and laparoscopic approach. The colonic mobilization is performed laparoscopically, while the rectal dissection is performed through a Pfannenstiel incision. A retrospective review established significantly longer hospital stay after hybrid procedures than after open procedures [27].

Another method is the hand-assisted laparoscopic surgery. A special access device for the hand is introduced in the abdomen. Compared with fully open techniques this method provides shorter operative time. High ligation of vessels, splenic flexure takedown, and lateral mobilization may be accomplished in a shorter period time with a hand-assisted technique. In hand-assisted laparoscopic surgery, rectal exposure and dissection can be either performed directly through the incision using the open techniques or laparoscopically with manual assistance [28]. This method combines the excellent laparoscopic view and the dissection techniques in open surgery and provides tactile sensation.

By performing distal rectal division directly through the incision using the open surgical staplers, hand-assisted laparoscopic rectal surgery may result in a lower anastomotic leakage rate.

15. Summary

After rigorous evaluation the laparoscopic surgery for colon cancer has become the gold standard. Laparoscopic colon resection for cancer, in experienced hands, can be performed safely and reliably with many short-term benefits to the patients while resulting in at least equivalent long-term outcomes as open surgery, which is supported by level 1 data. In conclusion, RCTs have demonstrated that laparoscopy does not adversely affect cancer related survival in patients with adenocarcinoma of the colon. Concerns about the technical difficulty of TME may have contributed to the exclusion of rectal cancer patients from most of these large multicenter RCTs resulting in little data on oncologic outcomes with laparoscopic rectal cancer resection. Laparoscopic rectal dissection is technically more demanding than open and constraints of a narrow pelvis may result in difficulty assessing and obtaining adequate surgical margins. However, there are several proposed benefits of laparoscopic rectal resection. A clear and magnified view of the pelvis provided by the improved optics of laparoscopy may aid sharp dissection for TME and assist in identification of vital pelvic structures including the ureters and autonomic nerves. In addition, pneumoperitoneum may separate the parietal and visceral fascia of the mesorectum facilitating dissection in this plane. Laparoscopic rectal cancer resection has a steep learning curve but increased experience with both open and laparoscopic TME will lead to shorter operating times and decreased morbidity. Current data suggests that laparoscopic rectal cancer resection may benefit patients because of reduced blood loss, earlier return of bowel function, and shorter hospital length of stay. Concerns that laparoscopic rectal cancer surgery may compromise short-term oncologic outcomes including number of lymph nodes harvested and CRM positivity do not appear to be supported by the available literature. However, there is a paucity of data concerning long-term oncologic outcomes and complications with laparoscopic rectal cancer surgery. There are two large, multicenter RCTs that are currently being conducted: the COLOR II trial in Europe and the ACOSOG-Z6051 trial in the United States. Both of these studies are comparing the laparoscopic and open approach for treatment of resectable rectal cancer. Results from these trials will provide information on the long-term outcomes of laparoscopic rectal cancer resection and are eagerly awaited. In view of the lack of level one data on oncologic outcomes, laparoscopic TME for locally advanced, curable rectal cancer should only be performed within the confines of a RCT.

Other potential, but less conclusively demonstrated benefits include better preservation of cell-mediated immune function and reduced tumor cell proliferation. Although a similar level of evidence does not yet exist for the laparoscopic rectal surgery for cancer, the evidence to date suggests that it is likely that the ongoing large randomized trials will demonstrate clinical benefits of laparoscopic rectal cancer surgery. New devices for minimizing of the abdominal trauma are being developed. The steep learning curve, cost and difficult training are still hindrance to the wide use of laparoscopic colon surgery.

Author details

Anton Tonev[1], Nikola Kolev[1], Valentin Ignatov[1], Vasil Bojkov[3], Tanya Kirilova[2] and Krassimir Ivanov[1]

1 Department of General and Operative Surgery, University Hospital "St. Marina", Varna, Bulgaria

2 Department of Gastroenterology, University Hospital "St. Marina", Varna, Bulgaria

3 Department of Surgery, University Hospital "St. Marina", Varna, Bulgaria

References

[1] Reynolds Jr., W. "The first laparoscopic cholecystectomy, " Journal of the Society of Laparoendoscopic Surgeons, vol. 5, no. 1, pp. 89–94, 2001.

[2] Jacobs M., J. C. Verdeja, and H. S. Goldstein, "Minimally invasive colon resection (laparoscopic colectomy), " Surgical Laparoscopy & Endoscopy, vol. 1, no. 3, pp. 144–150, 1991.

[3] Berends F. J., G. Kazemier, H. J. Bonjer, and J. F. Lange, "Subcutaneous metastases after laparoscopic colectomy, " Lancet, vol. 344, no. 8914, p. 58, 1994.

[4] Buunen M. et al., "Survival after laparoscopic surgery versus open surgery for colon cancer, long-term outcome of a randomized clinical trial, " The Lancet Oncology, vol. 10, no. 1, pp. 44–52, 2009.

[5] Fleshman J., D. J. Sargent, E. Green et al., "Laparoscopic colectomy for cancer is not inferior to open surgery based on 5-year data from the COST Study Group trial, " Annals of Surgery, vol. 246, no. 4, pp. 655–662, 2007.

[6] Jayne D. G., P. J. Guillou, H. Thorpe et al., "Randomized trial of laparoscopic-assisted resection of colorectal carcinoma: 3-year results of the UK MRC CLASICC trial group, " Journal of Clinical Oncology, vol. 25, no. 21, pp. 3061–3068, 2007.

[7] Lacy M., S. Delgado, A. Castells et al., "The long-term results of a randomized clinical trial of laparoscopy-assisted versus open surgery for colon cancer, " Annals of Surgery, vol. 248, no. 1, pp. 1–7, 2008.

[8] Cima R. R., J. Pattana-arun, D. W. Larson, E. J. Dozois, B. G. Wolff, and J. H. Pemberton, "Experience with 969 minimal access colectomies: the role of hand-assisted laparoscopy in expanding minimally invasive surgery for complex colectomies, " Journal of the American College of Surgeons, vol. 206, no. 5, pp. 946–950, 2008.

[9] Froghi F., M. H. Sodergren, A. Darzi, and P. Paraskeva, "Single incision laparoscopic surgery (SILS) in general surgery: a review of current practice, " Surgical Laparoscopy, Endoscopy and Percutaneous Techniques, vol. 20, no. 4, pp. 191–204, 2010.

[10] Pigazzi A., F. Luca, A. Patriti et al., "Multicentric study on robotic tumor-specific mesorectal excision for the treatment of rectal cancer, " Annals of Surgical Oncology, vol. 17, no. 6, pp. 1614–1620, 2010.

[11] Zimmern A., L. Prasad, A. Desouza, S. Marecik, J. Park, and H. Abcarian, "Robotic colon and rectal surgery: a series of 131 cases, " World Journal of Surgery, vol. 34, no. 8, pp. 1954–1958, 2010.

[12] Dozois E. J., D. W. Larson, S. C. Dowdy, V. P. Poola, S. D.- Holubar, and R. R. Cima, "Transvaginal colonic extraction following combined hysterectomy and laparoscopic total colectomy: a natural orifice approach, " Tech Coloproctol. 2008 Sep;12 (3):251-4. doi: 10.1007/s10151-008-0428-4. Epub 2008 Aug 5

[13] Heald RJ, Moran BJ, Ryall RD, Sexton R, MacFarlane JK. Rectal cancer: the Basingstoke experience of total mesorectal excision, 1978-1997. Arch Surg 1998;133 (8):894–899

[14] Southall JC, Lee SW, Allendorf JD, Bessler M, Whelan RL. Colon adenocarcinoma and B-16 melanoma grow larger following laparotomy vs. pneumoperitoneum in a murine model. Dis Colon Rectum 1998;41 (5):564–569

[15] Clinical Outcomes of Surgical Therapy Study Group. A comparison of laparoscopically assisted and open colectomy for colon cancer. N Engl J Med 2004;350 (20): 2050–2059

[16] Bonjer HJ, Hop WC, Nelson H, et al; Transatlantic Laparoscopically Assisted vs Open Colectomy Trials Study Group. Laparoscopically assisted vs open colectomy for colon cancer: a meta-analysis. Arch Surg 2007;142 (3): 298–303

[17] Aziz O, Constantinides V, Tekkis PP, et al. Laparoscopic versus open surgery for rectal cancer: a meta-analysis. Ann Surg Oncol 2006;13 (3):413–424

[18] Hughes ESR, McDermott FT, Polglase AL, Johnson WR. Tumor recurrence in the abdominal wall scar tissue after large-bowel cancer surgery. Dis Colon Rectum 1983;26 (9): 571–572

[19] Veldkamp R, Khury E, Hop WC, et al. Colon Cancer Laparoscopic or Open Resection Study Group (COLOR). Laparoscopic surgery versus open surgery for colon cancer;short-term outcomes of a randomized trial. Lancet Oncol 2005;6:477–484

[20] Noel JK, Fahrbach K, Estok R, Cella C, Frame D, Linz H, Cima RR, Dozois EJ, Senagore AJ. Minimally invasive colorectal resection outcomes: short-term comparison with open procedures. J Am Coll Surg. 2007 Feb;204 (2):291-307. Epub 2006 Dec 12.

[21] Stucky CC, Pockaj BA, Novotny PJ, Sloan JA, Sargent DJ, O'Connell MJ, Beart RW, Skibber JM, Nelson H, Weeks JC. Long-term follow-up and individual item analysis of quality of life assessments related to laparoscopic-assisted colectomy in the COST trial 93-46-53 (INT 0146). Ann Surg Oncol. 2011 Sep;18 (9):2422-31.

[22] Moloo H, Mamazza J, Poulin EC, Burpee SE, Bendavid Y, Klein L, Gregoire R, Schlachta CM. Laparoscopic resections for colorectal cancer: does conversion survival? Surg Endosc. 2004 May;18 (5):732-5. Epub 2004 Apr 6.

[23] Leroy J, Jamali F, Forbes L, et al. Laparoscopic total mesorectal excision (TME) for rectal cancer surgery: long-term outcomes. Surg Endosc 2004;18 (2):281–289

[24] Liang JW, Zhang XM, Zhou ZX, Wang Z, Bi JJ. Learning curve of laparoscopic-assisted surgery for rectal cancer].Zhonghua Yi Xue Za Zhi. 2011 Jun 28;91 (24):1698-701.

[25] Araujo SE, da Silva eSousa AH Jr, de Campos FG, Habr-Gama A, Dumarco RB, Caravatto PP, Nahas SC, da Silva J, Kiss DR, Gama-Rodrigues JJ. Conventional approach x laparoscopic abdominoperineal resection for rectal cancer treatment after neoadjuvant chemoradiation: results of a prospective randomized trial. Rev Hosp Clin Fac Med Sao Paulo. 2003 May-Jun;58 (3):133-40.

[26] Gao F, Cao YF, Chen LS. Meta-analysis of short-term outcomes after laparoscopic resection for rectal cancer. Int J Colorectal Dis. 2006 Oct;21 (7):652-6.

[27] Allendorf JDF, Bessler M, Kayton ML, et al. Increased tumor establishment and growth after laparotomy vs laparoscopy in a murine model. Arch Surg 1995;130 (6): 649–653

[28] Lee SW, Feingold DL, Carter JJ, et al. Peritoneal macrophage and blood monocyte functions after open and laparoscopic-assisted cecectomy in rats. Surg Endosc 2003; 17 (12):1996–2002

[29] Martin JK Jr, Goellner JR. Abdominal fluid cytology in patients with gastrointestinal malignant lesions. Mayo Clin Proc 1986;61 (6):467–471

[30] Shantha Kumara HM, Feingold D, Kalady M, et al. Colorectal resection is associated with persistent proangiogenic plasma protein changes: postoperative plasma stimulates in vitro endothelial cell growth, migration, and invasion. Ann Surg 2009;249 (6): 973–977

[31] Law WL, Lee YM, Choi HK, Seto CL, Ho JW. Impact of laparoscopic resection for colorectal cancer on operative outcomes and survival. Ann Surg 2007;245 (1):1–7

[32] Lee SW, Gleason NR, Bessler M, Whelan RL. Port site tumor recurrence rates in a murine model of laparoscopic splenectomy decreased with increased experience. Surg Endosc 2000;14 (9):805–811

[33] Milsom JW, Bo°hm B, Hammerhofer KA, Fazio V, Steiger E, Elson P. A prospective, randomized trial comparing laparoscopic versus conventional techniques in colorectal cancer surgery: a preliminary report. J Am Coll Surg 1998; 187 (1):46–54; discussion 54–55

[34] Marcello PW, Fleshman JW, Milsom JW, et al. Handassisted laparoscopic vs. laparoscopic colorectal surgery: a multicenter, prospective, randomized trial. Dis Colon Rectum 2008;51 (6):818–826

[35] Lacy AM, Garcı´a-Valdecasas JC, Delgado S, et al. Laparoscopy-assisted colectomy versus open colectomy for treatment of non-metastatic colon cancer: a randomised trial. Lancet 2002;359 (9325):2224–2229

[36] Leung KL, Kwok SP, Lam SC, et al. Laparoscopic resection of rectosigmoid carcinoma: prospective randomised trial. Lancet 2004;363 (9416):1187–1192

[37] Ng SS, Leung KL, Lee JF, Yiu RY, Li JC. MRC CLASICC trial. Lancet 2005;366 (9487): 713; author reply 713–714

[38] Wexner SD, Cohen SM. Port site metastases after laparoscopic colorectal surgery for cure of malignancy. Br J Surg 1995; 82: 295-298

[39] Milsom JW, Böhm B, Hammerhofer KA, Fazio V, Steiger E, Elson P. A prospective, randomized trial comparing laparoscopic versus conventional techniques in colorec-

tal cancer surgery: a preliminary report. J Am Coll Surg 1998; 187: 46-54; discussion 54-55

[40] Kemp JA, Finlayson SR. Outcomes of laparoscopic and open colectomy: a national population-based comparison. Surg Innov 2008; 15: 277-283

[41] Breukink S, Pierie J, Wiggers T. Laparoscopic versus open total mesorectal excision for rectal cancer. Cochrane Database Syst Rev 2006; (4): CD005200

[42] Kim SH, Park IJ, Joh YG, Hahn KY. Laparoscopic resection for rectal cancer: a prospective analysis of thirty-month follow-up outcomes in 312 patients. Surg Endosc 2006; 20: 1197-1202

[43] Laurent C, Leblanc F, Gineste C, Saric J, Rullier E. Laparoscopic approach in surgical treatment of rectal cancer. Br J Surg 2007; 94: 1555-1561

[44] Quirke P, Steele R, Monson J, Grieve R, Khanna S, Couture J, O'Callaghan C, Myint AS, Bessell E, Thompson LC, Parmar M, Stephens RJ, Sebag-Montefiore D. Effect of the plane of surgery achieved on local recurrence in patients with operable rectal cancer: a prospective study using data from the MRC CR07 and NCIC-CTG CO16 randomised clinical trial. Lancet 2009; 373: 821-828

[45] Nagtegaal ID, Quirke P. What is the role for the circumferential margin in the modern treatment of rectal cancer? J Clin Oncol 2008; 26: 303-312

[46] Rullier A, Gourgou-Bourgade S, Jarlier M, Bibeau F, Chassagne-Clément C, Hennequin C, Tisseau L, Leroux A, Ettore F, Peoc'h M, Diebold MA, Robin YM, Kleinclaus I, Mineur L, Petitjean C, Mosnier JF, Soubeyran I, Padilla N, Lemaistre AI, Bérille J, Denis B, Conroy T, Gérard JP. Predictive factors of positive circumferential resection margin after radiochemotherapy for rectal cancer: The French randomised trial ACCORD12/0405 PRODIGE 2. Eur J Cancer 2012 Aug 18

[47] Marijnen CA, Nagtegaal ID, Kapiteijn E, Kranenbarg EK, Noordijk EM, van Krieken JH, van de Velde CJ, Leer JW. Radiotherapy does not compensate for positive resection margins in rectal cancer patients: report of a multicenter randomized trial. Int J Radiat Oncol Biol Phys 2003; 55: 1311-1320

[48] Braga M, Frasson M, Vignali A, Zuliani W, Capretti G, Di Carlo V Laparoscopic resection in rectal cancer patients: outcome and cost-benefit analysis. Dis Colon Rectum. 2007 Apr;50 (4):464-71.

[49] Kehlet H. Multimodal approach to control postoperative pathophysiology and rehabilitation. Br J Anaesth 1997; 78: 606-617

[50] Lassen K, Soop M, Nygren J, Cox PB, Hendry PO, Spies C, von Meyenfeldt MF, Fearon KC, Revhaug A, Norderval S, Ljungqvist O, Lobo DN, Dejong CH. Consensus review of optimal perioperative care in colorectal surgery: Enhanced Recovery After Surgery (ERAS) Group recommendations. Arch Surg 2009; 144: 961-969

[51] Spanjersberg WR, Reurings J, Keus F, van Laarhoven CJ. Fast track surgery versus conventional recovery strategies for colorectal surgery. Cochrane Database Syst Rev 2011; (2): CD007635

[52] Teeuwen PH, Bleichrodt RP, de Jong PJ, van Goor H, Bremers AJ. Enhanced recovery after surgery versus conventional perioperative care in rectal surgery. Dis Colon Rectum 2011; 54: 833-839

[53] Arumainayagam N, McGrath J, Jefferson KP, Gillatt DA. Introduction of an enhanced recovery protocol for radical cystectomy. BJU Int 2008; 101: 698-701

[54] Gustafsson UO, Hausel J, Thorell A, Ljungqvist O, Soop M, Nygren J. Adherence to the enhanced recovery after surgery protocol and outcomes after colorectal cancer surgery. Arch Surg 2011; 146: 571-577

[55] Lowell JA, Schifferdecker C, Driscoll DF, Benotti PN, Bistrian BR. Postoperative fluid overload: not a benign problem. Crit Care Med 1990; 18: 728-733

[56] Lobo DN, Bostock KA, Neal KR, Perkins AC, Rowlands BJ, Allison SP. Effect of salt and water balance on recovery of gastrointestinal function after elective colonic resection: a randomised controlled trial. Lancet 2002; 359: 1812-1818

[57] Tambyraja AL, Sengupta F, MacGregor AB, Bartolo DC, Fearon KC. Patterns and clinical outcomes associated with routine intravenous sodium and fluid administration after colorectal resection. World J Surg 2004; 28: 1046-1051; discussion 1051-1052

[58] Brandstrup B, Tønnesen H, Beier-Holgersen R, Hjortsø E, Ørding H, Lindorff-Larsen K, Rasmussen MS, Lanng C, Wallin L, Iversen LH, Gramkow CS, Okholm M, Blemmer T, Svendsen PE, Rottensten HH, Thage B, Riis J, Jeppesen IS, Teilum D, Christensen AM, Graungaard B, Pott F. Effects of intravenous fluid restriction on postoperative complications: comparison of two perioperative fluid regimens: a randomized assessor-blinded multicenter trial. Ann Surg 2003; 238: 641-648

[59] MacKay G, Fearon K, McConnachie A, Serpell MG, Molloy RG, O'Dwyer PJ. Randomized clinical trial of the effect of postoperative intravenous fluid restriction on recovery after elective colorectal surgery. Br J Surg 2006; 93: 1469-1474

[60] Conway DH, Mayall R, Abdul-Latif MS, Gilligan S, Tackaberry C. Randomised controlled trial investigating the influence of intravenous fluid titration using oesophageal Doppler monitoring during bowel surgery. Anaesthesia 2002; 57:845-849

[61] Liu S, Carpenter RL, Neal JM. Epidural anesthesia and analgesia. Their role in postoperative outcome. Anesthesiology 1995; 82: 1474-1506.

[62] Park WY, Thompson JS, Lee KK. Effect of epidural anesthesia and analgesia on perioperative outcome: a randomized, controlled Veterans Affairs cooperative study. Ann Surg 2001; 234: 560-569; discussion 560-569

[63] Rodgers A, Walker N, Schug S, McKee A, Kehlet H, van Zundert A, Sage D, Futter M, Saville G, Clark T, MacMahon S. Reduction of postoperative mortality and mor-

bidity with epidural or spinal anaesthesia: results from overview of randomized trials. BMJ 2000; 321: 1493

[64] Wu CL, Cohen SR, Richman JM, Rowlingson AJ, Courpas GE, Cheung K, Lin EE, Liu SS. Efficacy of postoperative patient-controlled and continuous infusion epidural analgesia versus intravenous patient-controlled analgesia with opioids: a meta-analysis. Anesthesiology 2005; 103: 1079-1088; quiz 1109-1110

[65] Levy BF, Tilney HS, Dowson HM, Rockall TA. A systematic review of postoperative analgesia following laparoscopic colorectal surgery. Colorectal Dis 2010; 12: 5-15

[66] Levy BF, Scott MJ, Fawcett W, Fry C, Rockall TA. Randomized clinical trial of epidural, spinal or patient-controlled analgesia for patients undergoing laparoscopic colorectal surgery. Br J Surg 2011; 98: 1068-1078

[67] Virlos I, Clements D, Beynon J, Ratnalikar V, Khot U. Shortterm outcomes with intrathecal versus epidural analgesia in laparoscopic colorectal surgery. Br J Surg 2010; 97: 1401-1406

[68] Meylan N, Elia N, Lysakowski C, Tramèr MR. Benefit and risk of intrathecal morphine without local anaesthetic in patients undergoing major surgery: meta-analysis of randomized trials. Br J Anaesth 2009; 102: 156-167

[69] Charlton S, Cyna AM, Middleton P, Griffiths JD. Perioperative transversus abdominis plane (TAP) blocks for analgesia after abdominal surgery. Cochrane Database Syst Rev 2010; (12):CD007705

[70] Marret E, Remy C, Bonnet F. Meta-analysis of epidural analgesia versus parenteral opioid analgesia after colorectal surgery. Br J Surg 2007; 94: 665-673

10

Screening for Colorectal Cancer

Syed Naqvi and Syeda Farah Nazir

1. Introduction

It has become an acknowledged fact that Colorectal Cancer (CRC) is a worldwide problem, with an annual incidence of approximately 1 million cases and an annual mortality of more than 500,000. Furthermore, the absolute number of cases will increase over the next two decades as a result of the aging and expansion of populations in both the developed and developing countries.

Apparently, CRC is the second most common cause of cancer related mortality among men and women in the world; so, most CRCs arise from sporadic adenomas, and a few from genetic polyposis syndromes or inflammatory bowel disease (IBD). The term "polyp" refers to a discrete mass that protrudes into the intestinal lumen. Therefore, the reported prevalence of adenomatous polyps, on the basis of screening colonoscopy data, is in the range of 18–36%.

The fact is that the risk for CRC varies from country to country and even within countries; the risk also varies among individual people based on diet, lifestyle, and hereditary factors. The most common neoplastic outcome of colorectal cancer screening is the adenoma. After having removed, patients need to be placed in a follow-up surveillance programme, very much similar to the patients with identified and treated cancer.

In the western world, we are very much aware that colorectal cancer has become an important health problem as each year, over 380,000 persons are diagnosed with colorectal cancer; bout half of these, patients die of the disease making colorectal cancer the second leading cause of cancer deaths in Europe. An estimated figure reveals that almost one million people suffering from colorectal cancer are going through cost – intensive treatments putting a huge burden on the healthcare system.

Screening is defined as population based testing in an asymptomatic individual to identify particular disease. The aim of screening is to lower the burden of cancer in the population by discovering latent disease in its early stages and treating it more effectively than diagnosed later when symptoms have appeared. As such, screening is a commendable method to reduce the burden of the disease. However, population screening targets a predominantly healthy population, and should therefore only be conducted after a careful consideration of both harms and benefits.

In 1968 the World Health Organization [1] (WHO) defined the first set of principles of population screening (Wilson &Junger 1968). These principles are still valid today.

The desirable features for community screening program for any disease are:

1. The disease should be an important health problem
2. Natural history of the disease must be known
3. The disease should be detectable at an early stage
4. Benefits of early detection should be there
5. Simple test should be available at early stage
6. The test should have high sensitivity and specificity and should be safe, effective, acceptable, inexpensive, and repeatable after an interval
7. Services should be in place to treat the early disease
8. Benefits of decrease mortality and morbidity should be there

Recommendation for action- general:

- Develop and disseminate structured educational programme for members of the public, providers, health-care systems, and policy-makers/political leaders. Effective educational programmes should be directed to each of the important participants in an acceptable manner.
- Develop evidence-based standards for quality throughout the screening process.
- Develop and disseminate inexpensive, easy-to-use clinical management systems.
- Advocate screening through national and local venues.
- Promote colorectal cancer screening as a part of comprehensive clinical preventive care.

Recommendation for action –Programme design:

Planning the screening programme:

- A target population should identify-asymptomatic men and women, age, risk factors (e.g., familial)
- The decision to implement colorectal cancer screening should be based on the relative burden of the colorectal cancer in the population to be screened.
- The screening strategy (test, interval, age range) should be based on medical evidence (guidelines), availability of resources, level of risk, and cultural acceptance by population.

- Support by influential professional and patient advocacy groups and from the media is essential.
- Evaluate the feasibility of the proposed programme. Address the development and allocation of the resources (financial, personnel, facilities).
- Evaluate the specific cultural and language needs of the population.

Implementation of screening programme:

- Identify the target unit for implementation, and ensure communication (training and education) with providers (general practitioners and others) and the target population.
- Develop and disseminate guidelines on screening, diagnosis, treatment, and surveillance in a patient friendly and culture sensitive manner.
- Develop methods for initial patient enrollment and follow-up.

Monitoring the Screening program:

- Careful, timely monitoring of following rates: screening uptake, re-screening, and follow-up of the positive test.
- Compliance with surveillance recommendations.
- Measurement of the programme quality should be in place, and evaluated regularly.
- Outcomes, including detection rates, cancer stage distribution, adenoma detection, complications, and finally, the effect on the population incidence and mortality.

2. Colorectal cancer risk assessment tools and referral system in different countries in the world

It is believed that colorectal cancer risk varies regionally according to geographical distribution of the population. As we will see in following sections, colorectal screening is yet to be implemented fully in general population of developed countries of the world. So in different regions, colorectal cancer risk assessment tools has been introduced to identify the high risk patients needs to be screened in general population of the society. Usually these risk assessment tools are for GPs and primary care units to identify the high risk patients to be screened.

2.1. Hamilton risk assessment tool for colorectal cancer

The risk assessment tool was based on work done by Professor Willie Hamilton in the CAPER studies (Cancer Prediction in Exeter), a series of case control studies which identified symptoms of common cancers that were presented to primary care and quantified the risk of cancer associated with them. The tool acts as reminder to GPs to consider the likelihood of an individual patient aged 40 or over having lung or bowel cancer given the symptom or combination of symptoms they present with. It is presented as three tables (colorectal cancer, lung cancer for non smokers and lung cancer for smokers) containing the risk values for each symptom in isolation or combination and is available as mouse mat or a desk easel so as to be easy to hand.

The parameter used in Hamilton risk assessment tool are: constipation, diarrhoea, rectal bleeding, loss of weight, abdominal pain, abdominal tenderness, abnormal rectal examination and haemoglobin <10g/dl.

2.2. USA National Cancer Institute (NCI USA TOOL)

A recent online tool for calculating colorectal cancer risk in men and women age 50 or older was launched, based on a new risk assessment model developed by researchers at the National Cancer Institute (NCI), part of the National Institute of Health. This new tool may help health care providers and their patients in making informed choices about when and how to screen for colorectal cancers and can be used in designing colorectal cancer screening and prevention trials.

So, by using easily obtainable information (e.g., personal and family medical history, lifestyle behaviours, and age), the tool provides an estimate of an individual`s risk of developing colorectal cancer over certain time periods (within five years, ten years, and over the course of lifetime). This risk-assessment model is first to provide an absolute risk estimate for colorectal cancer (i.e., the probability of developing colorectal cancer over a given period of time) for general non –Hispanic white population age 50 or older in United States.

In order to develop the risk assessment model, the researcher used data from two large- based case control studies. Several factors that have been previously associated with colorectal risk were shown to be predicted of a colorectal cancer diagnosis in those two studies including age; family history of colorectal cancer; consumption of vegetables; body mass index; cigarette smoking; use of aspirin or other non-steroidal anti inflammatory drugs; physical activity; use of hormone replacement therapy; previous history of sigmoidoscopy and/or colonoscopy; and history of polyps. Estimates of relative risk (comparisons of risk in one group to another) from the case-control studies were combined with population based data on colorectal cancer incidence from NCI`sSEER (Surveillance, Epidemiology and End Results) cancer registries to make the model broadly applicable in United States. [2]

"This colorectal cancer risk model should provide physicians and their patients a new tool to help in making informed decisions about cancer screening and other cancer prevention strategies. It may also assist policy makers in evaluating the usefulness of current and future population colorectal cancer screening approaches" said Andrew Freedman,Ph.D., lead author of the paper that describes the development of the risk-assessment model.

It has been observed that the majority of participants in the two case-control studies used to develop the model were non-Hispanic whites aged 50 or older, the researchers were unable to estimate relative risks for other age and racial/ethnic groups. However, there are plans to expand the tool to include these populations in the future. In addition, the tool is not applicable to individuals with certain gastrointestinal disorders (such as ulcerative colitis or Crohn`s disease), certain inherited genetic conditions, such as familial adenomatous polyposis or hereditary nonpolyposis colorectal cancers) or a personal history of colorectal cancer. These conditions are known to carry a high risk of colorectal cancer.

2.3. Asia-Pacific Colorectal Screening (APCS) score

From a development set of 860 asymptomatic subjects undergoing screening colonoscopy, multiple logistic regression was applied to identify significant risk factors advanced colorectal neoplasia defined as invasive carcinoma or advance adenoma. Odd Ratios for significant risk factors were utilised to develop risk score ranging from 0 to 7 (Asia- pacific Colorectal Screening (APCS score). Three tiers of risk were arbitrarily defined:0-1 `average risk` (AR); 2-3 `moderate risk` (MR); 4-7 `high risk` (HR). In this study performance of the APCS score in predicting risk of advanced neoplasia was evaluated

3. Current tests for colorectal screening and emerging screening tools

The following screening methods are currently used globally:

Guaiac-Based faecal occult bleeding test (gFOBT) is at present the most frequently used method in screening programme throughout the world. It detects the peroxidase reaction of Hemoglobin, which causes the detection paper impregnated with guaiac resin to turn blue. As it can react with animal haemoglobin, dietetic restrictions are necessary to exclude the false- positive results. A number of studies showed limited sensitivity of this test for both, advanced adenomas (11%) and carcinomas (13%). With gFOBT, a decrease in mortality for colorectal cancer by 15 to 33% has been proved.

Immunological faecal occult bleeding test (iFOBT) reacts exclusively to human haemoglobin, so no dietetic restrictions are seen as necessary.Taking and assessing the stool samples are easier than the case with gFOBTs, which may explain a higher participation in the target population. A wide range of qualitative and quantitative tests are available, with varying levels of sensitivity and specificity. The advantage of quantitative tests is the possibility to set cut-off limits; the most frequently used values are 75 or 10 ng/ml. The disadvantage of iFOBT is its cost. It is, no doubt, an expensive test as compared to gFOBT. But, presently, the price is approaching that of gFOBT for qualitative tests. As this test has higher sensitivity and specificity as compared to gFOBT, iFOBT is being increasingly used in screening programmes.

New screening methods include tests which examine the stool for the presence of abnormal DNA. Generally, these tests have higher sensitivity but lower specificity than gFOBT. They are expensive tests and a major obstacle in their implementation is their price. [3]

Flexible sigmoidoscopy is an endoscopic examination with maximum reach to splenic flexure. On the basis of emerging evidence---this is a promising screening test. A number of studies are under progress to accumulate enough evidence for usage of flexible sigmoidoscopy as a screening test based on WHO guidelines. Recommended interval varies from 3 to 5 years. A recent pilot study carried out in Darby UK* [36]. In the UK flexible sigmoidoscopy trial, 90% of all CRC detected at screening was found in the distal colon. According to one report by Sophie White et al from university of Sheffield, more than 60% adenomas are detected in left side of colon at screening age of the population and more than 70% CRC detected by flexible sigmoidoscopy at the screening age of the population.

Colonoscopy is another screening tool used in diagnostic and therapeutic endoscopic procedure which also detects lesion in proximal colon. It is more sensitive in detecting both adenomas and carcinomas. This is an established screening procedure for synchronous and metachronous tumours and surveillance of polyposis and non polyposis hereditary colorectal cancers. This is also a primary surveillance tool for multiple polyps according to guidelines. The risk of serious adverse events is higher than any other screening test with one in five hundred colonic perforation rate in expert hands. In spite of being gold standard, colonoscopy will not establish itself as an ideal population screening test due to its cost and adverse events and a lack of wide spread skills available.

Computed tomographic colonography (virtual colonoscopy) can detect lesions in the colon and rectum by reconstructing two-and three-dimentional images. To date, there is no evidence of reduction in incidence and mortality of colorectal cancer by this method in comparison with other screening tools. In cases, where caecum is not reached during colonoscopy due to patient related factors, CT colonography is the preferable screening tool to complete the examination. According to current NICE guidelines, the evidence of meta-analysis of data of 14 studies with a total of 1324 patients concluded that for CT colonography, the pooled per-patient sensitivity for polyps 10mm or larger was 88%, for polyps 6-9mm it was 84% and for polyps 5mm or smaller it was 65%. The pooled per-polyp sensitivity for polyps 10mm or larger was 81%, for polyps 6-9mm it was 62% and for polyp 5mm or smaller it was 43%. The overall specificity for the detection of polyps 10mm or larger was 95%. No significant complications were reported in the studies

Double contrast barium enema shows entire colon and rectum, although with significantly lower sensitivity and specificity than colonoscopy. The percentage of undetected carcinomas is upto 22%. This test is no longer widespread and in clinical practice due to its low sensitivity and specificity and availability of other better screening tools. Despite the fact, it still has a role in the areas in the world where colonoscopy and flexible sigmoidoscopy resources are severely limited.

It is quite obvious that Colorectal Screening is a complex process which in order to function requires the coexistence of number of factors such as a functioning invitation-reminder system, media campaigns targeted at the general public, the development of recommendations for general practitioners, patients compliance, sufficient funding, stratification of risks, and last but not least the election of the most suitable screening test. Among all available screening tests, only Fecal Occult Blood Test meets the WHO criteria.

4. Current global colorectal cancer screening pathways

4.1. Europe

Until 2007 Colorectal Cancer Screening was running or being established in 19 of 27 European countries [4] The target group contains approximately 136 million individuals suitable for colorectal screening (aged 50 to 74 years). Of this number, 43% individual come from 12 countries where colorectal population screening is performed or being prepared on either national or regional level; 34% come from the five countries where national population screening has been implemented (Finland, France, Italy, Poland and United Kingdom).

In 2007,gFOBT (which in 2003 was the only test recommended by the council of the European union) was used as the only screening method in twelve countries (Bulgaria, Czech republic, Finland, France, Hungary, Latvia, Portgal, Romania, Slovena, Spain, Sweedon, and United Kingdom). Colonoscopy was the only screening method used in Poland. In six countries, two types of the tests were used: i FOBT and flexible sigmoidoscopy in Italy, and g FOBT and colonoscopy in Austria, Cyprus, Germany, Greece, and Slovak republic. In the remaining 8 states, (Belgium, Denmark, Estonia, Ireland, Lithuania, Luxembourg, Malta, and the Netherlands), colorectal cancer screening has not been implemented yet. The age limit for target population varies across EU countries.

After 2007 Report, EU countries progressed toward the implementation of population screening programme. Recently, new EU guidelines for screening of colorectal cancers have been introduced.

In United Kingdom, a screening programme was announced in 2004 and initiated in 2006, with prospects of national coverage in 2009. It has been designed in two stages: with gFOBT tests at two yearly intervals with colonoscopy for positive tests. In 2007, the compliance was 52%. The program is carried out through regional centres falling under one of the five national hubs. The role of general practitioners is less significant here. [5]

The NHS Bowel Cancer Screening has achieved nation-wide coverage by 2010. The programme hubs operate a national call and recall system to send out FOBT kits, analyse samples and dispatch results. Consequently, each hub is responsible for coordinating the programme in their area and works up-to 20 local screening centres. The screening centres provide endoscopy services and specialist screening nurse clinics for people receiving abnormal results. Screening centres are also responsible for referring those requiring treatment to local hospital multidisciplinary team (MDT).

In Ireland, colorectal screening programme was launched in 2009 after National Screening Board Report which was published in December 2008 [6] A summary of the screening programme highlights:

- An immunochemical faecal occult blood test (iFOBT) is the primary screening tool for population-based colorectal screening programme.
- A target population for screening of all men and women aged 55 and 74 years with a screening interval of two years.

- Colonoscopy to be offered to those individuals who test positive with iFOBT

In France, Screening program was initiated in 2003, based on gFOBT tests at 2 years intervals with colonoscopy for positive result [7]. The role of general practitioners as coordinators is of crucial importance. The major advantage of French program is its good organization, with a call-recall system comprising central management at national level and individual steps taken by centres in individual departments. Asymptomatic individuals aged from 50-70yrs are mailed gFOBT tests, with the reminder at three monthly intervals for nonparticipants. Compliance in referred districts achieved 42%, and overall positive test rate was 2.7%. The screening programme has been generalised to the whole French territory since 2008.

In Italy, a nation-wide campaign was initiated in 2005; the implementation was entrusted entirely to 21 regional centres, including choice of the testing method. In Piedmont region, flexible sigmoidoscopy is the method of choice, in other regions iFOBT, with colonoscopy for positive tests. [8]

In Spain, the main obstacle to its implementation was the highly heterogeneous healthcare system, in terms of organization and insurance coverage in individual self governing units. That is why they are behind in implementation of screening program as compared to the UK, Germany, France, Italy and Finland.

In Finland, a structured screening programme was initiated in 2004. The target population, aged from 60 to 69 years (106000 individuals), was randomised into two groups. Individuals in the screening group were mailed a gFOBT test at intervals of 2 years. The finish program shows a high level compliance of the target population (70.8%), particularly for females [9]

Poland is the only state at the moment using colonoscopy as the only screening method, without the alternative of of FOBTs. An opportunistic screening programme was initiated in 2000, and by 2005, this had grown to 57 centres across Poland. The program is financed by ministry of health, independent of the overall healthcare system. The target population (Asymptomatic individuals aged 55-66 years) is recruited through general practitioners. High emphasis is placed on the quality control of the colonoscopies, with complications reported for 0.1% of the procedures, and no patient mortality. The advantage of the programme is through monitoring and evaluation, including monitoring of interval cancers. [10]

Germany was the first country to introduce a population screening program (in 1976) based on annual gFOBT for individuals more than 44 year of age. Since 2002, it has been offering participants a choice between colonoscopy at 55 year of age and FOBT at annual intervals between 50 and 55 year of age. After 55 year of age, examinations are carried out at 2 year, if the test results are positive colonoscopy is indicated. Those who undergo a screening colonoscopy with no neoplasia detected at initial examination are recommended re-examination at 10 years time if the first colonoscopy was carried out before they were 65. The positive feature of screening and data gathering is the emphasis on staging the disease at the time of its diagnosis. [11]

In the Czech Republic, CRC screening has many years of tradition. The country was the second in the world to start screening nation-wide, in 2000. In the initial years, gFOBT was offered to asymptomatic individuals more than 50 years of age by their general practitioners at preventative medical checks, followed by colonoscopies if tests were positive. Now both gFOBT and iFOBT are being offered. The implementation of the newly designed programme is supported by intense media campaign. [12,13]

Recently, the following EU guidelines for Colorectal Screening are published:

4.2. Australia

According to a recent survey, one in 12 Australians are likely to develop the colorectal cancers in their lifetime. [14] In Australia, CRC is second most common cause of cancer-related mortality. [15] survival from colorectal cancer is stage-dependent, yet fewer than 40% of individuals are diagnosed at a localised stage. [16]

In Australia, clinical practice guidelines for the prevention, early detection and management of colorectal cancer (the national guidelines) recommend that asymptomatic people classified as "at or slightly above risk" receive FOBT screening biennially, commencing at 50 years of age, with sigmoidoscopy (preferable flexible) consider every 5 yrs. [17]. Colonoscopy screening is endorsed only for asymptomatic people who are considered to be at "moderately increased risk" or "potentially high risk" due to risk features including personal or family history of CRC, adenoma and chronic ulcerative colitis. The recently re-funded National Bowel Cancer Screening Programme (NBCSP) offers one-off Immunochemical FOBT screening to people turning 50, 55 or 65 years of age.

Implementation of biennial CRC screening in Australia for all those aged 50-74 years could prevent up to 500 deaths per year, [18] with cost effectiveness comparable to breast and cervical cancer screening Programs. [19]

4.3. United States

In USA, men and women who are 50 to 75 year old should be screened for colorectal cancer in one of the following three ways; [20]

- A high-sensitivity faecal occult blood test (FOBT) every year.
- Sigmoidoscopy every five years and a high-sensitivity FOBT every three years.
- A colonoscopy every10 year.

Colorectal screening rates rose for both men and women. The rate for women increased slightly faster, so that the rates for men and women were about the same in 2010 [58.5% for men and 50.8%for women.The colorectal cancer screening was 58.6%, below the target of 70.5%.

4.4. Asia

In Asia colorectal screening percentage is at its lowest level and research revealed that colorectal cancer burden rapidly increasing in Asian countries [21]. A study to evaluate the cost-effectiveness of FOBT, flexible sigmoidoscopy and colonoscopy in Asian countries indicated that FOBT is cost-effective compared to flexible sigmoidoscopy or colonoscopy for colorectal screening in average risk population. [22]

The Increasing rate of colorectal cancer in Asia means that we need to take action immediately to prevent colorectal cancer and to diagnose the disease at early stages. The cost-effectiveness of screening programmes must be assessed in each individual country and research should be done to elucidate the epidemiology, genetic and environmental factors in development of colorectal cancer. [21]

5. Management of screening detected polyps

It is now widely accepted that the majority of colonic cancers arise from pre-existing adenomatous polyps (adenoma-carcinoma sequence).The supporting evidence being as follows: [23]

1. The prevalence of adenomas correlates well with that of carcinomas, average age of adenoma patients being around 5 years younger than patients with carcinomas.
2. Adenomatous tissue often accompanies cancer, and it is unusual to find small cancers with no contagious adenomatous tissue.
3. Sporadic adenomas are identical histologically to the adenomas of familial adenomatous polyposis (FAP), and this condition is unequivocal premalignant.
4. Large adenomas are more likely to display cellular atypia and genetic abnormalities than small lesions.
5. Distribution of adenomas throughout the colon is similar to that of carcinomas.
6. Adenomas are found up to one-third of all surgical specimens resected for colorectal cancers
7. The incidence of colorectal cancer has been shown to fall with long-term screening programme involving colonoscopy and polypectomy.

The patients who have undergone colonoscopy and had adenomas removed are at increased risk of developing colorectal cancer (CRC) in future, and therefore might benefit from colonoscopic surveillance. [24]

Surveillance Guidelines about colorectal adenomas are established by British Society of Gastroentrology. According to these guidelines surveillance of the colorectal adenomas depends upon ; number of polys, size of polyps and grade of dysplasia present in histology. Risk of colorectal cancer and adenomas with advanced pathology (>1cm or severely dysplastic) is greater. Risk can be stratified according to the findings at baseline and refined at each subsequent surveillance examination.

A Summary of surveillance guidelines [25] is:

- Low risk Patients with only 1-2 small <1cm) adenomas. No follow up or five yearly until one negative examination.

- Intermediate risk; Patients with 3-4 small adenomas or at least one >1cm.Three yearly colonoscopy until two consecutive negative examinations.
- High risk; Patients with >5 adenomas or > 3 adenomas at least one of which >1cm. An extra examination should be undertaken at 12 months before returning to three yearly surveillance.

The cut off age for stopping surveillance is usually 75 years but should also depends upon patients wishes and comorbidity.

Patients with incomplete examinations due to failed colonoscopies, for whatever reasons, should undergo repeat colonoscopy or alternative complete colonic examination (ct colonography). These guidelines are based on accurate detection of adenomas; otherwise risk status will be under estimated.

Large sessile adenomas removed piecemeal should be re-examined every three months. Small areas of residual polyp can be retreated endoscopically, for further check for complete eradications in three months. If extensive residual polyp is seen, open surgical resection needs to be considered. If there is complete healing of polypectomy site, then there should be sigmoidoscopy or colonoscopy at one year before returning to three yearly Surveillance. India ink tattooing aids recognition of the polypectomy site at follow up.

Stopping Surveillance.

The cut-off age for stopping surveillance is usually quoted as 75 years as the remaining life expectancy is likely to be less than the average time required for new adenomas to become malignant. After this age, it is unlikely that the benefits of surveillance will outweigh the potential risk of the procedure. However, this should not preclude further surveillance in a fit and motivated person who has a tendency to produce multiple or advanced adenomas at follow up.

The risk and benefit of adenoma surveillance needs to be balanced at all ages, particularly in patients who have significant co morbidity.

The decision to undertake each colonoscopy examination at follow up should depend not only on the number and type of adenomas, but also on the patient's age and wishes, and the presence of significant co morbidity. The Patient status should be established prior to attendance for each examination possibly by questionnaires.

6. Importance of audit in screening and screening relating colonoscopies

In any screening programme, as with any other medical service programme, adequate steps must be taken to ensure that the original objectives are being met and that methodology meets appropriate standard. The importance of maintaining the quality of screening programmes should never be under estimated. Evaluation, audit and quality control should be an integral part of any screening programme to ensure that it is achieving what it meant to be.

Colonoscopy is gold standard in important ultimate diagnostic tool in population screening programmes. Skilful colonoscopy with more then 95% caecal intubation rate is requirement for effective colorectal screening.

In the UK, before rolling out of the National Bowel Cancer Screening Programme, a large-scale study of colonoscopy practice was carried out. [26] The study demonstrated disappointing results with poor caecal intubation rates (76.95) and higher than expected complication rates. Since then there has been significant investment in endoscopic training, a quality assurance framework for endoscopic units has been implemented and National Bowel Screening Programme (NBSP) has been rolled out.

A nationwide audit of colonoscopy practice was conducted over a 2-weeks periods from 28 February 2011 until 11 March 2011. [27]. The study was performed prospectively, with the data entry occurring electronically through the purpose built website. All units performing >100 colonoscopies annually on NHS patients were included. Data on 20085 colonoscopies and 2681 colonoscopists were collected from 301units. Results showed 95.8% adjusted caecal intubation, 32.1% polyp detection rate, 92.3% resected polyps were retrieved and 90.2% o procedures achieved acceptable level of comfort. A total of 8 perforations and 52 significant haemorrhages were reported. Eight patients underwent surgery as a consequence of a complication.

The audit confirms that there has been significant improvement in performance of colonoscopy in UK since the last study reported 7 Years ago (caecal intubation rate 76.9%) and the performance is above the required national standard. But there is continuous need for assessment and audit of screening tools to keep the required national standard.

7. Colonoscopy capacity, training and accreditation

Most colon cancers are assumed to have adenomatous polyp phase. Therefore, colonoscopic detection and polypectomy provides the opportunity for cancer prevention [25]. So, colonoscopy is gold standard in high risk patients and patients with FOBT positive in population screening program. As we have discussed in previous sections, effective colorectal screening depends on available colonoscopy expertise in different part of the world

The aim of colonoscopy is to visualize whole of the colonic mucosa in order to identify pathology. A systemic review [28] of back-to-back studies has shown polyp miss rate at colonoscopy of 22% even in expert hands, especially polyps less than 1cm. Available data about polyp miss rates have shown a variation in performance between endoscopists, but this can be wider in very expert endoscopists. This shows that there is link between individual technical skill and polyps detection rate [29]. The single most important factor in the technique is withdrawal time after caecal intubation. The current recommendation is that colonoscopists should spend 6-10 minutes during withdrawal inspecting the colonic mucosa [30].

Skills in colonoscopy technique and coecal intubation rates are directly proportional to adenoma detection rate. In a standard endoscopy unit, single adenoma detection rate should not be less than 20%. Inadequate skills in colonoscopy can also lead to higher percentage of the procedure related complications.

In 2004, the largest prospective study of colonoscopic practice in UK revealed poor outcome in terms of completion and perforation rate, as well as deficiencies in all aspect of training. The guidelines on training have been published both in UK and the USA. [30-31]

Colonoscopy training and its accreditation is a challenging task. Structured colonoscopy training is lacking in most of the countries. The NHS Bowel Cancer Screening Programme (NHS BCSP) commenced in July 2006 and recruited expert colonoscopists to carry out colonoscopies in the programme. Owing to the known variability in colonoscopy skills, strict criteria have been developed for the accreditation of screening endoscopists to minimize the risk of the complications and inaccurate and incomplete examinations.

The Joint Advisory Group of GI Endoscopy (JAG) was established under the Academy of Medical Royal Colleges and now has a number of colleges and societies with an interest in endoscopy as members who are responsible for agreeing and setting policy and strategy and advising its constituent bodies and organizations (such as GMC and NHS)on standard and in endoscopy. The Jag office manages the administrative functions of the screening Assessor Accreditation System process on behalf of the NHS BCSP which is a web-based application process.

There are several advantages of this accreditation process, to both the unit and the individual endoscopists involved. Accreditation is an essential part of preparation for the implementation of local screening programme in UK. It also provides opportunities to demonstrate high level colonoscopic skills and improve the local endoscopy service. In addition it helps clinicians who wish to teach colonoscopy locally or on courses. The accreditation process leads to the Joint Advisory Group on GI Endoscopy (JAG) certificate of competency to perform screening derived colonoscopy.

8. Hereditary risk cancer and colorectal cancer screening protocol

Inherited bowel cancer comprises of 5% of the total colorectal cancers. Based on risk of Inherited bowel cancer population can be divided into three groups: Low risk group, Moderate risk group and High risk group based on family history. Approach for screening surveillance is different in three groups:

8.1. Low risk group

It includes the individuals with:

1. No personal history of bowel cancer: no confirmed family history of bowel cancer; or
2. No first degree relative (i.e. parent sibling or child) with bowel cancer; or
3. One first degree relative with bowel cancer at or above the age of 40 years.

In this group, the risk of bowel cancer may be twice the average risk [31] and there is no evidence to support invasive surveillance in his group [24]. These individuals should be explained that they are atonly marginally increased risk of developing colorectal cancer, and that this risk is not sufficient to outweigh the disadvantages of colonoscopy. They should be educated regarding symptoms of colorectal cancer, and importance of reporting if further members of the family develop cancers. And they should be encouraged to take part in the population screening for colorectal cancer.

8.2. Moderate risk group

Individuals are included in this category if there is:

1. One first-degree relative with colorectal cancer below the age of 45 without any feature of high risk group.
2. Two first-degree relatives with bowel cancer diagnosed at any age without any of the feature of high risk group.

In this group there is three to six fold relative risk of colorectal cancer. [31]. There is only marginal benefit from invasive surveillance (colonoscopy). Current recommendations are that individuals should be offered colonoscopy at 35-40 year of age (or at presentation if they are older), and again at the age of 55 years. [24]. Coecal intubation is mandatory, as neoplasms in individuals with a strong family history are often proximal; if the caecum is not reached, virtual colonoscopy should be performed.

8.3. High risk group

In this group, hereditary non-polyposis colorectal cancer (HNPCC) and various polyposis syndromes are included. Criteria for inclusion in this group includes:

1. Family member of familial adenomatous polyposis (FAP) or other polyposis syndrome; or
2. Member of family with known lynch syndrome; or
3. Pedigree suggestive of autosomal dominantly inherited colorectal (or other lynch syndrome associated) cancers.

In this group the individuals have one upto a 1 in 2 chance of inheriting a lifetime risk and more than 50 % chances of developing colorectal cancers. They must be referred to a clinical genetics service.

According to World Gastroenterology Organisation, the low risk group and population without obvious inherited colorectal cancer history are labelled as average risk population, while moderate rick and high risk groups are considered as one group with increased risk of colorectal cancer. Global screening guidelines cascades are established in 2007 based on these risk groups.

8.4. Lynch syndrome or Hereditary Non Polyposis Colorectal Cancers (HNPCC)

Lynch syndrome is inherited as an autosomal dominant fashion. It comprises of 2% of the colorectal cancers and is commonest of inherited bowel cancers. It is associated with endometrial carcinoma (30-70%), gastric carcinoma (5-10%), ovarian carcinoma in females (5-10%), urothelial carcinoma (5%) and others (small bowel pancreas and brain)< %5

Predictive genetic testing should be offered. These individuals should have first colonoscopy at the age of 25 years or five years before earliest colonoscopy in the family and gastroscopy at the age of 50 or five years before earliest gastric cancer in family. [24]. Colonoscopy and gastroscopy should be done two yearly.

Screening for extracoloic cancers in Lynch syndrome is available. There is little evidence of benefit. Recommendation varies from centre to centre, but surveillance is advised if there is family history of particular cancer. Recommended options for extracolonic surveillance [32] are;

- Annual transvaginal ultrasound, colour flow Doppler imaging and endometrial sampling.
- Annual CA125 level and clinical examination (pelvic and abdominal).
- Upper gastrointestinal endoscopy every two years.
- Annual urinalysis /cytology.
- Annual abdominal ultrasound of renal tracts, pelvis, and pancreas.
- Annual liver function tests,CA19-9,CEA

Familial adenomatous polyposis (FAP)

It is less common than Lynch syndrome. In FAP risk of colorectal cancer is 100%.

FAP is characterised by:

- Hundred of colorectal adenomatous polyps at a young age (second or third decade of life);
- Duodenal adenomatous polyps;
- extra-intestinal manifestation;
- Mutation in the APC gene at chromosome5q

If family mutation is known, at risk family member should be offered predictive genetic testing in their early teens. If this is not possible, then clinical surveillance is required. Usually, polys develop in teenage. Colonoscopy should only be performed in symptomatic children before teenage years. Otherwise annual flexible sigmoidoscopy starting at 13-15 years of age is recommended. If no polyps are detected, 5 yearly colonoscopy at the age of 20 years with annual flexible sigmoidoscopy in the intervening years. [24]. Flexible sigmoidoscopy should be performed carefully to avoid false negative results. Chromo-endoscopy is an option in doubtful cases.

9. Future research for improvement of screening programme

Although most of the screening programme based on research has shown improved survival in patients whose tumours are detected by screening, all population screening studies are prone to biases.

Selection bias arises from the tendency of people who accept screening to be particularly health conscious and therefore atypical of population as a whole.

Length bias indicates the tendency for screening to detect a disproportionate number of cancers which are slow growing, which thereby has good prognosis.

Lead-time bias results from the time between the date detection of cancer by screening and date when it would have been diagnosed had the subject not been screened. As survival is measured from time of diagnosis, screening advances the date at which diagnosis is made, thus lengthening the survival time without necessarily altering the date of death.

Because of these biases effectiveness of any screening can be assessed only by well designed randomized trials comparing disease –specific mortality in a population offered screening with that in an identical population not offered screening.

Initially three large randomized trials, using FOBT (Minnesota, Nottingham, in Funen Denmark) [33,34,35] showed reduction in mortality. These trials provided solid ground to initiate colorectal screening programme in western countries and US.

Randomized controlled trials are expensive and difficult to manage and may be ethically questionable in situations where control group is denied treatment for the condition in question. Despite this, UK National Screening Committee will only recommend the introduction of any new programme after assessing the findings of a properly conducted randomized controlled trial. The committee also keeps all screening programmes under regular review to ensure that they continue to perform in the way intended and continue to be effective.

9.1. Bowel cancer screening programme research committee

The research committee considers the feasibility and scientific value of research projects that arises from the screening programme in UK. It encourages collaboration between researchers and tries to prevent duplication.

The committee, chaired by Professor John Scholefield, meets quarterly and has considered over 60 research applications. The area of research considered by the committee included uptake/acceptability of screening test, epidemiology/histopathology and screening technologies. Here we will mention some important research project in relation with screening.

9.2. False positive research study

A research project to investigate the causes of false positive results on Foecal Occult Blood (FOB) testing is now under way. The five year project, funded by cancer research UK is a collaboration between university of Oxford and newly formed NHS cancer screening programmes` Research unit, which is based in the university` cancer epidemiology unit.

The pilot studies started early in 2008 and the study will eventually involve over 200,000 screening programme participants, including about 2,500people with a positive FOB test result who are categorized as normal following a colonoscopy.

9.3. UK flexible sigmoidoscopy screening trial

This trial looked at bowel cancer incidence and mortality reduction 11 years after a single screening examination with flexible sigmoidoscopy [36]

It examined the efficacy and duration of effect of ;

- A once only flexible sigmoidoscopy screen between ages 55 and 64 years.
- Removal of small polyps (<10m) during screening
- Colonoscopy only for high risk adenomas.

170,000 people were entered into the trial. Cumulative incidence, including prevalent cancers detected at screening, was reduced by 50% for the cancers in the rectum and sigmoid colon, and 33 percent for bowel cancer overall. Bowel cancer mortality was reduced by 43 percent.

The trial concluded that flexible sigmoidoscopy screening-with removal of small polyps at the examination is safe and, when offered only once between the ages 55 and 64, confers a substantial and long lasting benefit.

9.4. HTA: Frequency of follow-up for patients with intermediate grade colorectal adenomas

Beginning in September 2006, this study examined the effort of extending intervals between follow-up colonoscopies in people found to have intermediate adenomas, as defined by the British Society of Gastroentrology guidelines. It is using data from hospitals ad from bowel cancer screening initiatives to identify groups of patients with intermediate adenomas. The risk of cancer and severe adenomas will be assessed according to the interval between examinations and the number, size and features of adenomas detected.

Firstly, the study will identify whether all patients with intermediate adenomas require surveillance; secondly, whether the intervals are of the appropriate length; thirdly, it should also demonstrate how many follow-up examinations are needed. Finally, it will determine whether informing patients they need to have colonoscopy distresses them or whether they feel reassured as a result. A health economist will analyze the cost to individual patients and to the NHS and compare these with any potential benefit.

9.5. NHS bowel cancer screening programme evaluation group

The NHS Bowel Cancer Screening Programme Evaluation Group reviews and develops criteria used for evaluation and monitoring the progress of the Bowel Cancer Screening Programme.

It Includes representatives from all the professional groups in the programme as from the Cancer Screening Evaluation Unit, the Health and Social Care Information Centre and Bowel Screening Wales.

10. Current screening percentage of at risk world population and future of colorectal screening

World Gastroenterology Organization (WGO), in affiliation with International Digetive Cancer Alliance (IDCA), launched guidelines for international colorectal screening programmes after indicating the low percentage of screening programme in place in different coutries of the world. In these guidelines, they emphasise the need of some kind of screening programme in place based on locally available screening facilities

As mentioned earlier, the risk for colorectal cancers varies from country to country and even within countries. The risk also varies among individual people based on diet, lifestyle, and hereditary factors. Colorectal cancer screening is particularly challenging, as reflected in current low screening rates in most countries where there is high risk for colorectal cancer. Colorectal cancer screening is complex as there are multiple options, it requires considerable patient effort (Fecal Occult Blood Slides, Colonoscopy Preparation etc.), and it requires sedation and health-care partner for some tests (colonoscopy). [37]

It is an acknowledged fact that the lowest screening percentage of on risk population for colorectal cancer is in Asia and Africa. In most Asian and African countries, National Health Care systems and Health Insurance cover only a minority of people. So, access to healthcare facilities is limited in many rural areas and communities of low socio-economic status. In Asian countries, there is little health authority support for colorectal cancer screening and very low public awareness for this emerging epidemic in Asia. [38]

For the screening programme to be successful, multiple steps need to be taken correctly, beginning from awareness and recommendation from the primary-care physician, patient acceptance, financial coverage, risk stratification, screening test, timely diagnosis, timely treatment and appropriate follow-up. If any one of these steps is left faulty or not of high quality, the screening programme will certainly fail. (WGO)

10.1. International colorectal screening cascade

According to WGO guidelines, colorectal screening cascade consist of set of recommendations based on availability of resources in different countries of the world beginning with 1 (highest resources available) and ending with 6 (minimal resources available. [37]

10.1.1. Cascade Level 1

This is a set of recommendations for countries where high level of resources (Financial, professional, facilities) available.

For average- risk 10 yearly colonoscopies starting at 50 years.

For increased- risk patients more frequently two yearly or five yearly colonoscopies starting at 40 yrs of age.

10.1.2. Cascade Level 2

Recommendations are same as cascade level 1 but they apply when colonoscopy resources are more limited.

For average- risk once in life time colonoscopy at the age of 50.

For increased risk recommendations are same as cascade1.

10.1.3. Cascade Level 3

Recommendation are same as cascade level 1 but apply when colonoscopy resources are more limited but flexible sigmoidoscopy resources are available.

For average- risk flexible colonoscopy 5 yearly starting from 50 years of age with diagnostic workup with full colonoscopy in case of positive flexible sigmoidoscopy.

Recommendations for increased- risk are same as level 1 cascade.

10.1.4. Cascade Level 4

Recommendations are same as level 3 but they apply when flexible sigmoidoscopy and colonoscopy resources are more limited.

For average-risk screening flexible sigmoidoscopy once in life time at the age of 50 years. Diagnostic colonoscopy workup for positive flexible sigmoidoscopy or neoplasia depending on availability of resources.

Recommendations for increased risk are same as level 1 cascade.

10.1.5. Cascade level 5

Recommendations are same as resource level 4 but they apply when diagnostic colonoscopy is severely limited.

For average- risk population flexible sigmoidoscopy is recommended once in a life time at the age of 50 years. Diagnostic colonoscopy only when advanced neoplasia is detected.

Recommendations for screening increased-risk patients depend on colonoscopy resources available.

10.1.6. Cascade Level 6

Recommendations are same as for level 1 but they apply when flexible sigmoidoscopy and colonoscopy resources are severely limited.

For average -risk population, Faecal Occult Blood Testing (FOBT) should be done every year starting at the age of 50 years. The type of test used depends upon colonoscopy resources available and dietary habits of the population. The diagnostic work-up can be done either with colonoscopy, if available or barium enema, if colonoscopy is not readily available.

Therefore, recommendations for increased risk individuals are to identify them separately for special screening (level 1) and the decision depends on available colonoscopy resources. If not available, these people can be screened with average-risk individuals.

These guidelines are established considering a lack of resources in poor socioeconomically countries and can provide a base for the structured global screening programme. We hope the world will take measures to implement population screening programmes to save mankind from the cruel hands of colorectal cancer.

Author details

Syed Naqvi* and Syeda Farah Nazir

FRCS Colorectal surgery, RCSI, Dublin, Ireland

References

[1] Wilson JMG, JungerG (1968). Priciples and practice of Screeningfor Disease. Geneva: World Health Organization.

[2] Freedman AN, Slattery ML, BallardBarbash R, Willis G, Cann BJ, Pee D, Gail MH, and Pfeiffer RM. A Colorectal Cancer Risk Prediction Tool for White Men and Women Without Known Susceptibility. JCO. Online December 29, 2008.

[3] Ahlquist DA, Sargent Dj, Loprinzi cL et al. Stool DNA and occult blood testing for screen detection of colorectal neoplasia. Ann Intern Med.2008:149:441450,W81

[4] Von Karsa L, Anttila A, Ronco G et al. Cancer screening in European Union. Report on the implementation of the council recommendation on cancer screening. First report ISBN 9789279089343.European communities (publ.) Printed in Luxembourg by services of European commission.Lyon:IARC Press; 2008.

[5] West NJ, Boustiere C, Fischbach W, Parente F, Leicester RJ. Colorectal cancer screening in Europe, differences in approach; similar barriers to overcome. \int J Colorectal Dis.2009; 24:731740.

[6] National Cancer Screening Services, recommendation for colorectal screening programme in Ireland. 3, December 2008

[7] Goulard H, BoussacZarebska M,AncellePark R, Bloch J. French colorectal cancer screening pilot programme. : results of first rounds.J MED Screen. 2008;15:143148.

[8] Zorzi M, Falcini F, Fedato C, Grazini G et al. Screening for colorectal cancer in Italy.: 2006 survey.Epidemiol prev.2008;32:5568.

[9] Malila N, Oivanen T, Malminiemi O, Hakama M. Test, episode, and programme sensitivities of screening for colorectal cancers as a public health policies in Finland. Experimental design.BMJ. 2008;337:a2261

[10] Regula J, Rupinski M, Kraszewska E, Polkowski M, et al colonoscopy in colorectal-cancer screening for detection of advanced neoplasia. N Eng J Med. 2006;355:18631872.

[11] Pox C, Schmiegel W, Classen M. Current status of screening colonoscopy in Europe and in united states. Endoscopy.2007;39:168173

[12] Fric P, Zavoral M, Dvorakova H, Zoubek, et al. An adapted programme of colorectal cancer screening – 7 years experianceand cost benefit analysis. Hepatogastroentrology. 1994:41:413416

[13] Zavoral M, Zavada Filip, Salek C, Czech society of gastroenterology: colorectal cancer screening in Czech republic. Endoscopy. 2006;38:7480

[14] Australian institute of health and welfare. Australian cancer incidence and mortality (ACIM) books. Bowel Cancer for Australia Canberra:AIHW, 2011. http://www.aihw.gov.au/acimbooks

[15] Australian institute of health and welfare. Cancer in Australia 2010:An Overview.Canberra :AIHW,2010 (AIHWCat No.CAN 56. Cancer Series No. 60. http://www.aihw.gov.au/publicationdetail/?id=6442472459

[16] National Cancer Institute.Surveilance epidemiology and end results. SEER Stat Fact Sheets: colon and rectum. (http://seer.cancer.gov/statfacts/html/colorec.html.

[17] Australian Cancer Network Colorectal Guidelines revision Comittee. Guidelines for prevention, early detection and management of colorectal cancer. Sydney: The cancer council Australia and Australian Cancer Network.,2005. http://www.nhmrc.gov.au/filesnhmrc/publications/attachments/cp106 0 pdf

[18] Pignone MP, Flitcroft KL, Howard K et al. Costs and cost effectiveness of full implementation of biennial foecal occult blood test screening program for bowel cancer in Australia. Med J Aust 2011;194:180185.

[19] Anderson R, Haas M, Shanahan M. Cost –effectiveness of cervical screening in Australia:what is the inpact of screening in different intervels or over a different age range.Aust N ZJ Public Health 2008:32: 4352.

[20] .Centre for Disease Control and Prevention (CDC). Cancer screening –United states. 2010 MMWR2012;61 (3):4145

[21] .M Amin P, increased burden of colorectal cancer in asia.World J Gasrointest Oncol 2012 April15;4 (4):6870.

[22] .Tsoi KK, Ng SS, Leung MC, Sung JJ. Cost–effectiveness analysis on screening for colorectal neoplasm and management of colorectal cancer in Asia. Aliment pharmacol ther 2008;28:353363

[23] Leslie A, Carey FA, Pratt NR et al. Colorectal adenomacarcinoma sequence. Br J Surgery2002;89:84560

[24] Dunlop MG. Guidance on large bowel surveillance for people with two first degree relatives with colorectal cancer under 45 years. Gut 2002;51 (SupplV):1720

[25] W S Atkin, B P Sounders. Surveillance guidelines after removal of colorectal adenomatous polyp. Gut2002;51:v6v9doi:10.1136/gut.51.suppl_5.v6

[26] Bowels CJ, Leicester R, Romaya C, et al. Prospective study of colonoscopic practice in the UK today:are we adequately prepared for national colorectal cancer screening tomorrow.

[27] OC007 The national colonoscopy audit : a nationwide assessment of the quality and safety of colonoscopy in the UK. Gut2012;61: A3doi:10.1136 / gutjnl2012

[28] Van Rijn JC,reitsma JB, Stoker J et al. Polyp miss rate determined tandem colonoscopy: a systemic review.Am J Gastroenterol 2006;101 (2):34350

[29] Rex DK, Cutler CS, Lemal GTet al. Colonoscopic miss rate of adenoma determined by backtoback colonoscopies.Gastroentrology 1997 ;112 (1):248

[30] Bond J, Winawer S et al. Quality in the technical performance colonoscopy and continuous quality improvement process for colonoscopy. Recommendations of US MultiSociety Task Force on colorectal cancer.Am J Gastroenteral 2002;97 (6):1296308

[31] Houlston RS, Murday V,Harocopos C et al. Screening and genetic counselling for relatives of patients with colorectal cancer in a family cancer clinic.Br Med J 1990:301:3668

[32] Vasen HFA, Moselein G, Alonso A et al.Guidelines for clinical management of Lynch Syndrome (Hereditary Non Polyposis Colorectal Cancers). J Med Genet 2007;44:35362

[33] Mandel JS, Church TR, Ederer F et al. Colorectal cancer mortality: effectiveness of biennial screening for fecal occult blood. J Natl Cancer cancer inst199;91:4347

[34] Hardcastle JD, Robinson MHE,Moss SM et al. randomized controlled trial of fecal occult blood screening for colorectal cancer. Lancet 1996;348;14727

[35] Kronborg O, Fenegar C Olsen J et al. Rndomised study of screening for colorectal cancer with fecal occult blood test at Funen in Denmark. Lancet 1996.;348:146771.

[36] Prof Wendy S Atkin, Rob E, Ines K H, et al.Onceonly flexible sigmoidoscopy screening in prevention of colorectal cancer: a multicentricrandomised control trial.Lancet, Volume 375, issue 9726,pages 16241633 8 May 2010.

[37] World gastroenterology organization (WGO)/International Digestive Cancer Alliance. Practice guidelines for colorectal cancer screening ; 2007.

[38] Sung J. Colorectal Cancer Screening: Its time for action in Asia. Cancer Detect Prev 2007;31:12

Permissions

All chapters in this book were first published in CCSDT, by InTech Open; hereby published with permission under the Creative Commons Attribution License or equivalent. Every chapter published in this book has been scrutinized by our experts. Their significance has been extensively debated. The topics covered herein carry significant findings which will fuel the growth of the discipline. They may even be implemented as practical applications or may be referred to as a beginning point for another development.

The contributors of this book come from diverse backgrounds, making this book a truly international effort. This book will bring forth new frontiers with its revolutionizing research information and detailed analysis of the nascent developments around the world.

We would like to thank all the contributing authors for lending their expertise to make the book truly unique. They have played a crucial role in the development of this book. Without their invaluable contributions this book wouldn't have been possible. They have made vital efforts to compile up to date information on the varied aspects of this subject to make this book a valuable addition to the collection of many professionals and students.

This book was conceptualized with the vision of imparting up-to-date information and advanced data in this field. To ensure the same, a matchless editorial board was set up. Every individual on the board went through rigorous rounds of assessment to prove their worth. After which they invested a large part of their time researching and compiling the most relevant data for our readers.

The editorial board has been involved in producing this book since its inception. They have spent rigorous hours researching and exploring the diverse topics which have resulted in the successful publishing of this book. They have passed on their knowledge of decades through this book. To expedite this challenging task, the publisher supported the team at every step. A small team of assistant editors was also appointed to further simplify the editing procedure and attain best results for the readers.

Apart from the editorial board, the designing team has also invested a significant amount of their time in understanding the subject and creating the most relevant covers. They scrutinized every image to scout for the most suitable representation of the subject and create an appropriate cover for the book.

The publishing team has been an ardent support to the editorial, designing and production team. Their endless efforts to recruit the best for this project, has resulted in the accomplishment of this book. They are a veteran in the field of academics and their pool of knowledge is as vast as their experience in printing. Their expertise and guidance has proved useful at every step. Their uncompromising quality standards have made this book an exceptional effort. Their encouragement from time to time has been an inspiration for everyone.

The publisher and the editorial board hope that this book will prove to be a valuable piece of knowledge for researchers, students, practitioners and scholars across the globe.

List of Contributors

Valentin Ignatov, Nikola Kolev, Anton Tonev, Shteryu Shterev, Georgi Ivanov, Alexander Zlatarov and Krassimir Ivanov
Department of General and Operative Surgery, University Hospital "St. Marina" - Varna, Bulgaria

Elitsa Encheva
Department of Radiology, University Hospital "St. Marina" - Varna, Bulgaria

Tanya Kirilova
Department of Gastroenterology, University Hospital "St. Marina"- Varna, Bulgaria

Tsvetelina Teneva
Department of Image diagnostics, University Hospital "St. Marina"- Varna, Bulgaria

C. Alberto Blanco
Hospital Santos Reyes, Aranda de Duero (Burgos), Spain

R. Sánchez
Health Care Centers of Aranda de Duero (Burgos), Ávila, Spain
F. Piniella, D. Pescador, G. Borobio, A. García and C. Cano Health Care Centers of Aranda de Duero (Burgos), Salamanca, Spain

Teodoro Palomares and Ignacio García-Alonso
Dpt. of Surgery and Radiology and Physical Medicine, Faculty of Medicine and Dentistry, University of the Basque Country, Leioa, Spain

Ana Alonso-Varona
Dpt. of Biology and Histology, Faculty of Medicine and Dentistry, University of the Basque Country, Leioa, Spain

Vicente Portugal
Unit of Colorectal Surgery, Hospital Galdakao-Usansolo, Galdakao, Spain

Tanya Kirilova
Department of Gastroenterology, University Hospital "St. Marina", Varna, Bulgaria

Roberta Fusco
Department of Diagnostic Imaging, Radiant and Metabolic Therapy, "Istituto Nazionale dei Tumori Fondazione G. Pascale" - IRCCS, Naples, Italy

Mario Sansone
Department of Electrical Engineering and Information Technologies University 'Federico II' of Naples, Italy

Mario Petrillo, Paolo Delrio and Fabiana Tatangelo
Department of Radiology, Second University of Naples, Italy

Antonio Avallone
Gastrointestinal Medical Oncology, "Istituto Nazionale dei Tumori Fondazione G. Pascale" - IRCCS, Naples, Italy

Antonella Petrillo
Department of Diagnostic Imaging, Radiant and Metabolic Therapy, "Istituto Nazionale dei Tumori Fondazione G. Pascale" - IRCCS, Naples, Italy

Fabio Cianchi, Fabio Staderini and Benedetta Badii
Department of Surgery and Translational Medicine, Center of Oncological Minimally Invasive Surgery, University of Florence, Italy
Unit of Endocrine and Minimally Invasive Surgery, AOU Careggi, Florence, Italy

Robert Partyka
Department of Anesthesiology, Intensive Treatment and Emergency Medicine, Medical University of Silesia, Katowice, Poland

Ray Swayamjyoti, Jim Khan and Amjad Parvaiz
Portsmouth Hospitals NHS Trust, Queen Alexandra Hospital, Portsmouth, UK

Anton Tonev, Nikola Kolev, Valentin Ignatov and Krassimir Ivanov
Department of General and Operative Surgery, University Hospital "St. Marina", Varna, Bulgaria

Vasil Bojkov
Department of Surgery, University Hospital "St. Marina", Varna, Bulgaria

Tanya Kirilova
Department of Gastroenterology, University Hospital "St. Marina", Varna, Bulgaria

Syed Naqvi and Syeda Farah Nazir
FRCS Colorectal surgery, RCSI, Dublin, Ireland

Index

www.ingramcontent.com/pod-product-compliance
Lightning Source LLC
LaVergne TN
LVHW080636210926
848485LV00003B/273